PSYCHIATRY AND THE CINEMA

Second Edition

Glen O. Gabbard
and
Krin Gabbard

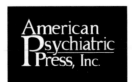
American
Psychiatric
Press, Inc.

Washington, DC
London, England

Copyright © 1999 Glen O. Gabbard and Krin Gabbard
ALL RIGHTS RESERVED
Manufactured in the United States of America on acid-free paper
05 04 03 02   6 5 4 3
Second Edition

American Psychiatric Press, Inc.
1400 K Street, N.W., Washington, DC   20005
www.appi.org

Library of Congress Cataloging-in-Publication Data
Gabbard, Glen O., 1949–
    Psychiatry and the cinema   /   Glen O. Gabbard and
  Krin Gabbard.   —   2nd ed.
        p.   cm.
    Filmography: p.
    Includes bibliographical references and index.
    ISBN 0-88048-826-3
    1. Psychiatry in motion pictures. 2. Motion pictures—
  Psychological aspects. I. Gabbard, Krin, 1948–   . II. Title.
PN1995.9.P78G3 1999
791.43′653—dc21   98-34017
                                                                              CIP

British Library Cataloguing in Publication Data
A CIP record is available from the British Library.

To Our Parents

Contents

About the Authors ix

Illustrations xi

Foreword xv
  Irving Schneider, M.D.

Preface to the First Edition xvii

Preface to the Second Edition xix

Introduction xxi

PART ONE

THE PSYCHIATRIST IN THE MOVIES

1 Typology, Mythology, Ideology 3

2 The Alienist, the Quack, and the Oracle 35

3 The Golden Age 75

4 The Fall from Grace 107

5 The Female Psychotherapist in the Movies 147

6 Clinical Implications 171

PART TWO

THE PSYCHIATRIST AT THE MOVIES

7 Methodology and Psychoanalytic Film Criticism 189

8 Play It Again, Sigmund: Psychoanalytic Approaches
to the Classical Hollywood Text 205

9 3 *Women:* Robert Altman's Dreamworld 221

10 Narcissism in the Cinema I:
The Cinematic Autobiography 233

11 Narcissism in the Cinema II: The Celebrity 251

12 *Alien* and Melanie Klein's Night Music 277

13 "Phallic" Women in the Contemporary Cinema 293

Epilogue 309

A Filmography for the Depiction of Psychiatry
in the American Cinema 315

Chronology 353

References 363

Subject Index 375

Film Index 401

About the Authors

Glen O. Gabbard, M.D., is Bessie Walker Callaway Distinguished Professor of Psychoanalysis and Education in the Karl Menninger School at the Menninger Clinic. He is also Director and Training and Supervising Analyst at the Topeka Institute for Psychoanalysis and Clinical Professor of Psychiatry at the University of Kansas School of Medicine in Wichita. Dr. Gabbard is the author or editor of twelve books, including *Psychodynamic Psychiatry in Clinical Practice: The DSM-IV Edition* (1994). He is also the film review editor for the *International Journal of Psycho-Analysis*.

Krin Gabbard, Ph.D., teaches film, literature, and cultural studies at the State University of New York at Stony Brook. He is author of *Jammin' at the Margins: Jazz and the American Cinema* (1996) and editor of *Jazz among the Discourses* (1995) and *Representing Jazz* (1995). He is currently working on a book about movies, masculinity, and music.

Illustrations

1. Ginger Rogers with Barry Sullivan in *Lady in the Dark* (1944). [p. 10]

2. Judd Hirsch with Timothy Hutton in *Ordinary People* (1980). [p. 19]

3. Katharine Hepburn imprisoned by Freudian quack (Fritz Feld) in *Bringing Up Baby* (1938). [p. 20]

4. Herbert Grimwood attempts to drive Douglas Fairbanks to suicide in *When the Clouds Roll By* (1919). [p. 38]

5. Claudette Colbert and Theodore von Eltz minister to Nick Shaid in *Private Worlds* (1935). [p. 45]

6. Murderer (Chester Morris) arouses the curiosity and the sympathy but not the malice of oracular Ralph Bellamy (with Rose Stradner) in *Blind Alley* (1939). [p. 46]

7. Fred Astaire treats Ginger Rogers in *Carefree* (1938). [p. 48]

8. Claude Rains, in *Now, Voyager* (1942), joins Bette Davis for a hot dog. [p. 52]

9. Tyrone Power about to be outsmarted by Helen Walker in *Nightmare Alley* (1947). [p. 58]

10. Lew Ayres probes the mind of Olivia de Havilland and her "evil twin" in *The Dark Mirror* (1946). [p. 60]

11. Olivia de Havilland with caring, effective psychiatrist (Leo Genn) in *The Snake Pit* (1948). [p. 62]

12. Olivia de Havilland with incompetent quack (Howard Freeman) in *The Snake Pit* (1948). [p. 64]

13. Jimmy Piersall (Anthony Perkins) and his wife (Norma Moore) with faceless psychiatrist (Adam Williams) in *Fear Strikes Out* (1957). [p. 80]

14. Joanne Woodward as Eve Black, one of *The Three Faces of Eve* (1957), with Lee J. Cobb and Edwin Jerome. [p. 82]

15. Ginger Rogers with husband (Dan Dailey) and analyst (David Niven) in *Oh, Men! Oh, Women!* (1957). [p. 84]

16. Howard da Silva as Dr. Swinford in *David and Lisa* (1962). [p. 87]

17. Sidney Poitier, as the movies' first black psychiatrist, overcomes the racism of Bobby Darin in *Pressure Point* (1962). [p. 89]

18. Young Sigmund Freud (Montgomery Clift) with Cecily (Susannah York) in John Huston's *Freud* (1962). [p. 98]

19. Montgomery Clift's dream in *Freud* (1962). [p. 100]

20. Peter O'Toole details his sex life for Dr. Fritz Fassbender (Peter Sellers) in *What's New, Pussycat?* (1965). [p. 117]

21. McMurphy (Jack Nicholson) at odds with Nurse Ratched (Louise Fletcher) in *One Flew Over the Cuckoo's Nest* (1975). [p. 134]

22. Bibi Andersson heals Kathleen Quinlan in *I Never Promised You a Rose Garden* (1977). [p. 138]

23. Saul Benjamin (Dudley Moore) succumbs to the spell of his patient (Elizabeth McGovern) in *Lovesick* (1983). [p. 139]

24. Dr. Hannibal Lecter (Anthony Hopkins) is interviewed by Clarice Starling (Jodie Foster) in *The Silence of the Lambs* (1991). [p. 142]

25. Matt Damon engages in unconventional therapy with Robin Williams in *Good Will Hunting* (1997). [p. 145]

26. Ingrid Bergman nurtures Gregory Peck while her ex–training analyst (Michael Chekhov) looks on in *Spellbound* (1945). [p. 150]

27. Muckraking journalist Tony Curtis about to expose Natalie Wood, before falling in love with her, in *Sex and the Single Girl* (1964). [p. 153]

28. Hope Lange copes with Elvis Presley's transference in *Wild in the Country* (1961). [p. 155]

29. Barbra Streisand basks in the glow of Nick Nolte in *The Prince of Tides* (1991). [p. 158]

30. Madeleine Stowe and Bruce Willis in *12 Monkeys* (1995). [p. 160]

31. Sissy Spacek and Shelley Duvall in Robert Altman's *3 Women* (1977). [p. 224]

32. Edgar (Robert Fortier) teaching Pinky (Sissy Spacek) how to kill in *3 Women* (1977). [p. 229]

33. Roy Scheider, Ben Vereen, Ann Reinking, and unidentified dancer in Bob Fosse's modernist, allegorical musical *All That Jazz* (1979). [p. 237]

34. Joe Gideon (Roy Scheider) choreographs his own death in Bob Fosse's *All That Jazz* (1979). [p. 238]

35. Woody Allen as Sandy Bates in *Stardust Memories* (1980). [p. 240]

36. Woody Allen with Anne de Salvo and Jaqui Safra in *Stardust Memories* (1980). [p. 247]

37. Robert De Niro in Martin Scorsese's *The King of Comedy* (1983). [p. 257]

38. Zelig (Woody Allen) with Coolidge and Hoover in *Zelig* (1983). [p. 263]

39. Mia Farrow as Dr. Eudora Fletcher, the savior and lover of Leonard Zelig, in Woody Allen's *Zelig* (1983). [p. 264]

40. Jeff Daniels and Danny Aiello in *The Purple Rose of Cairo* (1985). [p. 269]

41. Mia Farrow with Jeff Daniels in *The Purple Rose of Cairo* (1985). [p. 271]

42. The crew of the *Nostromo* wakes up in Ridley Scott's *Alien* (1979). [p. 285]

43. Kane (John Hurt) explores the maternal body of a derelict ship in *Alien* (1979). [p. 286]

Foreword

If psychiatry had not existed, the movies would have had to invent it. And in a sense they did. *Psychiatry and the Cinema* tells the story of how the movie industry took the profession of psychiatry—its patients, theories, and explanations—and transformed it into a hybrid that joined the fantasies of the public with its own quest for profit in ways that were sometimes wondrous, but more often disappointing.

One could pair the history of the movies with the history of any profession, say an account of how the movies have depicted lawyers. Or a history of the cinema and dentistry could be traced from Gibson Gowland's painless dentist in Eric von Stroheim's *Greed* to Laurence Olivier's sadistic one in *Marathon Man*, with glances along the way at W. C. Fields, Bob Hope, and Alan Arkin, among many other screen practitioners. These histories would provide interesting and amusing insights into the vicissitudes of American film, the changes in the profession depicted, and the influence of popular culture on both.

But none would have the resonance and power of psychiatry and the movies, for to an uncommon extent the two have shared the same subject matter. Both movies and psychiatry have had as their prime focus human thought, emotions, behavior, and, above all, human motivation. In pursuit of their common subject, movies and psychiatry have frequently intersected. The two most explicit encounters are the subject of this book: psychiatrists have studied the movies, and the movies have depicted psychiatry.

The study of movies by psychiatrists has taken two major directions. Early in the history of the cinema, there was an attempt to understand the appeal and the power of the motion picture medium itself, apart from the specific content of any individual film. The outstanding example of this effort was Hugo Münsterberg's 1916 classic *The Film: A Psychological Study*. His central statement bears repeating: "The photoplay tells us the human story by overcoming the forms of the outer world, namely, space, time, and causality, and by adjusting the events to the forms of the inner world, namely, attention, memory, imagination, and emotion."

Ten years later, in 1926, the eminent psychoanalyst Hans Sachs acted as consultant in Germany to the first movie on psychoanalysis, *Secrets of a Soul*. He went on to pursue his interest in movies in a series of articles in the English film journal *Closeup*. In a 1928 article he took Münsterberg one step further: "The film seems to be a new way of driving mankind to conscious recognition . . . by making the inexpressible expressible by means of displacements on to a small incidental action."

A number of interesting analyses have continued this approach, but the more popular direction in the psychiatrist's interest in movies has consisted of the uncovering of the covert message in individual movies or in film genres. This emphasis has clearly risen from the psychoanalytic approach to art and literature, much of it pioneered by Freud, not a movie fan himself, but an avid interpreter of the arts. In recent years the semiologists, with their merging of linguistic and psychoanalytic method, have come to occupy a central position in the effort to uncover the hidden messages in popular movies. The second part of *Psychiatry and the Cinema* presents illuminating examples of the interpretive methods that psychoanalysts have brought to the study of the movies.

It is the movies' interest in psychiatry, however, that occupies the major part of this study, and it makes for a fascinating story. From the comic Dr. Dippy in the nickelodeons of 1906 to the heroic or evil psychiatrist in the movie currently playing in the nearest multiplex shopping mall theater, an interesting parade of mental health professionals has appeared on our screens. Their multiple personalities grace the pages of this volume. But above and beyond the depiction of psychiatrists themselves, one wonders what movie scriptwriters would have done without dreams, amnesia, or homicidal maniacs, or where films, or psychiatrists for that matter, would have been without the ubiquitous traumatic event.

The French filmmaker Jean-Luc Godard once commented that "the cinema is neither art nor life, but something in between." Certainly very few psychiatric films have aspired to art, and even fewer have represented real life, but as Glen and Krin Gabbard so effectively demonstrate, that in-between area has yielded a series of films of great fascination, entertainment, dismay, and, one must even admit, educational value.

Irving Schneider, M.D.

Preface to the First Edition

This book has been a cooperative project by writers from distinctly different intellectual backgrounds. The result has been a truly integrative effort to synthesize the relevant dimensions of film scholarship with those of psychiatry and psychoanalysis. Not only have we been able to avoid the all-too-obvious problems that might have confronted brothers engaged in a collaborative project of this kind, but we have also been able to reach a consensus on the many controversial issues raised by our study. Although both of us have contributed significantly to every chapter in this book, our own specialties have required each of us to contribute more to certain sections than to others. If readers occasionally find differences of style or emphasis in the text, they may be sure these differences reflect no substantive disagreement between us.

The illustrations for this book also require a word of explanation. Many recent works about film have included frame enlargements from actual prints of movies. This convention puts on the page the exact image that audiences momentarily see during a screening of a film. We have chosen instead to rely on the still photographs that studios have traditionally provided for promotional purposes. Although these stills seldom reproduce exact scenes from movies, they often reveal specific relationships among characters that the filmmakers—or, just as important, the studio executives—have tried to establish. In most cases we have chosen a still because it offers a striking example of how a film wishes to portray psychiatry, even if the precise contents of the photograph never appear in the film.

Psychiatry and the Cinema could not have been written without the generous contributions of many friends and colleagues. We would especially like to thank Irving Schneider, Gerald Mast, Daniel M. Fox, Paul Fink, Robert

XVIII PSYCHIATRY AND THE CINEMA, SECOND EDITION

Mugge, Penelope Russianoff, Donald F. Muhich, Andrea Walsh, James Castrataro, Harriet Meier Castrataro, Jacob Lipkind, Louise Vasvari, and Carrol Lasker. We owe a special debt of gratitude to the staff of the University of Chicago Press. Like the authors of what must be 90 percent of the books about movies today, we received invaluable assistance from Charles Silver and Mary Corliss of the Museum of Modern Art. We also appreciate efforts on our behalf by the staff at the Library of Congress. Mrs. Faye Schoenfeld patiently typed numerous versions of the manuscript and was of invaluable assistance in organizing an enormous amount of correspondence. The State University of New York at Stony Brook and the Menninger Clinic provided both moral and financial support for portions of the project. Finally, we have been fortunate to receive exceptional tolerance and steadfast encouragement from two remarkable women, Paula Beversdorf Gabbard and Joyce Davidson Gabbard.

A shorter version of chapter 10, "Narcissism in the Cinema I: The Cinematic Autobiography," was published in *Psychoanalytic Review* 71:319–28, 1984. Copyright 1984, The Guilford Press. Reprinted with permission. Parts of chapter 12, "*Alien* and Melanie Klein's Night Music," appeared in *Psychoanalytic Approaches to Literature and Film*, ed. Maurice Charney and Joseph Reppen (Madison, N.J.: Fairleigh Dickinson University Press, 1987). Reprinted with permission of Associated University Presses. An earlier version of chapter 9, "*3 Women*: Robert Altman's Dreamworld," was published in *Literature/Film Quarterly* 8:258–64, 1980. Publication rights held by *Literature/Film Quarterly*, Salisbury State University. Reprinted with permission.

Preface to the Second Edition

Requests for a new edition of *Psychiatry and the Cinema* have come from colleagues in clinical practice as well as in colleges and universities. Since the book is still the only resource to attempt a thorough survey of the subject, we have decided to update, contribute some new chapters, and, in a few cases, rewrite entire chapters. We have been consistently amazed in this undertaking at how much we have been obliged to add to the book. First, we have expanded our discussion of the female therapist in the movies that was originally a subsection within chapter 1; it now stands separately as chapter 5. The chapter on the myth of the "phallic" woman and the chapter on *Casablanca* represent completely new additions. We have expanded chapter 6 to consider more broadly the clinical implications of how the movies portray psychotherapists, and we have substantially enlarged chapter 7 to discuss some of the new trends in psychoanalytically oriented film theory. This survey of new developments has been painted with broad strokes because it would be impossible to acknowledge all of the many important books and articles that have appeared in print since 1986.

We have been even more amazed by the proliferation of films that deal with psychiatry or psychotherapy in some way or another. Our original 1986 filmography topped out at approximately 300 films. It now approaches 450. We wonder if more psychiatrists are represented in American movies than are surgeons or practitioners of any other medical specialty. This surfeit of representations alone demanded a new edition.

Since the appearance of our first edition in 1987, psychiatry has continued to distance itself from psychoanalysis and psychotherapy. Nevertheless, in the cinematic world, the emphasis remains on the talking cure, and the effective prescribing of medication is rarely depicted. Hence, we continue to use the term *psychiatry* in the broadest possible sense to encompass all mental health professionals, especially those who practice psychotherapy.

Chapter 8, "Play It Again, Sigmund: Psychoanalytic Approaches to the Classical Hollywood Text," was originally published in the *Journal of Popular Film and Television* 18(1):6–17, 1990. Reprinted with permission of the Helen Dwight Reid Educational Foundation. Published by Heldref Publications, 1319 18th St., N.W., Washington, DC 20036-1802. Copyright 1990. An earlier version of chapter 13, "'Phallic' Women in the Contemporary Cinema," was published in *American Imago* 4:421–39, 1993. Copyright 1993, The Johns Hopkins University Press. Reprinted with permission.

Once again we are deeply grateful to the many friends and colleagues who made contributions, large and small, and helped this book grow. We would like to thank in particular Michael I. Levy, Keren Pomp, and Abigail Gabbard. We also owe a large debt of gratitude to Faye Schoenfeld for her careful work on the manuscript. We thank the editors at American Psychiatric Press for believing in the project from the outset. As before, we dedicate the book to two extraordinary people who taught us to love the cinema as well as the life of the mind, Lucina Paquet Gabbard and Glendon Gabbard. And again, we thank the two women who have provided the atmosphere of love and concern that made this book possible, Paula B. Gabbard and Joyce Davidson Gabbard.

Introduction

They grew up together. Cinematic art and modern psychodynamic psychiatry, both still in their infancy, were brought to the United States from Europe at the turn of the century and were firmly established within a few decades. The relationship has been complementary and also hostile. As cooperative endeavors, both psychiatry and the cinema strive to cut through the seemingly random content of everyday life and reveal the secrets of the human character, and since curing and entertaining are often related in our culture, movies as well as psychiatry have been regarded as therapeutic. Psychiatry has provided filmmakers with abundant material, even if we consider only the psychoanalytically derived "motivations" that have driven actors in every genre of film, from musicals to westerns (Holland 1959). Movies have become the great storehouse for the images that populate the unconscious, the chosen territory of psychoanalytic psychiatry. Irving Schneider (1985) has pointed out that as early as 1900 a writer would describe his psychotic episode in terms of the "magic lantern" effects of the first nickelodeons. Early surrealist filmmakers even saw the production of dream images in the human unconscious as fundamentally analogous to the "cutting" process by which movies are made (Williams 1981), and the American film industry was being called a *Traumfabrik*, or "dream factory," as early as 1931 (Ehrenburg). More recently, psychoanalytically inclined students of film have made persuasive connections between the language of the cinema and Freud's account of the dream work (Metz 1982).

Because of the opportunities they have provided for filmmakers, psychiatrists and psychiatry have played roles in almost every type of film, including silent farces like *Plastered in Paris* (1928), gangster films like *Blind Alley* (1939), classic tearjerkers like *Now, Voyager* (1942), teen exploitation horror flicks like *I Was a Teenage Werewolf* (1957), Doris Day sex farces like *Lover Come Back* (1961), low-budget art films like *David and Lisa* (1962), and contemporary Hollywood biopics like *Frances* (1982). In fact, considerably more than four hundred films across the spectrum of Hollywood genres make some use of psychiatry. This figure does not include many English and Continental films in American circulation that deal with the subject, nor does it include innumerable B movies—forgotten quickies from the 1940s, nudies from the 1960s, and straight-to-video ephemera from the 1980s and 1990s—many of which have found a place for psychiatrists in their mise-en-scènes. Nevertheless, whether movies are A, B, or triple-X, they present few psychiatrists who do not belong to a fairly limited range of stereotypes. In addition, only a few basic conventions characterize how American films have dealt with psychiatry and its practitioners. Schneider (1985), for example, has divided all movie psychiatrists into three categories: Dr. Dippy (after a film we will discuss in chapter 2), Dr. Evil, and Dr. Wonderful.

Even though these stereotypes and conventions offer filmmakers the opportunity to produce fantastic dream sequences or logical explanations for the otherwise inexplicable behavior of their characters, practitioners of psychiatry have seldom found reason to applaud the images of themselves appearing on the screen. For reasons that are not difficult to understand, the motion picture industry has shown only a passing interest in the more complex aspects of psychiatric treatment. The one hundred minutes of the average American film have only rarely provided an insider's view of World War II, space exploration, or even baseball. We can scarcely expect the medium to provide balanced insights into the multifaceted, constantly evolving questions of psychotherapy: any serious attempt at such an undertaking would probably bore audiences silly. Filmmakers and their audiences are, of course, much more interested in the compelling, arousing, or consoling entertainment that is usually characterized, perhaps unfairly, as "escapist." For a variety of reasons, many of which are addressed in this work, psychiatry has regularly been exploited for purposes largely inconsistent with the profession's loftier goals.

In our attempts to sort out the various relationships between movies and psychiatry, we often will be concerned with the stereotypical characters and conventions that dominate the presentation of movie psychiatrists. We have found that the predominance of certain stereotypes changes, often dramatically, from one historical moment to the next, and the portrayal of psychiatrists is best understood in terms of the largely mechanical needs of the films in which they appear, particularly within the conventions of genre. Also, we are often able to identify a relationship between historical changes in the mental health profession and its image on the screen: some of the more negative portrayals can be blamed on psychiatrists themselves, and some cannot.

Chapter 1 is an overview of the most common stereotypes and of the film genres in which these stereotypical characters and plots are ensconced. Because we are primarily concerned with cultural/historical patterns in the American view of psychiatry in the movies, we have confined ourselves to theatrically released American-made films. In spite of their immense appeal and importance, we will not engage in extended analyses of Robert Wiene's *The Cabinet of Dr. Caligari*, G. W. Pabst's *Secrets of a Soul*, Fritz Lang's *The Testament of Dr. Mabuse*, Liliana Cavani's *The Night Porter*, or Ingmar Bergman's *Face to Face*. The discussion of psychiatrists in foreign films, as well as in American television programs, would require more elaborate methodologies and would expand our subject beyond manageable proportions. We will make reference to these only when our inquiry into the American cinema demands it. After we have established the familiar stereotypes and genres, along with the problems of their interpretation, we will devote three chapters to what appears to be a historical pattern in the evolution of cinematic depictions of psychiatry.

The term *psychiatrist* is used generically in this study to represent all mental health professionals, particularly psychotherapists. To attempt further distinction among the various mental health disciplines would be to go far beyond the efforts of filmmakers themselves. Significantly, American films have never completely succeeded in distinguishing psychiatrists from psychoanalysts, psychologists, social workers, and other therapists. In *The Dark Mirror* (1946), for example, the door to Lew Ayres's office bears the inscription "Dr. Scott Elliott, M.D., Ph.D., M.S., Psychologist." This confusion may also represent a more deeply rooted perception, one that effectively segregates movie psychiatrists from other medical doctors such as surgeons or pediatricians. Throughout our research for this study, we have found that the work of psychiatrists in the cinema is frequently indistinguishable from that of clergymen, caseworkers, school guidance counselors, or even newspaper advice columnists. At least since the 1930s, the American cinema has focused so heavily on simplified versions of the psychiatric "talking cure" that the profession has in effect become demedicalized in the movies.

In our survey of how movies have portrayed psychiatrists (chapters 2–4), we have attempted to tie these changing images to American cultural history. While it is true that the Hollywood cinema "reflects" American attitudes, it is also true that it reflects them selectively. We will attempt to identify both the popular notions that became manifest in films and those that appeared either belatedly or not at all. After we have completed this historical survey, we will devote a chapter to the cinema's representation of female therapists, a striking example of how patriarchal ideology continues to flourish, even (or especially) where science and medicine are involved. We will also devote a chapter to the clinical implications of our study, particularly the impact that the cinematic mythology of psychiatry has had and can have on the relationship between patient and therapist.

Part One of this study addresses how movies have looked at psychiatrists. We occasionally make use of the insights of Freud and his followers to account for these cinematic images, but our principal subject in Part One is the changing image of the psychotherapist in American movies, an image that may or may not accurately reflect American attitudes. In Part Two we adopt the reverse perspective and look at movies with psychiatrically informed eyes, thus completing our study of the complementary relationship between psychiatry and the movies. One reason for the ubiquity of psychiatrists in the American cinema may be their profession's relevance—in the imaginations of both moviemakers and movie consumers—to how film affects the mind. Even the most naïve statements about movies "warping" the minds of young people acknowledge the profound and mysterious impression that the cinema has on its viewers. We feel that an inquiry into images of psychiatry in films also ought to examine the relationship of movies to the workings of the unconscious. Further, we believe that psychoanalytically informed criticism can be an extremely important aid to understanding the special hold that the movies have on audiences.

Applying psychology to the movies is by now a familiar pursuit, one that goes back at least to 1916 when Harvard psychologist Hugo Münsterberg (1916/1970) published his thoughts on how "the photoplay" can replicate the actual workings of the mind more successfully than conventional narrative forms. Modern psychoanalytic film criticism probably began in 1950 when Martha Wolfenstein and Nathan Leites (1970) realized that films repay psychological scrutiny just as richly as the plays of Sophocles, Shakespeare, and Ibsen, to which Freud had once applied his substantial skills as a literary critic. Since the appearance of Wolfenstein and Leites's work, mental health professionals have frequently written about movies, and the bibliography of psychoanalytic film criticism is now much too expansive to summarize here. We mention only Harvey R. Greenberg's *Screen Memories* (1993) as an excellent and readable example of the psychiatrist at the cinema. In colleges and universities, psychoanalytic criticism, or something very much like it, is as familiar to students of film as the Odessa Steps or Rosebud.

In the first chapter of Part Two we will attempt a brief survey of the important developments in psychoanalytic film criticism that have taken place since the 1970s. The remarkable ascendancy of Jacques Lacan as a key figure in film theory has brought together a substantial community of scholars who draw upon linguistics, feminism, Marxism, and semiotics as well as psycho-analysis. Although we owe a debt to these writers, we have relied more upon the literature of clinical psychoanalysis and less upon semiotic theory for our analyses of the films addressed in Part Two. In particular, we have chosen to illustrate a number of methodologies based on different theoretical frame-works that we find particularly suited to several interesting films. All of the movies discussed in Part Two repay psychoanalytic scrutiny, although most of them have yet to be systematically illuminated in terms of this tradition.

Few of the movies that we discuss in *Psychiatry and the Cinema*, espe-cially in Part One, are masterpieces of the art. With the prominent exception of Alfred Hitchcock, few of the American "pantheon" directors are well rep-resented in our filmography: Orson Welles, Fritz Lang, John Ford, and Josef von Sternberg never made American films that deal directly with psychiatry, even though their mastery of character and mise-en-scène places them among the most psychologically sophisticated directors. In the chapters that follow, we are much more likely to encounter the films of Anatole Litvak, Mark Robson, Curtis Bernhardt, or Edward Dmytryk, directors whose works for the most part were long ago brushed aside into the relative oblivion of those directors considered to be studio journeymen. Perhaps the mere pres-ence of a psychiatrist in an American film signals that it contains a thematic shortcut, that the filmmaker has severed some Gordian knot by inserting the brief but authoritative pronouncements of a psychiatrist. The French critic Marc Vernet has made a somewhat different observation: "The great contri-bution of psychoanalysis has been to provide a new alibi for the structure of the American narrative film" (1975, 233). Even Hitchcock—some would say *especially* Hitchcock—has made awkward use of psychoanalytically engi-neered plot mechanics, for example, in *Marnie* (1964), a film that does not even include a psychiatrist in its cast of characters. We will have a good deal more to say about Hitchcock, whose use of psychiatry requires special atten-tion to the complex means by which his films are "enunciated." But most of the films we address in Part One are less challenging, inviting cultural/socio-logical treatment more often than close reading. By the same token, most of these films are relatively unsophisticated from a cinematographic point of view—inevitably employing the "invisible style" of classical Hollywood (Bordwell, Staiger, and Thompson 1985)—and do not demand the kind of shot-by-shot analysis that can illuminate more complex films.

The mediocrity or obscurity of most of the films we discuss in this book should in no way undermine the validity of our argument. If the questions of genre, historicity, and interpretation that we raise in chapters 1–4 are valid, we should be able to apply them to the whole range of American films, not

just to those that have been canonized by box-office receipts or critical acclaim.

Our principal interest in these movies is not, after all, whether they are
aesthetically or commercially successful. All of them were created with the
intention of returning at least some money to the studio, and all were tailored
to closely studied populations of ticket-buyers. With few exceptions, the
films were made according to well-established formulas that only a handful
of filmmakers were willing to modify to any substantial degree. Consequently, our interest is most aroused when the portrayal of psychiatrists
changes dramatically over a short period of time or when a certain character
type suddenly begins to appear more frequently. Our goal is, first, to identify
these changes in the movies and, second, to offer some means of accounting
for them. In doing so, we may mention the most cynical exploitation films in
the same sentence as an Academy Award winner (assuming for the moment
that the Oscar-honored film is qualitatively different from the former). But
by concentrating almost entirely on a film's relationship to psychiatry, we
may also develop new criteria for thinking about these films. Even when a
film touches only briefly on psychiatry, its treatment of the subject can tell
us a great deal about the film's attitudes and intentions, including those that
the film's makers may not have articulated elsewhere.

PART ONE

THE PSYCHIATRIST
IN
THE MOVIES

CHAPTER 1

Typology, Mythology, Ideology

The changing images of psychiatry during some ninety years of American cinema offer a unique opportunity to assess the complex interactions between different currents in twentieth-century American culture. Part One of this book addresses the strange relationship between movie "mythology" and the history of psychiatry in the United States. In chapters 2, 3, and 4 we will consider the history of cinematic representations of the psychiatrist in terms of three periods: one before, one after, and one during a Golden Age in the late 1950s and early 1960s when psychiatrists were almost consistently idealized. Negative stereotypes predominate during the periods before and after this Golden Age, though for sharply different reasons. To understand these historical changes, we must first consider the kinds of movies that have established themselves in our culture and the special needs in them that psychiatrists answered. We will see that the myths embedded in American movies have offered only a few highly conventionalized niches for doctors of the mind and that the generic therapies available to movie psychiatrists are equally limited. In chapter 5, we will consider the narrowly circumscribed role of the female psychiatrist in the movies. For now, in the present chapter, we are concerned with *continuity* in images of psychiatry throughout the twentieth century. Our thesis here is that a film's handling of psychiatry presents an especially useful stance for "decoding" that film, even when a psychiatrist appears to be a strictly marginal character.

In his consideration of movie mythology, Michael Wood (1975) has observed that American films, especially those made before the 1960s, involve frequently contradictory assumptions about our most important worries. He suggests that entertainment does not so much present an escape from problems as it does a "rearrangement of our problems into shapes which tame them, which disperse them to the margins of our attention" (18). Problems in movies, whether world wars or juvenile delinquency, can appear vividly real at times, though ultimately they may be revealed to have little importance. Wood continues: "The mythological function of the movies is to examine these problems without seeming to look at them at all. Movies assuage the discomforts of blurred minds; but they also maintain the blur" (21). One of the major blurs that Wood finds in the American spirit as reflected in movies is the indiscriminate equation of "assertions of the self" with issues of the greatest national or international importance. At the beginning of *Casablanca*, for example, Rick (Humphrey Bogart) is basically an American isolationist, unwilling to become involved in world politics. When he finally does take action and shoots Strasser (Conrad Veidt), he is acting from personal feelings for Ilsa (Ingrid Bergman) and Victor Laszlo (Paul Henreid) rather than from any patriotic motives. And yet the film is clearly intended as an endorsement of the policy that brought the United States into World War II.

Robert B. Ray (1985) has expanded this interpretation of *Casablanca*, applying to the film a methodology that has greatly influenced our argument in this book. Ray argues that *Casablanca* successfully transforms world conflict into the conventional problems of melodrama because it appropriates the traditional story of "the outlaw hero versus the official hero" that Americans knew well from years of being exposed to movies about the Old West. The character of Rick looks back to a tradition of uniquely American heroes (including, for example, Huck Finn) and ahead to the Shane of Alan Ladd and director George Stevens. All of these characters are reluctant heroes who exist on the fringes of society and the law, struggling with conflicts that approximate but eventually replace the larger political questions. Ultimately, "the self-determining, morally detached outlaw hero came to represent America itself" (Ray 1985, 91). The outlaw hero is usually at odds with an official hero, who represents a parallel tradition in American mythology with roots in parental figures such as George Washington and Abe Lincoln. Ray even points out the striking physical resemblance that Victor Laszlo (Henreid), the "official hero" of *Casablanca*, bears to George Washington (1985, 98). Although our sympathies are with the outlaw hero, American movies of the "classic" period (usually marked as 1930 to 1945) generally find ways of sparing the audience the psychological agony of choosing him over the official hero. At the climax of *Casablanca*, Rick and Laszlo find themselves working

CHAPTER I

toward the same goal, much in the same way that Shane avoids conflict with that film's putative hero (Van Heflin) by joining him in the fight against the bad guys. We will examine *Casablanca* more extensively in chapter 8.

We have simplified Wood's and Ray's readings of *Casablanca*, but their thesis should be clear: the most popular U.S. films frequently avoid answering the most troubling questions by displacing them into melodrama, where solutions are more easily found. Drawing upon the work of Charles Eckert (1974b), who has compared this displacement to Freud's account of displacement in the dream work, Ray finds reconciliation to be the most important psychological element in classical Hollywood's "thematic paradigm." Because melodrama throws a film's center of gravity onto the decisions of a single individual, American movies reinforce the often paradoxical belief that the answer—and, ultimately, the solution—to just about anything lies within ourselves. Wood (1975) cites the end of *The Best Years of Our Lives* (1946), in which the Dana Andrews character only has to pull himself together in order to get a job, even though the film grimly argues that no worthwhile jobs are open to him in the difficult years after World War II. Wood mentions psychoanalysis, "which is easily cast as a doctrine of self-help," as a means for preparing the self for the inevitable victory over what lies outside (1975, 38). But Wood does not discuss how psychoanalysis, which also says that deep-seated problems have been with us since childhood and may even be intractable, becomes an easy target for films that deny the realities behind our worries. The long-standing ambivalence toward psychiatry in American movies grows naturally out of an optimistic mythology that uses psychiatrists in two dissimilar ways.

Throughout this study, we will use the term *ideology* in much the same sense as does Louis Althusser (1977), who defines it as "a system . . . of representations (images, myths, ideas, or concepts, depending on the case)" (231). As many film critics have discovered, this definition is ideally suited to the study of movies. Although he is reluctant to use the term as prominently as other critics, Robert Sklar (1975) has convincingly traced the dominant ideology implicit in American films. Sklar observes that for all its affronts to traditional values, Hollywood's major contribution was essentially the affirmation of familiar American beliefs about, for example, "the virtues of deferred gratification and the assurance that hard work and perseverance would bring success" (196). He shares Michael Wood's thesis that American films made earlier than the 1960s seldom venture outside received cultural myths. However, Sklar is more interested in how these myths are related to economics and power than to the half-conscious workings of "blurred minds" that Wood addresses. Like Ray, Sklar quotes Roland Barthes, whose book

Mythologies describes "collective representations" such as movie myths, and he joins Barthes in the call to "go further than the pious show of unmasking them and account *in detail* for the mystification which transforms petit-bourgeois culture into a universal nature" (197). Sklar attempts such an accounting with the great master of these mystifications and transformations, Frank Capra. Following Sklar, we will show in chapter 2 how in *Mr. Deeds Goes to Town* (1936) Capra used an absurd psychiatrist from Vienna as a foil for that most natural of men, Gary Cooper, who in this film carries a name that suggests his uniquely American talents and desires, Longfellow Deeds.

Another way of thinking about psychiatrists in American movies suggests something other than the ideologically charged transformations of which Barthes speaks. Apart from what would seem to be an ideological function in the movies, psychiatrists have often provided a convenient means for effecting the mechanics of plot, regardless of what that plot may be. In one sense, the people who have written fiction, drama, and stories for television or the movies have found the psychiatrist to be as important an invention as the telephone. Before the telephone, dramatists had to go to great lengths to establish background information. In act 1 of Ibsen's otherwise gracefully crafted masterpiece of 1884, *The Wild Duck*, one by one each of the major characters crosses the stage as he is identified in the conversation of two servants. After Alexander Graham Bell made his contribution to civilization, a playwright could accomplish just as much with a phone call in the first scene. An actor could then stand alone on stage and quickly supply crucial information while talking to an imaginary character by phone. Amanda Wingfield's telephone conversations in Tennessee Williams's *The Glass Menagerie* present a good example of this technique: her unsuccessful attempts to sell magazine subscriptions are a poignant character revelation.

Like telephone conversations, psychiatric consultations have offered filmmakers the perfect device for unearthing dark secrets and simplifying exposition. As early as 1922, an individual resembling a psychiatrist sets up key scenes in *The Man Who Saw Tomorrow*, a silent film in which the hero goes to a psychologist/mesmerist to find out which of two women he should marry. Once the man is hypnotized, the film cuts to a pair of dream sequences foretelling events in the hero's life with each of the two women. Of course, psychiatrists are on hand for flashbacks much more frequently than flashforwards, as for example in Curtis Bernhardt's *Possessed* (1947). The film begins with an incoherent and delirious Joan Crawford wandering alone through city streets. Placed under the care of psychiatrists, who are initially incapable of learning her identity, she soon reveals the information that they (and the audience) require when she is injected with a truth drug, part of a process called "narcosynthesis," a favored technique in the films of the late 1940s. Although the psychiatrists make elevated pronouncements about what they learn of her story (and although their patriarchal account of the heroine's condition has a definite ideological component), their major function in the film is to provide a bridge into flashbacks containing the Crawford character's life story.

In more recent years, psychiatrists as movie characters have become subtler, though no less conventionalized, vehicles for exposition and character development. Playing the expensive call girl Bree Daniels in Alan J. Pakula's *Klute* (1971), Jane Fonda engages in two strikingly different styles of acting. As the plot of the film takes her through scenes of romance and suspense, she is confident and smooth. But in scenes with her female psychiatrist (Vivian Nathan), Fonda uses the improvisational techniques of method acting to express the inner thoughts of her character, and she becomes hesitant and uncertain. Psychotherapy offered Pakula the opportunity to reveal vulnerability and complexity in the self-confident Bree that might otherwise have been lost to the melodramatic demands of the scenario. In the same year as *Klute*, a psychiatrist performed a similar function while listening to the confessions of George C. Scott in the first moments of Arthur Hiller's *The Hospital* (1971). The psychiatrist (David Hooks) appears only in this introductory scene so that the audience can establish early on that Scott's character is depressed and contemplating suicide.

A formalist critic might say that a psychiatrist used in this fashion functions principally as what Henry James (1934) has called a *ficelle*. Literally the strings with which a puppeteer controls his puppets, a *ficelle* has the same role as the colorless confidants and confidantes to whom several centuries of stage heroes and heroines have explained their thoughts for the benefit of the audience. For James, a *ficelle* is of special importance in fiction when the author chooses to write in a self-effacing voice or to emphasize the complexity of the central characters by juxtaposing them with minor, one-dimensional characters. The invention of psychotherapy has presented filmmakers with the ideal *ficelle*, one that need not even speak, yet whose presence allows a character to engage in intense self-scrutiny before the cameras.

So far we have touched on the ideological and "mythological" forces that shape the role of the cinematic psychiatrist and on the less ideologically charged formal necessities that they often are called on to effect. We now offer a reading of a film that provides a good example of these and other forces in action as well as a model for interpreting them. Falling midway through the ninety years of psychiatry in American movies, Mitchell Leisen's *Lady in the Dark* (1944) unassumingly introduces conventions we will encounter repeatedly throughout this study: the "faceless" psychiatrist, the psychiatrist as plot expediter, the psychiatrist as spokesman for the dominant ideology, as well as the psychiatrist with the ability to effect a dramatic cure after the resurrection of a repressed trauma from childhood. *Lady in the Dark* was based on a 1941 Broadway musical hit (467 New York performances) written and directed by Moss Hart with music by Kurt Weill and lyrics by Ira Gershwin. The film version was also a box-office success, even though it omits many of the Weill/Gershwin songs, including the haunting "My Ship," which is only hummed a few times by the eponymous lady played by Ginger Rogers. The film, however, does not lack production numbers, almost all of which originate in Rogers's analytic sessions, much in the same way that the narcosynthesis sessions in *Possessed* provide the frame for flashbacks.

Lady in the Dark begins with Liza Elliot (Rogers) suffering a malaise for which her doctor can find no medical explanation. When he suggests that she see a "psychoanalyst," she interjects, "You're not serious. You don't really believe in that?" Liza is the editor of *Allure*, a popular fashion magazine, and although Rogers is made up to be an attractive woman, her character dresses in rather severe business attire. Charley Johnson (Ray Milland), an employee at the magazine who makes her the butt of his frequently cruel jokes, has suggested that holding down a man's job has made Liza too masculine and that he would like to have her position at the magazine. Two other men in Liza's life are Kendall Nesbitt (Warner Baxter), a wealthy older man who has given Liza her editor's job and who would marry her if his wife would give him a divorce, and Randy Curtis (Jon Hall), a popular young movie idol who much prefers Liza to the mobs of squealing women who crowd around him when he arrives for a photo session at Liza's office. She seems unwilling to accept his dinner invitation, however, and cannot even recall that they have met.

When Liza reluctantly arrives at the office of psychoanalyst Alexander Brooks (Barry Sullivan), her first session soon gives way to a balletic dream sequence that works several characters from her life into a highly stylized setting. In a second session, after Nesbitt has told Liza that his wife will divorce him and that they can marry, Liza dreams up a wedding that is an elaborately costumed medieval pageant. After a long dance number featuring Munchkin-like figures, the royally clad Liza and Nesbitt approach the altar, but before the dream is over, she has embraced not Nesbitt but Randy, the movie star.

The analyst's interpretation of Liza's dream ignores the Munchkins and goes right to the resemblance between Nesbitt and Liza's father. In a surprisingly frank exposition of psychoanalytic theory (and one that suggests

Freud's 1916 reading of Ibsen's *Rosmersholm)*, the psychoanalyst tells Liza that she is reluctant to marry Nesbitt because she fears violating the oedipal taboo. Liza bristles at the suggestion, but Dr. Brooks authoritatively speaks.

> BROOKS: If it's not true, then why do you reject Randy
> Curtis? . . . Most women would be very interested in Randy
> Curtis.
> LIZA: I am not most women . . . . I can think of nothing I'd hate
> more than a lot of men chasing after me making love to me.
> BROOKS: Aren't you rejecting his invitation because you're
> afraid of competing with other women?

We soon learn that Liza's beautiful but aloof mother had made Liza feel like an ugly duckling. Once when Liza tried to perform a song ("My Ship") that she had carefully prepared with her father, the mother ignored the child while flirting with one of her admirers. The mother died while Liza was still in her childhood, and one day the little girl put on a blue dress that was a favorite of her father's whenever her mother wore it. Still grieving over his beautiful wife's death, the father flew into a rage when he saw his daughter in the dress, an incident that Liza had repressed but that ultimately caused her to suffer anxiety and depression. After learning all of this repressed information, the psychoanalyst lectures Liza on her flight from femininity, finally concluding that she needs "some man to dominate" her.

Smiling, Liza walks out into the sun a changed woman. Almost immediately she encounters Randy, the boyishly handsome movie star who has already expressed more than a passing interest in her. Liza seems to enjoy his attentions, especially now that she can hold her own with a man whom many other women find attractive but who is not a surrogate father. Randy soon asks her to marry him, but only after he has unsettled her a little by telling her how much he needs her to run the new movie production unit he is planning. He concludes his marriage proposal with the words: "Don't worry. You're still going to be the boss." Liza is agonizing over a marriage proposal for the second time in a few days when Charley (Milland) enters her office to apologize for the numerous times he has insulted and ridiculed her. He explains that he behaved badly because he wanted power. Liza then realizes that Randy is much too submissive for her and that she has found the necessary dominant male in Charley. The film ends as they embrace.

Lady in the Dark is most memorable for its production numbers, despite its introduction of psychoanalytic dream interpretation into the unlikely genre of musical comedy. Perhaps as a result, the analyst who serves primarily as the triggering device for these set pieces is something of a cipher, detached from any other character, including the heroine (plate 1). However, Dr. Brooks's detachment need not characterize a film of this type. Compare, for example, Barry Sullivan's character in *Lady in the Dark* with the psychiatrist played by Yves Montand in Vincente Minnelli's *On a Clear Day You Can See Forever* (1970). The Montand character performs the same function of listening to the heroine, in this case Barbra Streisand, so that the film can cut to flashy production numbers, which illustrate the reincarnated heroine's past lives. But although Montand is frequently pushed into the penumbrae by the formidable Streisand, his suave, Continental character is much more substantial than Sullivan's. Montand even becomes a principal player in the reconstruction of Streisand's previous lives. The neutral attitude affected by Sullivan in *Lady in the Dark* is consistent with the professional conduct expected of "real-life" psychiatrists. In the movies, however, his colorlessness is unusual.

In one sense, Dr. Brooks in *Lady in the Dark* can be understood as a spe-

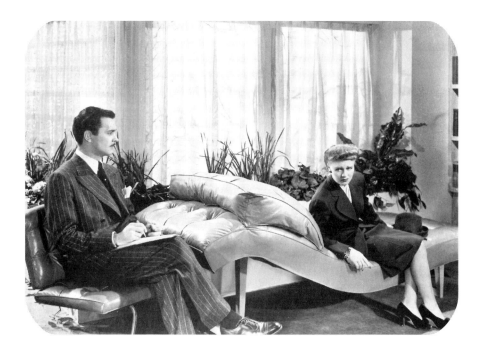

PLATE 1.   Ginger Rogers with Barry Sullivan in *Lady in the Dark* (1944). Paramount Pictures. The Museum of Modern Art/Film Stills Archive.

cial kind of *ficelle*—the analyst as plot mechanism—a recurrent phenomenon in American films before and after this one. His flat character would seem to result logically from his perfunctory presence as a device for facilitating plot and exposition. We call this character type *the faceless psychiatrist* after his peculiar lack of identifying traits. Even facelessness, however, can be understood in terms of the historical interactions between movies and psychiatry. In earlier films such as *The Front Page* (1931), the problem of how to present an interesting psychiatrist in a bit part was solved (as it had been in the stage play of 1928) by introducing the stereotypical Viennese with tails, pince-nez, and a vaudeville version of a *Mittel Europa* accent. Although this figure has persisted to the present, Americanized psychiatrists first began to appear in the mid-1930s, especially when the presentation was intended to be positive. Hollywood was acknowledging that psychoanalytic psychiatry was no longer the exclusive province of European—that is, "foreign"—immigrants.

Schneider (1977) has reported that Moss Hart wrote *Lady in the Dark* as a tribute to his own analyst, and perhaps for this reason the handsome and poised Barry Sullivan was given the part in the film. The work of a sympathetic psychiatrist, however, is somewhat more obscure than that of a Viennese quack, and many people, then and now, believe that therapists deliberately wear expressionless masks for their patients. Consequently, Dr. Brooks has few of the distinguishing qualities that characterize bit players such as the wisecracking cab drivers, the diplomatic policemen, or the effeminate sales clerks who regularly populated films of this period. Sullivan, working in film for only the second time in *Lady in the Dark*, is almost a stand-in for the *idea* of a psychiatrist. He has moments of compassion as well as authority, but unlike almost every other character in the film, he has few, if any, human qualities. We have no idea what kind of husband or father he is, or even if he *is* a husband or father. Nor do we have any idea what personal feelings he may hold for his patient.

Facelessness has continued to be part of the typology of the movie psychiatrist, even though the significance of this kind of character seems to have changed. In more recent films the facelessness of psychiatrists is often a function of their ineffectiveness: if they had more character, they might be able to help people. In Michael Pressman's *Some Kind of Hero* (1982), Richard Pryor plays a returning prisoner of war whose best friend was killed in Vietnam, whose wife has just left him, and who laughs hollowly when a faceless shrink lamely asks him if he has "any problems." An almost identical scene occurs in a more serious film, Michael Cimino's *The Deer Hunter* (1978), when an Army psychiatrist mechanically asks dehumanizing questions of Christopher Walken, who responds with grim humor. This myth of

the ineffectual or out-of-touch psychiatrist has been especially well represented in movies during the last twenty years. In chapter 4 we will discuss
the various ideologies that emerged from the 1960s along with this character
type.

The psychiatrist in *Lady in the Dark*, however, is characteristic of very different movie myths of the 1940s. We have quoted Michael Wood on the consoling function of classic American movies, which acknowledge our deepest
anxieties while at the same time making them seem marginal. Liza Elliot's depression is rooted in painful childhood memories, but most of her therapy is
dramatized as charming musical pageantry. Even the Munchkins in one of her
dreams provide a consoling counterpoint, evoking the child's fantasy of *The
Wizard of Oz*, a film released just five years before *Lady in the Dark*. The
earlier film was about an orphan who, as Harvey Greenberg (1975) has persuasively argued, heroically overcomes her adolescent anxieties. Not only is
the rejection that Liza suffered at the hands of both her mother and her father softened by this reference to *The Wizard of Oz* and the possibilities of
transcending orphanhood, but the effects of this rejection are soon dispelled
entirely by her psychoanalyst.

The myth of psychiatry expressed in *Lady in the Dark*, as well as in other
films from the early and mid-forties such as *Now, Voyager, Spellbound*, and
Since You Went Away, is rooted in a cinematic romance with psychoanalysis
that looked forward to what we call the Golden Age (1957–63). During
World War II the wondrously soothing message that personal problems are
easily solved was well received, and all four of these films were box-office
winners. Psychiatry offered the perfect means for disposing of a problem by
wrapping it in mystifying, pseudoscientific trappings and then sending it
away cheerfully. The facelessness of Dr. Brooks in *Lady in the Dark*, as well
as his function as a kind of elaborate song cue, reflects the film's preference
for denying the pain of childhood rejection over a more unsettling inquiry
into how a patient comes to terms with the family romance.

Feminist analysis has concentrated on another side of Dr. Brooks's function in *Lady in the Dark*. Even women who have embraced few of the goals of
the women's movement might today object to the "you need a man to dominate you" message that *Lady in the Dark* offers. Molly Haskell (1974) has
found the film to be a good example of the limited and limiting roles that
women are asked to fill, even in what have been called "women's films." The
message of many Hollywood films from the thirties through the fifties is that
women cannot and should not have it all. According to Haskell, in the "sacrifice" category of women's film, a woman must give up "(1) herself for her
children—e.g., *Madame X, The Sin of Madelon Claudet;* (2) her children for

their own welfare—e.g., *The Old Maid, Stella Dallas, To Each His Own;* (3) marriage for her lover—e.g., *Back Street;* (4) her lover for marriage or for his own welfare—e.g., *Kitty Foyle* and *Intermezzo,* respectively; (5) her career for love—e.g., *Lady in the Dark, Together Again;* or (6) love for her career—e.g., *The Royal Family of Broadway, Morning Glory*" (163). As Haskell points out, the theme of these films is that women are only "complete" when they surrender to the roles that conventional middle-class ideology assigns to them. When a sophisticated Manhattan psychoanalyst verifies these attributes in *Lady in the Dark,* we have an excellent example of what Barthes (1972) means when he suggests that institutions such as movies can transform "petit bourgeois" homilies into "nature."

Andrea Walsh (1984), who characterizes *Lady in the Dark* as "rabidly" antifeminist, observes that the film was made in a decade that began and ended with the equally popular films *His Girl Friday* (1940) and *Adam's Rib* (1949), both of which suggested that achievement and femininity can be compatible. *Lady in the Dark,* presenting the opposite view, can nevertheless coexist with these films because all three compellingly address the same problems of social roles confronting women in the 1940s. Walsh has also brought the history of American psychoanalysis into a discussion of *Lady in the Dark,* specifically the "biologically determinist Freudianism à la Helene Deutsch and the notorious Lundberg and Farnham" (1984, 161). These last two authors used a popularized version of Freud's writings to discourage women from remaining in the workplace. Walsh argues that in spite of the new independence that women began to experience as they entered the workforce during World War II, the dominant ideology of the United States in the 1940s drifted toward a "feminine mystique" that was instrumental in justifying the massive demobilization of women after the war. This ideology, supported by American government and industry, found its intellectual validation in books such as Lundberg and Farnham's *Modern Woman: The Lost Sex* (1946). Walsh does not point out the extent to which the fear of a potentially explosive army of jobless male veterans lay behind the postwar demobilization of women. She is right, however, in refusing to characterize Freud's work as antifeminist, even though popularized Freudianism easily lends itself to the perpetuation of traditional female stereotypes. *Lady in the Dark* is an excellent case in point.

What then do we make of Dr. Brooks in this film? The film presents him much as Schneider (1985) has described him: "a compassionate, intelligent, sophisticated man." Through his efforts, we are told, the Ginger Rogers character overcomes her depression and lives happily ever after in a necessary surrender to domesticity. With a few changes, however, this same scenario can turn sinister, as in fact it does in a 1970 film, *Diary of a Mad Housewife*, the story of a frustrated woman (Carrie Snodgress) whose psychiatrist urges her to find fulfillment as a wife and mother, even though the film portrays his suggestions as grotesquely inappropriate to her actual situation.

Unlike the psychiatrist in *Diary of a Mad Housewife*, Dr. Brooks in *Lady in the Dark* invites entirely different interpretations. The question of his "meaning" becomes especially problematic when we are concerned with the ideologically explosive issue of the role of women, but also when the subject is embedded in a film such as *Lady in the Dark* that does not fit neatly into only one category. Both Haskell and Walsh have called it a "women's film," even though it may be the only musical that they include in that category. Musicals make different demands on their audiences than women's films, and any interpretation of *Lady in the Dark* ought to address the genre to which it belongs. Although Rogers had won an Academy Award in 1940 for her performance in an *echt* women's film, *Kitty Foyle*, she also had danced her way through no less than nine musicals with Fred Astaire—not to mention several other musicals, including two choreographed by Busby Berkeley—and in *Lady in the Dark*, she surely carried this musical comedy association for audiences. Following a pattern that Laura Mulvey (1975) has identified in musicals, *Lady in the Dark* often stops its "diegetic," or conventional, narrative flow for production numbers in which the audience is invited to examine Rogers's body. In women's films, stars such as Claudette Colbert, Joan Crawford, Katharine Hepburn, and Joan Fontaine usually carry less of the theatricalized glamour that Ginger Rogers possesses, and their bodies are seldom presented for the audience's visual pleasure outside a strictly narrative context. If *Lady in the Dark* exists primarily for its music and spectacle, we are even more inclined to see the psychiatrist simply as a *ficelle* and a means for introducing production numbers. If we focus more on the dilemma facing Rogers as the heroine of a women's film, his function is more important, and he becomes her liberator or her enslaver, depending on what Stanley Fish (1976) would call "the interpretive community" to which the viewer belongs.

We have begun this chapter with a discussion of *Lady in the Dark* because it easily invites several modes of analysis. An attempt to account for the psychoanalyst in *Lady in the Dark* raises historical questions not only about psychoanalysis itself but also about American movies, about American culture in general, and about American myths that underlie them. Coexisting with these historical questions, and to a certain extent overlapping them, are problems of film genres, styles, and stereotypes. Although it has its fascinations, *Lady in the Dark* critically fails as a film (Walsh is probably correct in calling it "an aesthetic disaster"), but it does introduce important conventions such as the faceless *ficelle,* the psychiatric agent for society, and the simple cure based on the recall of childhood memories. The rest of this chapter will be devoted to a survey of the character traits assigned to psychiatrists in American films and of the film genres that give life to these stereotypes.

Double-Edged Stereotypes

American movie myths have much in common with myths from worlds even more exotic than Hollywood. Film scholars interested in myth have appropriated some of the same methodologies used by classicists and anthropologists. Michael Wood (1975) cites the work of G. S. Kirk (1970), a classicist who has studied myth in a variety of cultures. Drawing on the binary analytic method of Claude Lévi-Strauss, Kirk sees myth as a mediation between opposites that allows for the coexistence of seemingly incompatible truths. For example, from the eighth through the fourth centuries B.C., the Greeks possessed two completely different myths about the centaurs—beasts, half-man and half-horse—that lived outside society in purely natural surroundings. Centaurs of one group were savages who routinely attempted to rape human women and battle their protectors. Those of another type, including Chiron, the tutor of heroes such as Achilles and Jason, were wiser and gentler than most mortals. Kirk suggests that the Greeks reconciled themselves to the paradox of a natural world that could be both fierce and gentle by creating two corresponding models of man existing literally *in nature,* that is, attached to an animal. Horses, after all, can be fierce in action but gentle in repose.

Kirk's structuralist model of mythmaking is fully compatible with the apparently paradoxical way in which movie myths treat our problems: "Myth offers an apparent way out of the problem, either by simply obfuscating it, or making it appear abstract and unreal" (1970, 21). The myths in American movies serve the ancient function of allowing us to live with the contradictory, to keep our illusions at the same time that we acknowledge our limitations. Or, as Robert Ray has observed, "the great Hollywood czars became naïve, prodigious anthropologists" (1985, 13).

Movie psychiatrists may offer the film student a privileged view of cinematic mythmaking in action. Each of their attributes can be divided into "good" and "bad" halves, producing complementary pairs of "good" and "bad" psychiatrists. Like the two classes of centaurs through four centuries of Greek civilization, paired stereotypes of psychotherapists have coexisted comfortably throughout the history of American cinema. We offer table 1 as a basic guide to movie stereotypes of psychiatrists, reserving for later a discussion of the more complex depictions. Each attribute in the far-left column is a constant that movies present differently in good and bad psychiatrists.

We have suggested that the idea of the "faceless" psychiatrist in American films since the later 1960s reflects his or her ineffectuality or helplessness before insuperable problems such as those experienced by the victims of the U.S. involvement in Vietnam. On the other hand, the ideology of Robert Mulligan's *Fear Strikes Out*, the 1957 film about baseball player Jimmy Piersall, clearly allows for the success of psychiatry, and the faceless doctor in that film (Adam Williams) seems to work his cure simply by being near. When a film is sympathetic to psychiatry, the faceless, functional psychiatrist (named Dr. Brown) usually accomplishes his work quickly, as if the filmmakers were anxious to get on with the business of the plot. This seems to be the case both in a comedy like Norman Jewison's *The Thrill of It All* (1963) and in a more earnest film such as Elia Kazan's *Splendor in the Grass* (1961): in both these films from the Golden Age, protagonists are put on the path of conquering their problems after a few minutes of screen time with their psychiatrists. The logical extension of the faceless psychiatrist is, of course, the invisible psychiatrist. *Diary of a Mad Housewife*, for example, ends with a tight close-up of the heroine as she listens quietly to a chorus of self-involved characters at what is apparently a group therapy session presided over by a therapist who is neither seen nor heard. The same practice of holding the camera on an actor's face while he or she talks to an invisible psychiatrist has been used by Woody Allen in *Interiors* (1978), by Ken Russell in *Crimes of*

TABLE 1.   Cinematic Stereotypes of the Psychiatrist

Attribute	Good Psychiatrist	Bad Psychiatrist
Faceless	Cures by presence	Ineffectual
Active	Effective and caring	Manipulative, criminal, or vindictive
Oracular	Omniscient; good detective	Arrogant but misguided
Social agent	Reconciling	Repressive and malevolent
Eccentric	Human and fallible	Neurotic and ridiculous
Emotional	Compassionate	Psychotic
Sexual	Healing lover	Exploitative lecher or libidinous clown

Passion (1984), and by Mike Figgis in *Leaving Las Vegas* (1995). In Arthur Hiller's *The Lonely Guy* (1984), Steve Martin speaks to his analyst exclusively through an intercom.

When "good" psychiatrists play more important roles, and the audience has the opportunity to see them working actively, they are deeply involved with their patients, and their cures usually work, even if the psychotherapists function as little more than advice-dispensing guidance counselors. Consider as examples the following films spanning four decades: classic forties' films, such as *Now, Voyager* and *Lady in the Dark;* Golden Age films, such as *The Three Faces of Eve* (1957) and *David and Lisa* (1962); and films of later vintage, such as *I Never Promised You a Rose Garden* (1977) and *Ordinary People* (1980). When we see "bad" psychiatrists actively pursuing their work, they can be manipulative, like James Earl Jones in Aram Avakian's *End of the Road* (1970); vindictive, like Lane Smith, the pencil-sharpening quack in Graeme Clifford's *Frances* (1982); avariciously crooked, like Helen Walker in Edmund Goulding's *Nightmare Alley* (1947); or easily corrupted, like the military psychiatrist in Tony Richardson's *Blue Sky* (1994), who hospitalizes a nuclear scientist so that his commanding officer can spend more time with the scientist's wife.

One of the most common charges made against psychiatrists is that they pretend to knowledge they do not have (Freedman and Gordon 1973). Accordingly, the movies have given us a great variety of oracular psychiatrists, although they too exist as mythological pairs. When a psychiatrist's oracularity is regarded as a positive trait, the psychiatrist will appear to know everything about a case in a dazzling display of brilliance. When asked to make discoveries outside the confined world of doctor and patient, psychiatrists can be intrepid detectives like Ralph Bellamy in Charles Vidor's *Blind Alley* (1939) and Simon Oakland in Alfred Hitchcock's *Psycho* (1960), who leave behind few mysteries for the police to solve. A negative psychiatrist with oracular pretensions is likely to be a pompous know-it-all, who is in fact misinformed or misguided.

The convention of the psychiatrist as society's agent deserves a more detailed discussion, especially when the films in which psychiatrists appear portray society negatively. In films such as *Lady in the Dark*, in which we are asked to accept the dominant ideology, psychiatry helps confused individuals to live more happily in a benevolent society. Much the same can be said of the supremely compassionate psychoanalyst bearing the formidable name Sigmund Gottlieb Golden in John Cromwell's *Since You Went Away* (1944), who heals the spirits of wounded veterans and helps Jennifer Jones find sense in her life after the death of her fiancé. The other side of this myth presents psychiatrists as co-conspirators and willing accomplices in crimes against sensitive and vital individuals. Milos Forman's Academy Award–winning *One Flew Over the Cuckoo's Nest* (1975) has become the most prominent among numerous films that portray psychiatry as a weapon in the substantial arsenal that society uses against its nonconforming members. The protagonist of *Cuckoo's Nest*, Randle McMurphy (Jack Nicholson), becomes a Christ figure for whom shock therapy is the crown of thorns and lobotomy the cross.

American movies frequently portray psychiatrists as eccentric or weird on the assumption that someone must be a bit crazy to become a psychiatrist. Many real-life psychiatrists have grown accustomed to hearing the double-edged compliment, "You don't act like a psychiatrist." Hence, the popular stereotype of the eccentric psychiatrist is well represented in the movies. If the psychiatrist is portrayed in a positive light, his tendency to be different becomes refreshing and human, as with Dr. Berger (Judd Hirsch) in Robert Redford's *Ordinary People*. Berger's messy office (plate 2), disheveled manner of dress, and informal, if not brusque, style of speaking make him a pleasant contrast to the orderly but sterile environment presided over by his patient's mother (Mary Tyler Moore). Berger is weird and "psychiatrist-like," but also human and fallible.

When eccentric psychiatrists are seen in a more negative light, they are portrayed as more neurotic than their patients and in need of treatment themselves. Ridiculous psychiatrists can be traced back at least to 1938, when Fritz Feld added a nervous tic to the Viennese stereotype in Howard Hawks's *Bringing Up Baby* (plate 3). The sanitarium doctor who menacingly wags his finger in the face of Olivia de Havilland (see plate 12 in chapter 2) in Anatole Litvak's *The Snake Pit* (1948) fits into the same category, as does the misguided doctor in Gilbert Cates's *Oh, God! Book II* (1980), who looks at his diplomas on the wall to shore up his fragile self-esteem. Later on, *Oh, God! Book II* features an entire roomful of self-inflated, humorless psychiatrists, at least one of whom recalls Fritz Feld from forty years earlier by displaying a pronounced tic.

If the movie psychiatrist departs from emotional neutrality, our scheme becomes slightly more complex. In *Agnes of God* (1985), Jane Fonda throws herself into her work, risking her professional and personal security for the sake of a naïve young nun (Meg Tilly) who believes that she was impregnated by an angel. Outside the office, a psychiatrist can get falling-down drunk, as does Gregory Peck in *Captain Newman, M.D.* (1963), and still be as charming as Peck's leading lady (Angie Dickinson) seems to find him as she lovingly sees him home. In *Starting Over* (1979), Charles Durning goes to great lengths to help his brother (Burt Reynolds) overcome a serious case of pre-

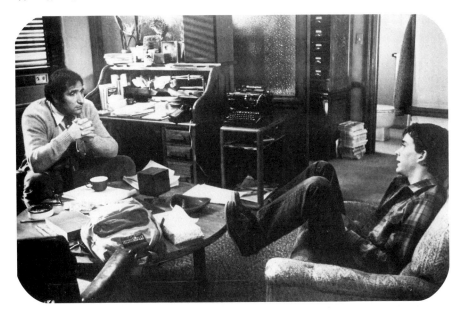

PLATE 2.   The disorder of this man's office reflects his ability to help his patients: Judd Hirsch with Timothy Hutton in *Ordinary People* (1980). Paramount Pictures. The Museum of Modern Art/Film Stills Archive.

marital anxiety. Just as often, however, the movies present negative images in which the emotional psychiatrist is substantially more disturbed than his patients, or he or she is simply psychotic. In addition to psychiatrists who actually murder their patients—Peggie Castle in *I, the Jury* (1953), Maximilian Schell in *St. Ives* (1975), and Michael Caine in *Dressed to Kill* (1980)—we might mention Rip Torn, who films his own breakdown in *Coming Apart* (1969). In one of the first cinematic depictions of psychiatrists, the mind doctor (Herbert Grimwood) in Victor Fleming's *When the Clouds Roll By* (1919) turns out to be an escaped lunatic (see plate 4 in chapter 2).

A psychiatrist's emotional life is judged less clearly in the movies in which he or she falls in love with a patient. It is much more difficult here to separate the "good" psychiatrists from the "bad" ones because audiences are seldom asked to find fault with therapists who help their patients by giving them love. However, as anyone familiar with psychiatric ethics knows, acting on countertransference sexual wishes is strictly forbidden. The prohibition is spelled out clearly to Ingrid Bergman in Alfred Hitchcock's *Spellbound* (1945), to Jason Robards, Jr., in Henry King's *Tender Is the Night* (1962), to Dudley Moore in Marshall Brickman's *Lovesick* (1983), and to Lena Olin in

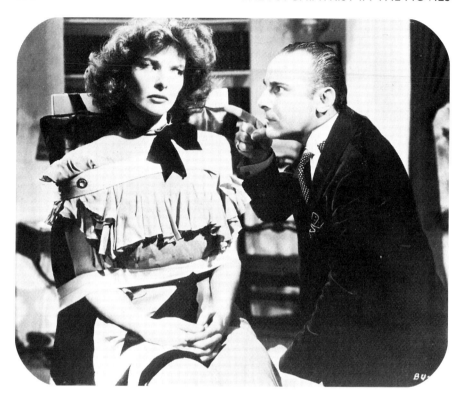

PLATE 3.   Even a quack like Fritz Feld in *Bringing Up Baby* (1938) can tell that Katharine Hepburn has been behaving strangely. RKO. The Museum of Modern Art/Film Stills Archive.

Mike Figgis's *Mr. Jones* (1993), films that span almost fifty years. In each case, a former mentor or colleague warns the romantically inclined psychiatrist about the dangers of falling in love with a patient. Yet in each film the audience is invited to sympathize with the lovers and to applaud the actions of the emotionally involved psychiatrist. These and other films contribute to the demedicalization of psychiatry, suggesting that disturbed people need only love and that if psychiatrists really care they can save their patients by supplying that love, even if they also must give up their profession and the possibility of healing anyone else.

When films portray psychiatry more negatively, the romantically inclined psychiatrist is often held up to ridicule—for example, the sexually jealous Richard Benjamin in Stan Dragoti's *Love at First Bite* (1979) and the lecherous Peter Sellers in Clive Donner's *What's New, Pussycat?* (1965) (see plate

20 in chapter 4). Even in a film such as Philip Dunne's *Blindfold* (1966), a tongue-in-cheek spy mystery about a psychiatrist (Rock Hudson) who uses psychiatric as well as detective skills to outsmart enemy agents, Hudson is shown to have been through a long list of failed relationships with women; as each engagement is announced in newspaper social columns and then called off, reporters begin referring to him as "Dr. Bluebeard." In a less comic setting, Tom Conway in Jacques Tourneur's *Cat People* (1942) attempts to seduce Simone Simon, even though her husband (Kent Smith) is his friend. The reverse situation is represented in Otto Preminger's *Whirlpool* (1950); although the psychoanalyst played by Richard Conte is idealized in every other way, he cannot devote enough attention to his troubled wife (Gene Tierney), who wanders into the clutches of a murderous hypnotist/astrologer (José Ferrer). But when it comes to a psychiatrist's romantic inadequacy, the sex of the psychiatrist is usually female, as we will show in chapter 5.

Psychiatry and Film Genres

Whether it's Ingrid Bergman in *Spellbound* from 1945 or Madeleine Stowe in *12 Monkeys* from 1995, a female therapist in love will do anything to save her lover. Both films suggest that the participation of women in the psychiatric profession, especially when psychiatry is divorced from scientific medicine and its technical trappings, can be an extension of women's nurturing instincts rather than an unseemly encroachment into a male profession. This view is rooted more in the unyieldingly patriarchal conventions of these films than in the films' historical contexts. Films such as *Knock on Wood*, *Sex and the Single Girl*, and *A Very Special Favor*, in which the heroines lose a good deal of the dignity they initially possessed, belong to a different genre: farce/comedy can afford to be less veiled in its antagonism to female achievement. Or, as Freud has written, we are often most serious when we are joking. We have suggested that the interpretation of a film such as *Lady in the Dark* can be strongly influenced by a priori assumptions about the genre to which it belongs. We will now attempt to catalog the various genres in which movie psychiatrists are likely to appear and to assess the effect that the concerns of these genres can have on how mental health professionals are portrayed.

Although movies of more recent vintage are sometimes more difficult to classify as "melodrama," "romantic comedy," "psychological thriller," or even "western" than are earlier films, the most financially successful movies still seem to lend themselves to one-sentence descriptions. Audiences would rather know that they are about to sit through a "romantic story of doomed love on a large, sinking ocean liner" or a "funny/inspirational film about a cute creature from outer space" than pay money for an experience they cannot comfortably label. As a consequence, Hollywood films almost always have fallen into easily identifiable categories, many of which were already available in dime-store novels, newspapers, and the theater when the first filmmakers began looking around for plots. This is not to suggest, however, that film genres are monolithic and unchanging. On the contrary, film genres have always responded to social change as well as to audience expectations, with firmly entrenched genres rising and falling in popularity and subgenres arising out of larger traditions (Braudy 1977). Moreover, in the last two decades, some kinds of films have moved from large screen to small screen, adapting themselves along the way to the demands of serial drama, commercial interruptions, smaller budgets, and varying production techniques. One example is the "mother film," a type of movie that makes heroic figures out of women who make sacrifices for their children and that has evolved from the likes of *Stella Dallas* (1937) to the numerous melodramas now seen almost exclusively on television, especially on the cable channel Lifetime, which is aimed at a female audience. Of course, even attempts by filmmakers such as Robert Altman to undermine genres can serve in the end to broaden and perpetuate those very traditions (Self 1984); and though these genres may continue to evolve, certain characters within them must continue to play stereotypical roles or else the pieces of a genre film, almost by definition, will not fit together.

Musicals and romantic comedies may seem not to take issues very seriously, but as we have seen when women therapists appear in these films, ideology can often operate most directly when it is softened by the film's lighter tone. As Leo Braudy (1977) points out, a major goal of musicals and comedies is to "puncture pretension," exactly what they do in films from *The Front Page* (1931) to *The Gay Intruders* (1948) to *Lover Come Back* (1961) to *High Anxiety* (1977) to *The Santa Clause* (1994). All of these films take comic advantage of the distinguished air that psychiatrists affect or that society has bestowed upon them. But when psychiatrists are central in comedies and musicals, they are usually united with a lover by the end, countertransference notwithstanding. The singing, tap-dancing psychiatrist played by Fred Astaire in Mark Sandrich's *Carefree* (1938) wins Ginger Rogers; the handsome psychiatrist played by Charles Drake is united with his nurse (Peggy Dow) in the conclusion to Henry Koster's *Harvey* (1950); and Dudley Moore gives up everything for Elizabeth McGovern at the end of *Lovesick* (1983).

In crime-and-detective movies, psychiatrists divide along the same lines that we identified for films emphasizing their oracular abilities. In films such as *Blind Alley* (1939), *The Dark Mirror* (1946), *High Wall* (1947), *Blindfold* (1966), and *Still of the Night* (1982), psychiatrists are as successful at their own profession as they are in detective work. In almost all of these films, the brave and ingenious hero also wins a lover at the end, just as we might expect from stories about all but the most hard-boiled private detectives. When psychiatrists are bad or misguided, they stand in the way of the detective work practiced by the heroes in films such as *I, the Jury* (1953 and 1982), *Mirage* (1965), *The Detective* (1968), *The Boston Strangler* (1968), and *Dead Bang* (1989). Needless to say, no romantic rewards flow to the psychiatrists in these films.

As we noted, films of the science fiction, horror, and fantasy traditions such as *The Medusa Touch* and *The Sender* put psychiatrists—often very sympathetic ones—up against supernatural obstacles. In Sidney J. Furie's *The Entity* (1983), Ron Silver plays one of several dedicated psychiatrists trying to help Barbara Hershey. If the film did not argue that the heroine actually is the victim of an invisible demon rapist, the efforts of the psychiatrists would seem perfectly valid if not heroic. Here, as in many films of this type, the scrupulously rational and earthbound work of psychiatrists makes them the perfect foil for the generic conceit of the unknown, the unseen, and the unimagined. This tradition may have begun with Jacques Tourneur's *Cat People* (1942), in which the suave English psychiatrist played by Tom Conway refuses to believe that Simone Simon can actually turn into a panther. However, we might want to go back even further to the naïve sanitarium doctor (Herbert Bunston) in Tod Browning's *Dracula* (1931), who, unlike the otherworldly-wise Professor Van Helsing (Edward Van Sloan), finds the vampire count to be a charming if eccentric aristocrat. Later on, the rational psychiatrist rendered impotent by the supernatural becomes a crucial ingredient in *Miracle on 34th Street* (1947), *Zotz!* (1962), *Oh, God! Book II* (1980), *The Terminator* (1984), and *Groundhog Day* (1993).

In Don Siegel's original 1956 version of *Invasion of the Body Snatchers*, as well as in Philip Kaufman's 1978 remake, a psychiatrist becomes one of the "pod people." We are never sure at what point the transformation takes place, but the well-established theme of the psychiatrist's inadequacy in the face of supernatural phenomena is enhanced by the suggestion that his familiar statements—the mind has the power to create illusions, etc.—originate not from professional conviction but from a conspiracy to conceal the horrible truth of an alien invasion. The psychiatrist played by Patrick Macnee in *The Howling* (1981) serves the identical function by first explaining the werewolf phenomenon in rationalist terms and then revealing himself to be one. John Boorman's *Exorcist II: The Heretic* (1977) is less than coherent on most levels, but it takes a clear position in juxtaposing the impotent gestures of a psychiatrist (Louise Fletcher) against the heroic posturings of the priest played by Richard Burton. The priest frequently responds to Fletcher's liberal humanist account of the world with Manichaean lectures about "Evil," the existence of which the film goes to some lengths to verify.

John Carpenter's *Halloween* (1978) may be unique in putting speeches about Evil in the mouth of the psychiatrist, played by Donald Pleasence. He alone has looked deeply into the eyes of the killer and seen the Devil, or, in the words of a terrified child, "the bogeyman." The police and the psychiatrist's nurse see the killer as just another crazy, but Pleasence's convictions are verified when the villain's corpse disappears after stopping five bullets from the psychiatrist's revolver. *Halloween* is a rare example of a horror/science fiction film in which a psychiatrist is not the last to recognize the existence of unnatural forces. This apparent anomaly has been explained by Robin Wood, who calls Pleasence's statements "surely the most extreme instance of Hollywood's perversion of psychoanalysis into an instrument of repression" (1986, 194). Wood's critique of *Halloween* involves the film's unwillingness to come to terms with the sexual and social themes that it clearly engages. The opening shots of the film, in which a confused six-year-old boy is revealed to be the killer of his sexually active older sister, contain the seeds for "the definitive family horror film": "the child-monster, product of the nuclear family and the small-town environment; the incest taboo that denies sexual feeling precisely where the proximities of family life most encourage it. Not only are those implications not realized in the succeeding film, their trace is obscured and all but obliterated" (Wood 1986, 194). When Pleasence identifies the killer as the Devil, an unchanging source of evil, *Halloween* has compromised the one figure who should be able to understand the forces of repression that drove a child to murder his sister. As the film stands, little in its treatment of the theme separates it from the mass of mad slasher films (a new wave of them in fact inspired by the box-office success of *Halloween*), which seem to argue that sex among teenagers ought to result in death. Although the plot suggests that the psychiatrist is uniquely aware of the nature of evil, *Halloween*'s subtext reveals that the psychiatrist is just as out of touch with the important issues as were his cinematic predecessors who denied the existence of vampires, invisible demons, and invading armies from outer space. Horror and science fiction films invariably suggest, in one way or another, that psychiatry cannot penetrate beyond the superficial.

Beginning with the first loosenings of the Production Code in the 1950s, the film industry found that psychiatrists could legitimize sexuality in films.

Before the new ratings system opened the floodgates of sexuality in 1968, a number of films appeared with titles like *Three Nuts in Search of a Bolt, Suburbia Confidential, The Twisted Sex, Ragina's Secrets*, and even *Loves of a Psychiatrist*. These films were part of a rash of "nudies" that used psychiatry largely to set up sex scenes but also to give the film some semblance of "redeeming social value." In at least one film, the offscreen words of a psychiatrist provided an easily ignored jargonistic sound track to go with the moans and cries of the actors. Not surprisingly, psychiatry became much less important to the adult film industry when the U. S. Supreme Court removed social redemption from its test for pornography.

Psychiatrists performed the same basic function on an only slightly more sophisticated level in the more socially acceptable "sex comedies" of the late fifties and early sixties. The profession gave a veneer of legitimacy to sexual leering in films such as *The Perfect Furlough* (1958), *Who's Been Sleeping in My Bed?* (1963), *Sex and the Single Girl* (1964), and *A Very Special Favor* (1965). However, Hollywood also created a genre of more serious "sex" films—more commonly referred to as melodramas—in which psychiatrists played a role. In *Splendor in the Grass* (1961), the audience knows that Deanie (Natalie Wood) is having a breakdown when she jumps out of a bathtub and exposes a good deal of her naked back. Presumably, the scene was a legitimate portrayal of mental illness and not subject to the same strictures as less ambitious subjects. George Cukor's *The Chapman Report* (1962), based on Irving Wallace's novel about Alfred Kinsey's research, cast Andrew Duggan as a faceless researcher doing psychoanalytically informed work in a community where the women (Jane Fonda, Claire Bloom, Glynis Johns, and Shelley Winters) engage in sexual activities not often suggested (and not actually seen even today) in family films. Duggan interviews the women from behind a room divider, thus exploiting the same voyeuristic fantasies that scenes in confessional booths had previously supplied to audiences. *The Chapman Report* provided titillation, but all in the inquiring spirit of social science. In case the psychiatric sanction was not sufficient, the film ended on the reassuring note that these women were not typical and that almost every other wife in the community was actually quite normal. A psychiatrist was also on hand to put the confessions of a prostitute into a more acceptable context in *Girl of the Night* (1960). Although it hardly fits into the genre of "sex film," John Huston's *Freud* (1962) was, after all, rereleased with the subtitle *The Secret Passion*, and Susannah York expresses more sexual energy in this film than was ordinarily permitted in the early 1960s.

Especially during the 1940s and 1950s, Hollywood turned its attention to the "social problem" film. Along with issues such as alcoholism, racism, and homosexuality, mental illness was explored and often exploited in this film genre, even though the subject was usually treated with deadpan earnestness. Consistent with the patterns of Hollywood mythmaking, films of this type often ended on an optimistic note so that audiences could leave the theater reassured, their anxieties eased. But as Robert Ray (1985) has written, many of these films were less convincing than their prewar counterparts, largely because Hollywood's thematic paradigm had lost much of its ability to effectively obscure the difficult questions that Americans confronted after World War II. Although social problem films about mental illness desperately needed psychiatric cures, and although mental health professionals became the most active participants in society's solution to its problems, the endings of these films were seldom satisfying. Faceless healers became a staple of the American cinema, beginning with Dr. Kik (Leo Genn) in *The Snake Pit* (1948) (see plate 11 in chapter 2). Within a few years, audiences could witness the achievements of psychiatry in *The Three Faces of Eve* (1957), *Fear Strikes Out* (1957), *The Mark* (1961), and *David and Lisa* (1962). Sometimes more than one social problem was addressed in the same film: for example, *Home of the Brave* (1949) and *Pressure Point* (1962), both produced by Stanley Kramer, explored mental illness and racism simultaneously, although, as we shall see, with varying degrees of equivocation.

Another type of motion picture, seldom acknowledged but ideally suited to our study, is the mental institution film, a subgenre of the prison movie. This subgenre has little in common with general hospital films, such as *Men in White* (1934) and *The Interns* (1962), which, with rare exceptions like *The Hospital* (1971), consistently idealize the healing powers of an institution's staff. The most famous example of the mental institution film is *One Flew Over the Cuckoo's Nest* (1975), in which an institution is explicitly portrayed as worse than a prison. In fact, almost all of the films in this genre suggest that institutions are the last place we should go if we wish to be "cured" of our emotional problems. Often the most sensational elements of psychiatric treatment are central in these films: *Shock Corridor* (1963), *Shock Treatment* (1964), *The Fifth Floor* (1980), and *Frances* (1982) as well as *Cuckoo's Nest* all make the most of electroconvulsive therapy (ECT) and insulin injection. *The Snake Pit* can fit into this category as well as the social problem genre, although it is one of the few mental institution films in which a patient actually recovers. Even when patients are not shocked or lobotomized in these films, they are not likely to benefit from their confinement. Like prison movies, institution films engage American myths of freedom, easily lending themselves to plots in which innocent people must face drastic curtailment of their liberties. This is certainly the case with the José Ferrer character in *The Shrike*

(1955), who, according to the film, never should have been committed in the first place. The years 1966 and 1967 saw the release of two completely different films that nevertheless belong to the institution film genre: in both the "theater of cruelty" *Marat/Sade* and the documentary *Titicut Follies,* there is little suggestion that the inmates of the asylums will benefit from their institutionalization.

The Cathartic Cure

Stereotyped portrayals of psychiatrists lead to stereotyped portrayals of psychiatric treatment. Consistent with their tendency to demedicalize psychiatry, movies have almost always presented a striking overrepresentation of "the talking cure" and an equally striking underrepresentation of treatments such as ECT and pharmacotherapy. Even though the introduction of effective medications has revolutionized American psychiatry, movie psychiatrists seldom prescribe them. In fact, American psychiatry during the last three decades has been characterized by a strong movement toward "remedicalization." Interest in psychoanalytic psychiatry has declined, while psychopharmacology, brain chemistry, and neurosciences have received more attention. There is no question, however, that psychotherapy is still portrayed as the predominant or exclusive therapeutic practice of the vast majority of movie psychiatrists. ECT has been depicted somewhat more often in movies, usually as punishment. In institution films such as *One Flew Over the Cuckoo's Nest* and *Frances,* ECT is used malevolently to produce socially appropriate behavior, lobotomy standing in reserve as the final solution to the nonconformist problem. In *The Snake Pit* (1948), ECT is made to appear grotesque by means of camera angles and orchestral crescendos on the sound track. To emphasize the excruciating pain of the process, the film focuses on the contraption forced into the mouth of the victimized patient (Olivia de Havilland), as if it were a bullet that cowboys bite during primitive surgery on the prairie with only a slug of whiskey for an anesthetic. However, after exploiting the melodramatic aspects of electroshock, *The Snake Pit* goes on to endorse its positive effects: after a few sessions, the patient's condition begins to improve, and soon she is able to reap the benefits of psychotherapeutic interventions. As we approach the Golden Age, and ECT is portrayed as effective, it usually occurs off-camera, as in *Fear Strikes Out* (1957), where we see the treatment room only from the outside.

The talking cure of psychotherapy and psychoanalysis seems more favored by moviemakers, even though it holds much less dramatic power than ECT.

Consequently, filmmakers have developed a convention that cuts across all periods of psychiatric films: the cathartic cure, the sudden and dramatic recovery from mental illness. This convention has also been noted by Vernet (1975) and Eber and O'Brien (1982), who emphasize that the formula lends itself well to the building of dramatic tension and its climactic release. No corresponding method exists by which a medical, rather than a mental, patient can dramatically recover from, say, an infectious disease unless the film appropriates more fantasy-oriented types of movie magic. Often a simple montage sequence can make a long period of recovery take up only seconds of screen time, but this convention cannot compete with the drama of the cathartic cure. As is the case with other conventions, the psychiatrist is not essential for these cathartic cures, variations of which appear frequently in films, even when some kind of therapist is completely absent. Consider the sudden recovery of Dorothy McGuire in *The Spiral Staircase* (1946), of Jane Wyman in *Johnny Belinda* (1948), or of Heather Sears in *The Story of Esther Costello* (1957). But when the recovering patient is not deaf, dumb, or blind, psychiatrists are frequently nearby.

Few practicing therapists report moments of catharsis such as those depicted in films. More importantly, real-life instances in which the sudden recovery of repressed memories is curative are even rarer. Many American films conventionally reflect one historical moment in the development of psychoanalysis, when Freud himself was attempting to cure his hysterical patients with this method. In his seminal 1895 work, *Studies on Hysteria*, Freud hypothesized that the conversion symptoms of hysterics were caused by repressed traumatic memories. The cure, in his view, was to derepress these memories. Hypnosis and suggestion were both means of removing the repression barrier and allowing these memories to surface. Freud soon learned, however, that the mere recovery of these memories was not in fact curative. He went on to develop the much more sophisticated and complex technique of analyzing resistances and transference as they developed in the analytic situation.

If filmmakers have studied the history of the psychoanalytic movement, it would seem that they stopped reading Freud's works at this particular historical point. Most of the positive portrayals of psychotherapy or psychoanalysis revolve around the derepression of a traumatic memory. The classic example is Nunnally Johnson's 1957 film *The Three Faces of Eve*. In this supposedly true story of a woman suffering from multiple personality (now called dissociative identity disorder), Joanne Woodward is cured by a caring and effective psychiatrist, Dr. Luther, played by Lee J. Cobb. As Dr. Luther becomes aware that he is dealing with a rare multiple personality syndrome, he searches the patient's past for an explanation of the illness. He apparently regards the cure and the discovery of the etiology of the illness as virtually synonymous. Dr. Luther laments how normal her childhood was and expresses a wish that he could find some shocking traumatic episode in her past, implying that such a trauma would be the key to unlock the mystery of both the etiology and the means of cure.

To assist the search, Dr. Luther employs hypnosis, another technique that is greatly overrepresented in the movies in proportion to its actual use by therapists and psychoanalysts. Prior to Dr. Luther's use of hypnotic methods, Joanne Woodward displays two personalities, Eve White, a depressed, withdrawn housewife, and Eve Black, a seductive, histrionic floozy (see plate 14 in chapter 3), whose emergence is usually accompanied by a jazzy clarinet on the sound track. When the psychiatrist begins to use hypnosis, Jane, a third personality, emerges as the integration of the two selves represented by Eve White and Eve Black. Woodward plays Jane by adopting better posture and, consistent with Hollywood's regional stereotyping, by dropping her Southern accent. Through further hypnosis, Jane is able to recover a repressed traumatic memory of an episode in her childhood when her parents forced her to kiss her dead grandmother in the coffin before her burial. After this memory is derepressed, Eve White and Eve Black are absorbed by the healthy and well-integrated personality of Jane, who discovers that she now has complete memory of her past. Jane's personality quickly becomes reconstituted after the emotional catharsis associated with recovering the memory and, as the film ends, she happily drives off with her new husband and her daughter. How the childhood trauma has caused the problem of multiple personality remains a mystery, as does the relationship between remembering the incident and curing the illness.

Although *The Three Faces of Eve* is based on a true account, it fits much more neatly into the mythological functions of psychiatry. Most psychiatrists rarely see a multiple personality, let alone anything approaching a cure as dramatic as this one. In fact, when the real-life "Eve," Chris Costner Sizemore, published her autobiography (1977), she revealed that the cathartic recovery of the repressed traumatic memory did not lead to a lasting resolution of her multiple personality syndrome. Following the treatment depicted in the film, more personalities appeared—twenty-two in all—over the ensuing years. Following a suicide attempt and intensive therapy, Sizemore finally achieved what she perceived to be a lasting recovery in 1974. Moreover, she reveals that other significant traumatic incidents occurred in her childhood besides the one depicted in the movie. This revelation is much more in keeping with our current understanding of multiple personality—that it is a pattern of repetitive incidents, rather than a single traumatic incident, that produces the syndrome.

Whether or not the depiction of the psychotherapeutic cure in *The Three Faces of Eve* is historically accurate, the point to emphasize here is that such a cure is the preferred account of the mechanism of psychotherapy in the movies. Sometimes cathartic cures do not even involve the derepression of a traumatic childhood memory. In the first scenes of Mark Robson's *Home of the Brave* (1949), a black serviceman named Moss (James Edwards) returns from a World War II battle and says that he cannot walk, even though doctors can find no physical disabilities. An Army psychiatrist (Jeff Corey) is introduced first for the familiar purpose of plot mechanics ("What happened on that mission?"), but he soon discovers the source of Moss's problem. In a series of flashbacks we learn that Moss was close friends with a white soldier, Finch (Lloyd Bridges), who eventually died on the mission. Just before he was shot, however, Finch called Moss "a dirty, yellow-bellied nig——" and then corrected himself by saying "nitwit." Moss becomes afflicted with hysterical paralysis because he cannot cope with the realization that he wanted Finch to die. Once all of this is explained to him, Moss says that he understands, but he still cannot walk. Finally, the psychiatrist begins taunting him, even calling him a "dirty nigger." This does the trick, and Moss rises to attack the psychiatrist only to realize that he has been cured. *Home of the Brave* was produced by Stanley Kramer, one of Hollywood's most outspoken liberals, and Carl Foreman's script was daring in its overt treatment of racism, especially for 1949. (The script was also inaccurate. No African Americans served in otherwise white platoons during World War II.) The cathartic cure is central to the film, and not just because it provides a dramatic climax. The way in which the cure is administered asks the audience to confront the harsh effects of racial prejudice upon black people while at the same time supporting the politically complementary idea that something can be done to heal the wounds inflicted by racial hatred. Nora Sayre (1982), however, is correct when she argues that the film badly confuses Moss's sensitivity to racism with racism itself and that by basing much of Moss's cure on the realization that he is "just like everybody else," the film denies the real problems of American racism, much as it submits psychiatry to the familiar optimistic conventions of movie myths. Consistent with the Hollywood paradigm of reconciliation, the cathartic cure in *Home of the Brave* provides an effective cinematic means for replacing the overwhelming problems of racism with an uplifting story of one soldier's dramatic recovery from paralysis.

Instant cures also appear in Charles Vidor's gangster film *Blind Alley*

(1939), as well as in its remake, Rudolph Maté's *The Dark Past* (1948). A good deal of primitive psychoanalytic theory is bandied about in the story of a gangster (Chester Morris in *Blind Alley*, William Holden in *The Dark Past*) who killed because of a desire to destroy his father. By coincidence, he finds himself in the house of a psychiatrist (Ralph Bellamy in the original, Lee J. Cobb in the remake) after escaping from jail. Holding the household hostage while waiting for members of his gang to arrive, the gangster is interrogated by the psychiatrist, whose interest in his captor seems purely scientific (see plate 6 in chapter 2). At first the gangster dismisses the doctor's questions with comments such as "Ah, you're a screwball," but he soon begins recounting a nightmare that has been keeping him awake for years. Using Freudian dream analysis, the psychiatrist identifies various displacements in the criminal's dream, finally explaining his antisocial behavior as a continuing desire to destroy his father. When he is finished, the doctor assures the gangster that he will no longer be able to kill, now that he understands his darker impulses. Like many other oracular psychiatrists in the movies, the doctor has done his job so well that when the police arrive, they easily shoot down the killer, who cannot bring himself to return their fire.

It is tempting to dismiss the preeminence of the cathartic cure as simply emblematic of a particular historical period in the cinematic treatment of psychiatry, but a quick look at an Academy Award–winning movie from 1980 reveals that this is not the case. The sudden recovery of Conrad Jarrett (Timothy Hutton) in *Ordinary People* is closely related to a moment of catharsis. Released from an institution after a suicide attempt, Conrad is brought closer to health by the parallel efforts of Dr. Berger (Judd Hirsch) and his girlfriend (Elizabeth McGovern). He cannot, however, overcome the hostility of his mother (Mary Tyler Moore), and when he learns that a girl he knew in the institution (Dinah Manoff) has killed herself, he slips back into suicidal depression. In desperation, he calls Dr. Berger in the middle of the night and arranges to meet him at the psychiatrist's office. In a few minutes, Berger has fixed on the guilt that afflicts Conrad over the death of his brother—also his mother's favorite child—when both boys were involved in a boating accident. Conrad is out of control in Berger's office, screaming and crying as he thrashes about the room. Raising his own voice to get Conrad's attention, Dr. Berger forces him to confront the memory of the boating accident. He asks Conrad what he did wrong, and after resisting the question, Conrad shouts at him, "I hung on!" With this catharsis, Conrad's survivor guilt is relieved, but he tells Berger that being alive does not feel good. The intense but unsentimental monotone delivery of Judd Hirsch makes the following exchange particularly effective:

BERGER: It is good, believe me.
CONRAD: How do you know?
BERGER: Because I'm your friend.
CONRAD: I don't know what I would have done if you hadn't
    been here. Are you really my friend?
BERGER: I am. Count on it. (Conrad reaches out and they em-
    brace.)

Free of his depression, Conrad arrives at the house of his girlfriend with every
indication that he is prepared to start life anew. After this scene, the film
need only dispose of its villain, Conrad's mother, who soon drives away and
leaves her son with his father—a postfeminist revision of the *Stella Dallas*
cliché of the mother who abandons her child in order to save her child.

The unlikely cathartic cure in *Ordinary People* did not prevent the film
from receiving an Oscar for best picture. In fact, the movie's popularity probably resulted from positive feelings that audiences experienced after witnessing the swift and total exorcism of the film's two major demons—Conrad's
depression and Mary Tyler Moore. No one can discount the fact that Judd
Hirsch was portrayed as a caring and effective psychiatrist. Nor can one dismiss the curative power of a genuine relationship between therapist and patient where the patient feels he is valued. The more interesting dynamics of
Conrad's depression, however, such as the obvious sibling rivalry and his consequent but unconscious death wish toward his brother, are left largely unexplored in therapy. Similarly, as Robin Wood has observed, there is no
examination of the overtly oedipal process that replaces the mother with a
more compliant female (Elizabeth McGovern) in order to facilitate the patriarchal reconciliation of father and son—a process in which, at least on the
subtextual level, the psychiatrist is complicit (1986, 263). The cathartic cure
in *Ordinary People* may not have alienated filmgoers, but it did inspire a parody in Jerry Lewis's *Cracking Up* (1983). When the comic protagonist
(Lewis) and his analyst (Herb Edelman) finally solve the patient's problems,
analyst and patient bound across the office into each other's arms in slow motion, à la the 1967 art-house hit *Elvira Madigan*.

Electroconvulsive therapy and the cathartic cure are not the only treatments that have become conventionalized in American movies. Simple,
commonsense advice is also frequently depicted as essential to psychotherapeutic technique. In the popular film *Now, Voyager* (1942), Dr. Jaquith
(Claude Rains) is never actually seen in the act of psychotherapy although, as
in plate 8 (see chapter 2), he occasionally mixes with his patients on an ele-
mental level. Basically, he conceptualizes the problem of Charlotte Vale

(Bette Davis) as overexposure to an unsympathetic parent, and the therapy he recommends is a South American cruise. This kind of guidance counseling may take the form of telling a woman that she needs a man to dominate her, as in *Lady in the Dark*. Or it may be somewhat more sophisticated, as in *Fear Strikes Out*, which, like *The Three Faces of Eve*, was based on a true story, the psychiatric struggles of baseball player Jimmy Piersall, played by Anthony Perkins. The film, however, portrays the recovery of Piersall solely in terms of reconciliation with the male parent, arguing that Piersall's domineering father (Karl Malden) caused his son's eventual breakdown by withholding love from the boy in order to drive him to higher levels of athletic achievement. After Piersall's psychotic depression is relieved through ECT, we see a number of sessions between a faceless psychiatrist and Piersall (see plate 13 in chapter 3). The cure is a three-part process in which the psychiatrist first demonstrates that Piersall's father has pushed him into unhappiness and mental illness, then helps the patient to understand that he must keep his father out of his life until the treatment is over, and finally leads Piersall to forgive his father and to leave the institution in a spirit of reconciliation.

This treatment, which results in patients' blaming and then forgiving their parents, is an almost generic cure that movie psychiatrists dispense like aspirin. It is consistent with movie myths of self-help, but more specifically with the notion that patients have no responsibility for their illness. Psychiatric disorders are caused by bad parents, and cure is effected by convincing the blameless offspring that he must forgive either his father or mother. While variants of this view of mental illness have persisted in psychiatry in recent years—for example, Kohut's (1971) view that empathic failures of the mother result in narcissistic disorders in the child—etiological theories have for the most part abandoned the formula of the schizophrenogenic mother and the victimized child. Modern psychiatry is much more likely to view most mental illnesses in terms of a complex interplay among biological, intrapsychic, and environmental factors, with a particular emphasis on the adequacy of the "fit" between child and nurturing environment (Thomas and Chess 1984).

In this chapter we identified typological and generic patterns in the portrayal of psychiatry in the movies. Sometimes these patterns result from the simple solutions that they offer filmmakers who wish to cut from the present to the past. At other times they are tied in with rigidly prescribed conventions of specific genres that audiences seem content to encounter again and again throughout their lives as moviegoers. These patterns also are strongly related to cultural myths, many of which perform the seemingly contradictory functions of acknowledging our problems while simultaneously denying their importance. The mysterious curative powers of psychiatrists can help facilitate this kind of paradoxical mythmaking, but they also can become myths in themselves. The ability of cultural myths to tolerate diametrically opposed images accounts for parallel traditions of good and bad psychiatrists.

On the other hand, conventions of plot and character are not always evenly distributed throughout cinematic history. And, as we have seen with *Lady in the Dark*, questions of interpretation depend on the historical context of the film. We have been able to link some of the conventions of psychiatry in the movies to specific historical eras, dividing psychiatric films into three periods. The first stretches from the earliest turn-of-the-century caricatures in crude one-reelers about escaped lunatics to about 1957. The second and shortest period, from 1957 through 1963, is the Golden Age of psychiatry in the cinema, in which the effectiveness and benevolence of psychiatry fully realized its mythic potential. Third is the period of almost consistently negative depictions, beginning almost immediately after the Golden Age ended. In the next three chapters, we will chart the changes in the image of the movie psychiatrist and attempt to account for these historical patterns.

CHAPTER 2

The Alienist, the Quack, and the Oracle

So far as we can tell, a psychiatrist first appeared in an American film in 1906. *Dr. Dippy's Sanitarium*, the prototype for the genre of mental institution films, evoked vaudeville stereotypes of madness and portrayed a sanitarium as a bedlam subject to sudden takeovers by inmates. When Dr. Dippy's patients overwhelm a newly hired attendant in this twenty-minute feature, they gleefully torment him by rolling him down a hill in a barrel and then by hurling knives at him in the style of the familiar knife-throwers in the circus. The inmates are easily brought under control, however, when Dr. Dippy arrives with a picnic lunch of pie, and as the film ends they all turn their undivided attention to the lusty enjoyment of their meal.

This crude entertainment was probably not created in the interest of dramatizing the work of a psychiatrist. More likely the intention was to capitalize on the great success of a 1904 one-reeler, *The Escaped Lunatic*. A publicity bulletin for the film describes it as "the escapades of an insane man who imagines himself to be Napoleon I. He escapes from the asylum by a miraculous jump from a third story window, and is pursued across the country by the keepers through a series of ludicrous adventures, until finally disgusted at the chase, he jumps back into the window of the asylum, and is very comfortably reading a newspaper when the tired and mud-spattered keepers enter" (Niver 1971, 130). Irving Schneider (1985) has identified several other films that attempted to duplicate the success of this film, but *Dr. Dippy's Sanitarium* is the only one in which a mental health professional, other than a "keeper," actually appears. Dr. Dippy's role in this particular version of a lunatic's antics seems to have been an afterthought, and it may partially explain why we have been unable to locate another film with a psychiatrist until thirteen years later in *When the Clouds Roll By* (1919).

Some American physicians had specialized in the treatment of mental disorders since the 1830s, and idealized portraits of fictional psychiatrists appeared at least as early as 1861 in the novels of Oliver Wendell Holmes, Sr. (Guthmann 1969). If nothing else, the first identifiable psychiatrist in American movies reveals the vastly different audiences to which novels and early films appealed. *Dr. Dippy's Sanitarium* also serves as the earliest example of an ambivalence toward psychiatry that runs through the entire history of the American cinema: primitive as it is, the film establishes some basic patterns that regularly recur. Dr. Dippy's institution is clearly not designed for the cure of its patients, but the director does not abuse his patients, and in fact he treats them with a certain amount of respect when he politely introduces them one by one to the new attendant. He is also able to bring his charges under control with dispatch and effectiveness, even if his pie treatment is rather unorthodox. The doctor is "dippy" apparently because he lives and works around crazy people whose childish and erratic behavior he cannot always control, and also because the film's producers thought that the name itself sounded funny.

Dr. Dippy's Sanitarium also relies heavily on the received stereotypes of the day. Like the protagonist in *The Escaped Lunatic*, one inmate dresses as Napoleon, while another, a sleepwalker out of Gothic romance, is clad in a flowing white nightgown, a candle and its holder in her extended arm. Dr. Dippy himself is the embodiment of a nineteenth-century medical stereotype: he has a beard, a pince-nez, tails, and a portly bearing. Although this image could fit many middle-class American doctors at the turn of the century, it was soon to be associated almost entirely with psychiatrists, particularly those with foreign accents. The stereotype is still present, by the way, in a film as recent as Billy Wilder's 1974 remake of *The Front Page*.

With easily recognizable characters and with a plot designed for action, the film need not concern itself with the nature of psychiatry and the character of psychiatrists. In fact, even with the limited number of genres available to American filmmakers in the first decade of this century, a similar film could have been made about unruly children in a reform school, cannibals in the jungle, or Indians in the Old West. The real importance of the institution is that it provides a recognizable background for slapstick comedy. As critics since Aristotle have observed, ridiculous characters are suitable subjects for comedy, even when real danger and violence are possible, and the 1906 audience laughed at *Dr. Dippy's Sanitarium* knowing that nothing bad was going

to happen to anybody they really cared about. Crazy people were fair game as comic subjects, and so were their keepers. Insane asylums and their occupants easily met the demands of one of the earliest types of film comedy.

Exploration, Explanation, and Exploitation

For all its shortcomings, *Dr. Dippy's Sanitarium* was at least able to associate a certain kind of doctor with mentally disturbed patients in an institution. During the early days of the American cinema, however, the proper domain of psychiatrists was regularly confused with that of hypnotists, clairvoyants, and other assorted specialists with obscurely defined credentials, setting a pattern for the demedicalization of psychiatry in hundreds of films yet to be made. In 1919, the same year that the revolutionary *The Cabinet of Dr. Caligari* appeared in Germany, Douglas Fairbanks starred in *When the Clouds Roll By*, a film that is memorable if only as the first directorial effort of Victor Fleming, who would later receive credit for directing both *The Wizard of* Oz and *Gone With the Wind*. *When the Clouds Roll By* is tailored primarily to the jumping-jack exuberance of Fairbanks, but its plot also involves a mysterious "doctor of the mind" who seeks to drive the hero to suicide as part of a scientific experiment (plate 4). Dr. Ulrich Metz, played by Herbert Grimwood with what appears to be a large false nose, is first introduced lecturing to an audience of his colleagues. A title card reads, "Here he confirms the popular prejudice of the time against the mushroom growth of dubious psychologists." In one of the most interesting scenes in the film, Fairbanks is given a meal specially prepared by Dr. Metz and his valet to produce nightmares. The resulting dream sequence, probably inspired by Edwin S. Porter's *The Dream of a Rarebit Fiend* (1906), represents one of the first instances in American film of the creative use of special effects to replicate the dreamworld. The film concludes as Fairbanks triumphs over several villains, including the mind doctor, who is discovered to be an escapee from an insane asylum.

Only a handful of films appeared in the 1920s with characters resembling psychiatrists. *The Case of Becky* (1921) involves a "nerve specialist" who saves his daughter from an evil hypnotist so that she can marry a nice young man. In *The Man Who Saw Tomorrow* (1922) a psychologist uses hypnosis to enable his clients to see into the future. Also in 1922, Will Rogers played a mild-mannered psychology professor in *One Glorious Day*. He tells the spiritualist society that he chairs that he is about to leave his body and reappear as a spirit. Instead, an aggressive entity takes over his body and does basically what the hero would have done were he not too meek. In *Boomerang* (1925)

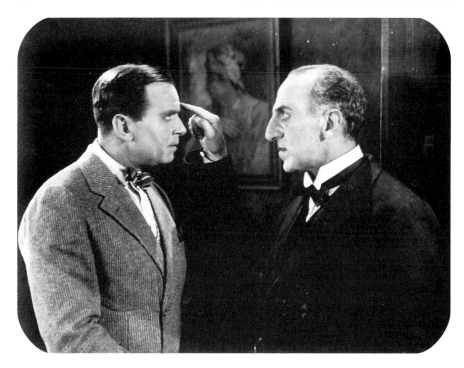

PLATE 4.   Herbert Grimwood is attempting to drive Douglas Fairbanks to suicide in *When the Clouds Roll By* (1919). The Museum of Modern Art/Film Stills Archive.

a doctor in need of patients sets himself up as the director of a mental institution, where he is joined by a female clairvoyant who signs on as his nurse. Surprisingly, the institution is a success, and the two get married. In the 1928 silent film *Plastered in Paris*, a "specialist" fails to cure a World War I veteran's kleptomania, an affliction that the film attributes to a war wound.

The scarcity of psychiatrists in films of the silent era does not, however, reflect their lack of importance in American culture. John Gach has chronicled the early history of psychiatry in the United States and concluded that "by 1920 the Freudian revolution had succeeded. Psychoanalysis . . . by then assured of its cultural niche . . . verged on orthodoxy" (1980, 155). Burnham (1979) has even unearthed a popular song of 1925 with the prolix title "Don't Tell Me What You Dreamed Last Night, for I've Been Reading Freud." Movies did not fully exploit the abundant cinematic possibilities offered by psychiatry, perhaps because of the producers' conservatism.   In spite of the success of a film like *When the Clouds Roll By*, the movie industry could flourish by continuing to rely on the conventions of vaudeville, the dime novel, and the stage melodrama, forms that had developed in the nineteenth century and that seldom needed psychiatry. Furthermore, the most ambitious producers, such as Cecil B. DeMille, found that the most lucrative formulas lay in biblical epics and spectacles rather than in genres like the social problem film, which might at this time have provided a niche for a psychiatrist. Even when psychiatrists began appearing more regularly in the talking films of the 1930s and 1940s, they were almost always embedded in scripts adapted from plays and novels. This may reflect the slow westward move of psychoanalysis; an accredited psychoanalytic institute was not established in the Los Angeles area until 1946. The playwrights and novelists in the Northeast may have been well acquainted with the profession of psychoanalysis, but the creative members of the movie industry were probably unfamiliar with the new breed of talking doctor because the film industry had been firmly based in the vicinity of Los Angeles since 1915.

However, even sophisticated playwrights like Ben Hecht and Charles MacArthur were willing to use psychiatry mostly for laughs, although Hecht, who would later contribute to Hitchcock's *Spellbound*, was clearly fascinated by the institution. Hecht and MacArthur's 1928 work *The Front Page* featured the appearance of an "alienist," as did the two film versions of the play, which mark both the beginning and the end of the 1930s. During the nineteenth century, "alienist" was one of several names variously assigned to doctors in mental institutions, including those accepted by courts to testify on the mental competence of defendants and witnesses. By the 1920s, psychiatrists had for some time been established as replacements for such experts. The Hecht and MacArthur stage play provided the basis for Lewis Milestone's 1931 film of the same title as well as for Howard Hawks's *His Girl Friday* (1940). In *The Front Page* of 1931 a motley collection of cynical reporters awaits the execution of Earl Williams (George E. Stone), the convicted, but unlikely, killer of a policeman in Chicago. One of the reporters (Edward Everett Horton) calls his editor to announce that an alienist named Max J. Egelhofer of Vienna has been called in to examine the convicted man. When the effeminate Horton character adds that Egelhofer has written a book called *The Personality Gland*, one of his colleagues adds, "And where to put it." The film also offers this exchange on the subject:

REPORTER 1: That doctor's the fourteenth pair of whiskers
   they've sent in on this case.
REPORTER 2: Say, those alienists make me sick. All they do is
   goose you and then send you a bill for five hundred bucks.

When we meet Egelhofer, he is directing a large dentist's light at the be-fuddled killer. His pince-nez is on a chain attached to his vest, and a medal hangs on a ribbon around his neck. The alienist also has a stylized beard and an accent that suggests Bela Lugosi more than a denizen of Vienna. When he interviews Earl Williams, he asks that he reenact his crime, even insisting that the sheriff hand the convict a gun for a more precise re-creation. When Williams reaches the crucial moment in his reenactment, Egelhofer asks, "And then what did you do?" Obligingly, the prisoner shoots him in the leg. As the alienist falls to the floor, he exclaims triumphantly, "Dementia praecox!" The movies had at last found a use for psychiatry.

Nine years later, in *His Girl Friday*, little has changed except that the alienist has become a beardless American. Still named Egelhofer, he is portly and wears a pince-nez, and the sheriff calls him both "Professor" and "Doctor," even though the filmmakers have also retained the obsolete title "alienist." For some reason the number of alienists in *His Girl Friday* who have been called to examine Earl Williams has been reduced by four. The relevant exchange between reporters is more typical of 1940, but the spirit is roughly the same as in *The Front Page:*

> REPORTER 1: Must be about the tenth alienist they've put on Williams. If he wasn't crazy before, he would be by the time ten of those babies got through psychoanalyzing him.
> REPORTER 2: Is this guy Egelhofer any good?
> REPORTER 3: Figure it out for yourself. He's the guy they sent to Washington to interview the brain trust. He said *they* were sane.

The 1940 version of Egelhofer also asks Earl Williams to reenact the shooting, but the audience does not actually see Williams shoot the alienist. However, we are told by the heroine (Rosalind Russell) that Egelhofer has been taken "to the County Hospital, where they're awfully afraid he'll recover."

The 1931 and 1940 versions of *The Front Page* make a fascinating comparison with chronologically parallel versions of Clemence Dane's play *A Bill of Divorcement*, George Cukor's original film adaptation dating to 1932, and John Farrow's faithful remake to 1940. Although this family melodrama raises biological questions about mental illness as well as moral questions about granting a divorce on the grounds of insanity, the only doctor in both films is a family physician. While the alienists in *The Front Page* and *His Girl Friday* are comic figures treating a completely sane individual, the crisis of mental illness in historically parallel versions of *A Bill of Divorcement* is presided over by a physician in general practice.

In spite of the ridicule and neglect suffered by the profession during this time, the 1930s also saw the first attempts to deal seriously with psychiatry in American film, *Reunion in Vienna* (1933) and *Private Worlds* (1935). These two films provide excellent examples of what Robert Sklar has called the two "golden ages" of the American cinema, one of "turbulence" and one of "order" (1975, 175). Inspired by the new possibilities of sound and determined to engage audiences with controversy, filmmakers spent the years 1930 through 1934 producing a body of work that succeeded so well in titillating and provoking Americans that it caused the creation of the Breen Office. Founded in 1934, the Breen (or Hays) Office strictly administered the movie industry's system of self-censorship, a production code that remained strong until the late 1950s. In his psychoanalytically astute study of the American cinema, Robin Wood has suggested that the code represented the purest example of how the forces of sexual repression operated on the powerful "drives" of the American cinema to produce a body of work consistent with dominant ideology (1986, 48). Although the code proscribed the sex and violence that had outraged religious groups since the earliest nickelodeon peep shows, it was also designed to bring back a lost audience of moviegoers who had been alienated by the film industry's fascination with social complexities during the early years of the depression. Almost immediately, vigilant enforcement of the Production Code worked alongside the New Deal administration to "boost the morale of a confused and anxious people by fostering a spirit of patriotism, unity and commitment to national values" (Sklar 1975, 175).

The social criticism and sexual license of Sidney Franklin's *Reunion in Vienna* (1933) is typical of what Sklar has called "the first golden age" (not to be confused with what we have called the Golden Age of psychiatry in the movies that began twenty-five years later). Based on Robert E. Sherwood's stage play, the film centers on the dilemma of Elena (Diana Wynyard), once the favorite mistress of Archduke Rudolf Maximillian von Habsburg (John Barrymore) but now the wife of the eminent Viennese psychiatrist Anton Krug (Frank Morgan). The action begins in 1929, ten years after the Habsburgs were expelled from Vienna. Elena first appears in the Schönbrunn palace, taking the official tour of rooms where she once carried on her affair with the charming but wildly irresponsible Habsburg aristocrat (Barrymore). When she returns home to her psychiatrist husband, we learn that she misses the romance that the practical and often didactic Dr. Krug openly preaches against. The therapeutic romance of Freud's Vienna cannot compare to the Old World romance of Habsburg Vienna.

The psychiatrist, however, is surprisingly tolerant when Rudolf flaunts Austrian law by returning from exile to resume his love affair with Elena. Krug clearly articulates the theme of the film, that the Habsburgs represent an obsolete order—a romantic dream—which has been replaced by rational values embodied most perfectly by psychoanalysis. When Rudolf arrives at Dr. Krug's door and offers to fight him for the favors of Elena, the psychiatrist's first impulse is to remove his glasses and fight the archduke with his fists. But the psychiatrist quickly comes to his senses and realizes that Rudolf has succeeded in making him appear a fool in the eyes of his wife. At this moment, Elena rises, apparently to choose between her two suitors. Before she can announce her choice, however, word arrives that the police are waiting outside to arrest Rudolf. Krug is unwilling to turn his rival over to the authorities and even departs to entreat the prefect of police to allow Rudolf to leave the country gracefully. In doing so, Krug intentionally leaves his wife alone with the archduke for the duration of the night, urging her to see him for what he is, a dream of her past.

Reunion in Vienna even suggests that Krug is willing to offer his wife a final sexual encounter with Rudolf—an opportunity she does in fact appear to seize—so that she can more easily bring to a close an old chapter in her life. The film ends the next morning with Rudolf gallantly taking his leave and Elena happily accepting her husband as the man most deserving of her love. The reunion of husband and wife becomes an allegory for the inevitable rise of reason, science, education, and psychoanalysis after the eclipse of Old World decadence. On the other hand, the film's rhetoric contradicts its own message, making Rudolf an infinitely more interesting figure than Krug. Similarly, the screenplay cannot resist applying religious, rather than rationalist, metaphors to psychiatry, even allowing Krug to refer to himself unashamedly as a "messiah." Yet *Reunion in Vienna* is primarily a lighthearted costume drama, which does not always spare psychiatry from the same satiric eye it directs toward the Habsburgs and their world. Krug's practice appears to be limited entirely to women who, as Krug's father (Henry Travers) explains, "tell him their dreams, and he tells them what to do about them."

A distinctly different brand of psychiatry is practiced in a more earnest film, *Private Worlds* (1935), directed by Gregory La Cava and produced by Walter Wanger. The seriousness of this film has much more to do with the Breen Office than it does with a dramatic change in American attitudes toward the profession. As Sklar has written (1975, 175), 1934 marked the beginning of "the second golden age of the American cinema." Turning away from satire and the sexual themes of early talking films such as *Reunion in Vienna*, Hollywood created a glamorous, consoling (and profitable) world of upbeat values, but it also attempted to shake off its somewhat disreputable image by connecting its product with highly respected and/or popular novels. This was the period of *The Barretts of Wimpole Street* (1934), *Les Miserables* (1935), and *A Tale of Two Cities* (1935).

It was also the period of *Private Worlds*, based on a novel by Phyllis Bottome, who later became Alfred Adler's biographer. In keeping with the new seriousness, the film was made with a Dr. Samuel Marcus acting as "technical adviser." Set in "Brentwood Hospital," *Private Worlds* involves the interactions of the staff with each other more than with their patients. The plot involves the love affair between the new director of the institution, Charles Monet (Charles Boyer), and the protagonist, a soon-to-be-familiar female psychiatrist who is out of touch with her emotions, played here by Claudette Colbert. Dr. Monet (Boyer) arrives at the sanitarium to tell Dr. Jane Everest (Colbert) that he strongly disapproves of women in the profession, thus arousing the anger of Jane's steadfast colleague, Alex MacGregor (Joel McCrea), who also dislikes the new director because he wanted the job for himself. MacGregor seeks revenge on Monet by carrying on an affair with Monet's sister (Helen Vinson), eventually causing his own wife, Sally (Joan Bennett), to attempt suicide. The main plot, however, focuses on the relationship between Colbert and Boyer, who proclaim their love for one another only after she has stepped down from her position at the hospital. Nevertheless, the film does not adhere completely to the antifeminist values we identified in chapter 1 as central to the ideology of the vast majority of American films with female psychiatrists. The McCrea character is capable of maintaining a professional and mutually respecting relationship with Jane Everest (Colbert) throughout the film, and in one early scene the female doctor even bids farewell to a male patient who heartily thanks her for curing him and then disappears for the duration of the film. Furthermore, Dr. Everest is not required to give up her profession for marriage; at the film's conclusion, the formerly misogynist Dr. Monet (Boyer) asks her to stay on at the institution after she has resigned. Perhaps Colbert's character was given greater latitude as a professional in 1935 because the American public and the film industry were not yet as concerned about the "proper" role of women as when female workers began leaving the home in great numbers in 1942.

Nevertheless, *Private Worlds* is primarily an awkward ninety minutes of melodrama, exploiting adultery as much as insanity, but always staying within the limits of the Production Code. The film even looks back to old silent films about escaped lunatics in several scenes with a violent patient whose outbursts can be controlled only by the soothing words of Dr. Everest. The film also offers an early example of the American cinema's difficulty in conceptualizing psychiatrists as medical doctors. Both Colbert and McCrea wear white coats throughout most of the film (plate 5) and carry on a long-term, though obscure, experiment involving microscopes, mathematical equations, and conversations about "neurons." They are scientific doctors in the same tradition as the medical paragons in the 1935 version of *Magnificent Obsession*, *The Story of Louis Pasteur*, and *Disputed Passage*, but when the psychiatrists actually treat patients, they are little more than "keepers," restraining the violent ones and consoling the depressed ones. McCrea even has a scene in which he successfully brings a smile to the face of a suicidal young woman by telling her that "life's a lot of fun when you find the joy of living." It did not take the movies long to learn that simplified talking psychiatry offers more drama and consolation than the scientifically technical aspects of the profession.

By 1939 the image of the oracular, demedicalized, and godlike psychiatrist had fully emerged in *Blind Alley* with Ralph Bellamy's portrayal of Dr. Shelby. Based on a play by James Warwick, the film begins as "Far Above Cayuga's Waters" plays on the sound track behind an establishing shot of a college campus. As the camera enters Dr. Shelby's classroom, he is lecturing authoritatively on the thin dividing line between madness and sanity. He even offers a kind of cultural relativism in his discussion of insanity by asking what Norwegians would think of "jitterbug jive" and what the Chinese might make of women's hats. He then turns Platonic and suggests that even love is a kind of madness. Returning home from the classroom that evening, his foreign-accented wife greets the doctor in their comfortable lakeside house. ("Cayuga's Waters" and the lake suggest Cornell, although its medical school is 350 miles away. Once again, the absence of medical imagery in a psychiatric film is striking.) The picture that emerges in the first minutes of this film suggests that Dr. Shelby combines two different roles that, according to John Burnham (1979), psychiatrists often filled in the 1930s. According to Burnham, the earliest American psychoanalysts saw themselves as "avant-gardists," disseminating Freud's revolutionary ideas, whereas later practitioners assumed a less controversial role as advocates for traditional Western values. The character that Ralph Bellamy plays in *Blind Alley* is both a professor and a psychiatrist; he upsets the parochial preconceptions of his students but argues for tolerance and pluralism; and he leads a traditional family life, although his wife is European. To use Burnham's terms, he is both a member of the social and intellectual avant-garde and a spokesman for "the rational and the humane," the second role having been "superimposed" on the first during the 1930s. Bellamy's Dr. Shelby represents a synthesis of the avant-garde psychiatrist (represented negatively in *The Front Page)* with images of psy-

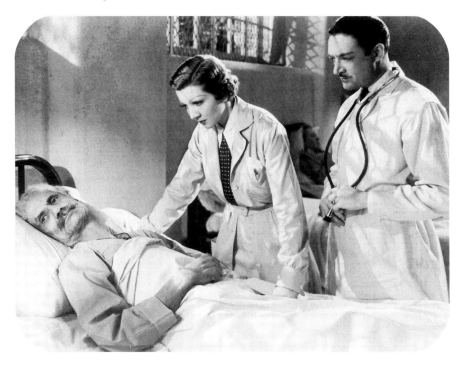

PLATE 5.   Two of the first—and last—medicalized psychiatrists in American movies: Claudette Colbert and Theodore von Eltz with Nick Shaid in *Private Worlds* (1935). Warner Brothers. The Museum of Modern Art/Film Stills Archive.

chiatry based on enlightened rationalism (as in *Reunion in Vienna* and *Private Worlds*).

Nevertheless, the doctor in *Blind Alley* is not out of place in the genre of gangster movies, maintaining his intellectual composure even when his house is invaded by an escaped killer (Chester Morris) (plate 6). Although the villain actually shoots down one of his students, fear and doubt never enter Dr. Shelby's mind. The cure that he administers, and that is responsible for the death of the gangster, seems to emerge from Shelby's scientific and professional mission rather than from any stratagems to eliminate his unwanted houseguest. Smoking the inevitable pipe, Bellamy lectures Morris on dream interpretation and unconscious motivation in the same spirit that he instructs his students. He even tells the killer, "You interest me."

The overall image of psychiatry that emerges in the movies of the 1930s is even more diffuse than *Reunion in Vienna*, *Private Worlds*, and *Blind Alley* might suggest. In fact, a comprehensive cinematic "myth" of psychiatry, built on a tension between diametrically opposed images, was already established by this time. For example, the idealizations in *Private Worlds* and *Blind Alley* must be understood alongside the negative portrayals of psychiatrists in *The Front Page* and in a film like Hobart Henley's *Free Love* (1930). Based on a play by Sidney Howard, *Free Love* introduces us to another avant-garde quack who is more out of touch with reality than his patients could possibly be. The constant bickering between Stephen and Hope Ferrier (Conrad Nagel and Genevieve Tobin) finally drives Hope to a psychiatrist. For a fee of $800, she learns that she is an "intuitive introvert" and that Stephen is an "in-fantile extrovert." This diagnosis is all Hope needs to collect her belongings and her children and leave her husband. She even goes to Atlantic City with her husband's best friend, thus inspiring Stephen to punch the man in the jaw. Stephen fails to bring his wife home until he recalls the advice of a casual acquaintance, a drunk he met in a speakeasy. "You should not have punched your best friend," the barroom philosopher tells him. "You should have

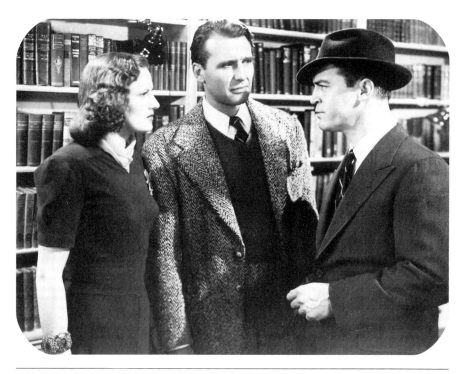

PLATE 6.   Murderer Chester Morris arouses the curiosity and the sympathy but not the malice of oracular Ralph Bellamy (with Rose Stradner) in *Blind Alley* (1939). Columbia Pictures. The Museum of Modern Art/Film Stills Archive.

punched your wife." When Stephen finally does exactly that, his wife recovers her senses and, without recriminations, falls into his arms as a repentant and faithful wife. Unlike *Lady in the Dark*, *Free Love* casts a psychiatrist as a force opposed to the received notions of femininity upheld by the film.

A blow to the jaw also plays a prominent role in one of Ginger Rogers's last films with Fred Astaire. As the dancing psychiatrist in *Carefree* (1938), Astaire is little more than a glorified hypnotist, but he is also one of the first stereotypical shrinks to save a patient by falling in love. Astaire even does a dance with Rogers in which he performs the conventional coaxing, arm-waving gestures of the show business hypnotist (plate 7). Ralph Bellamy is also in *Carefree*, but this time as Rogers's befuddled fiancé, who takes her to his friend the psychiatrist because she keeps breaking off their engagement. In accord with the Astaire/Rogers formula, she falls in love with the psychiatrist instead of with Bellamy although Astaire has yet to succumb to her allure. Quickly circumventing the problems raised by Rogers's passion for him, Astaire hypnotizes her and plants the conviction in her mind that she loves Bellamy. To make certain that she abandons her feeling for him, the psychiatrist even tells her that men like himself should be shot down like animals. Before Astaire can bring her out of the trance, however, she wanders out of his office, acquires a gun from her skeet-shooting fiancé, and does in fact attempt to shoot Astaire. By the time Astaire realizes that he is in love with Rogers, he is incapable of getting close enough to hypnotize and reprogram her. Finally, he crashes the ceremony just before Rogers and Bellamy's wedding, and after a blow to the jaw, Rogers returns to her trance. Astaire then quickly transforms her back into the woman who loves him. Clearly, there was no psychiatric adviser on the set of *Carefree*.

The pairing of Astaire and Rogers in *Carefree* must not, however, be dismissed so lightly. On the one hand, Ginger Rogers presents a curious case in the history of psychiatry in the movies, having played more analysands than probably any other actress: before *Carefree*, she appeared as an agoraphobic actress needing treatment in the comedy *In Person* (1935); later, she was analyzed in *Lady in the Dark* (1944) and, in 1957, *Oh, Men! Oh, Women!* Yet there is practically nothing in Rogers's screen persona that suggests anything but wholesome American normality. In *Carefree*, as in *Free Love* and *Reunion in Vienna*, psychotherapy is primarily a pastime for members of the idle rich who are a little short on common sense. Rogers ends up in Astaire's office because she only partially understands the not-so-awful truth that audiences at Leo McCarey's *The Awful Truth* (1937), Mitchell Leisen's *Hands Across the Table* (1935), and Howard Hawks's *His Girl Friday* would soon learn: marriage to Ralph Bellamy may offer security but certainly not excitement

(Cavell 1981b). On the other hand, the casting of Astaire as a psychiatrist suggests something a little different. While it is true that the great leading men of Hollywood—from John Wayne and Henry Fonda to Dustin Hoffman and Robert De Niro—have never played psychiatrists, it is also true that Astaire is, in the words of Michael Wood, "our enduring dream of the effortless conquest of recalcitrant circumstance" (1975, 150). When Astaire lends his aura to psychiatry, the profession becomes more than a little magical. Although *Carefree* was intended as just another container for the Astaire/Rogers formula, the tension between the perfectly healthy analysand and the perfectly graceful psychiatrist was an appropriate complement for the more fundamental tension in their relationship: "while the aristocratic, urbane Astaire was frequently called on to play musical versions of the outlaw hero . . . the saucy, down-to-earth Rogers appeared in parts that called for her to assume airs. . . . The plots that kept them apart, therefore, nearly always turned on mistaken identities, and it gradually became clear that the two were perfectly compatible" (Ray 1985, 166). On its subtextual level,

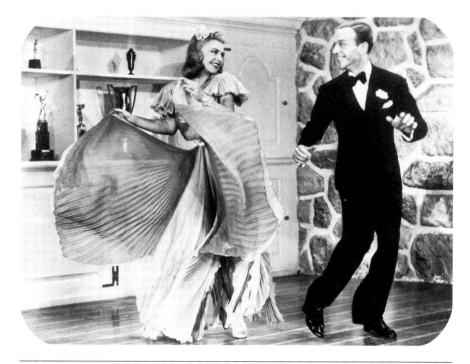

PLATE 7.   Therapy in the thirties: Fred Astaire treats Ginger Rogers in *Carefree* (1938). RKO. The Museum of Modern Art/Film Stills Archive.

Carefree also presents a perfect compatibility between Rogers's message that psychiatry is unnecessary and Astaire's that it is as graceful and effortless as his dancing. No better pair could have exemplified the split mythology of psychiatry that Hollywood had absorbed in the 1930s; the studios may not have understood the strange profession, but they knew exactly what to do with it.

Nevertheless, Astaire is regularly referred to as a "quack" in *Carefree,* even by some ducks he encounters near the lake in a bicycle tour of Central Park. More familiar stereotypes of the middle European quack in the 1930s are present in W. S. Van Dyke's *After the Thin Man* (1936), Ernst Lubitsch's *Bluebeard's Eighth Wife* (1938), Anatole Litvak's *The Amazing Dr. Clitterhouse* (1938), and Howard Hawks's *Bringing Up Baby* (1938). In the second of the *Thin Man* features, George Zucco plays "a crackpot psychologist" with thick glasses who at one point accuses a seemingly pleasant young man (James Stewart) of being crazy. When Nick Charles (William Powell) reveals that the Stewart character is a murderer, Stewart bursts into a wild confession of his hatred for various characters, deceased and otherwise, revealing himself, in fact, to be mad. In one of the film's final shots, the camera closes on Zucco, who exclaims, "Good heavens, I was right. The man is crazy." In *Bluebeard's Eighth Wife,* Lawrence Grant plays Professor Urganzeff, another bespectacled, goateed middle European eccentric, who runs a sanitarium to which Gary Cooper is briefly committed. When one of the doctor's patients is released, presumably after being cured of the conviction that he is a chicken, the patient takes one look at the stock market quotations in the newspaper and exclaims, "Cock-a-doodle-doo." Even more ridiculous is the psychiatrist in *The Amazing Dr. Clitterhouse,* who appears briefly in a courtroom scene and succeeds in confusing everyone, including himself. In chapter 1 we discussed the comic figure played by Fritz Feld in *Bringing Up Baby:* although the psychiatrist does offer the heroine (Katharine Hepburn) and the audience a crucial bit of psychological information ("The love impulse in men very frequently reveals itself in terms of conflict"), he is eventually shown to be as easily deluded as the bumbling sheriff he assists. In all three of these 1938 films, as in many to come, the audience can sustain ambivalent attitudes toward psychiatry by watching exotic psychiatrists demonstrate competence and then be deflated.

This kind of mythmaking is used to greatest effect in Frank Capra's *Mr. Deeds Goes to Town* (1936), written by Capra's regular collaborator Robert Riskin from a short story by Clarence Budington Kelland. Gary Cooper plays the "Capracorn" hero from a small town who embodies the American values that Robert Sklar (1975) has called "Jeffersonian agrarian." When Deeds decides to distribute his multimillion-dollar inheritance among the depression army of common men like himself, the New York bankers and lawyers protect their investments by enlisting the services of Emile von Haller (Wyrley Birch), "the most eminent psychiatrist in the world." Complete with pince-nez and thick accent, von Haller testifies in court that Deeds is insane and therefore not fit to spend his own money. Even though von Haller has never examined Deeds, he demonstrates the hero's "manic-depressive" qualities with a chart showing that Deeds vacillates in and out of a "sane and normal" range into "abnormal" and "subnormal" extremes.

Mr. Deeds's enemies in the film argue that his hobby of playing the tuba proves that he is insane. When the hero rises to defend himself, he argues that tuba-playing helps him to relax and concentrate in much the same way that other people are served by their nervous habits. Von Haller, as Deeds points out, is a doodler. When the court confiscates the psychiatrist's notepad, the camera reveals that von Haller has doodled a childish rendering of a grotesque face. In spite of his august stature, the doctor's more revealing practices show that he is strikingly different from what he pretends to be. His credibility destroyed, the doctor petulantly throws down his pencil.

The Viennese fraud in *Mr. Deeds Goes to Town* is the perfect foil for the virtues that Capra endorses in this film. Sklar describes the director's vision: "Capra's social myth, it's true, required turning back the clock to an imagined past social stability founded upon an image of the American small town, with comfortable homes, close-knit families, friendly neighbors—a modest but prosperous community with bountiful farms and a benign wilderness nearby" (1975, 210). Capra knew that audiences could accept this myth when presented with a world in which the only dissenting voices are easily discredited. At one point during his testimony, Dr. von Haller turns to one of the other court psychiatrists and asks if he recalls "the case of the young nobleman." How can we believe a man who comes from a world so distant and socially askew that it can include "a young nobleman"? As the psychiatrist continues to spout jargon and mystification, Capra's camera shows a courtroom gallery full of humbly dressed but respectfully silent spectators, one of whom scratches his head in confusion. As the film's audience regards itself in this mirror, it can believe that mental illness and the doctors who treat it are entirely out of place in America. In fact, the craziest people in the film are the charming and harmless Faulkner sisters from Deeds's hometown, who are convinced that everyone except themselves is "pixilated."

The 1930s end with a curious example of psychiatry in the cinema, *Children of Loneliness*. Filmed in 1939 but denied a license for exhibition until the 1950s because of its attention to forbidden subjects, *Children of Lone-*

liness uses a psychiatrist to link two vignettes about homosexuality. A psychiatrist who "aids the police in cases of abnormal sexuality" narrates the film and appears in both episodes when characters concerned about their sexuality visit him. In the first episode, the doctor tells a young woman not to submit to the sexual advances of her girlfriend, and in the second he counsels a male painter who fears that the "femininity" of his work reveals sexual abnormality. This plot summary, however, does not capture the tone of the film, which is closer to *Reefer Madness* than to *Making Love* and was clearly intended to exploit the issue of homosexuality rather than to educate the public. Nevertheless, the film is one of the first to present a psychiatrist entirely without avant-garde or exotic associations and in the new role as a spokesman for "normality." *Children of Loneliness* was eventually resurrected and released in the same year as *Glen or Glenda?* (1953) to capitalize on the enormous publicity surrounding the sex change operation of Christine Jorgensen in 1952 (Russo 1981).

The Forties: Dr. Jaquith, Dr. Kik, and the Sinister Dr. Ritter

One of the most influential cinematic psychiatrists from the 1940s was Dr. Jaquith (Claude Rains) in *Now, Voyager* (1942). The character looks back to the pipe-smoking oracle played by Ralph Bellamy in *Blind Alley*, but like many of the idealized psychiatrists of the early 1940s, he is entirely rooted in a straightforward rationalism with none of the avant-garde trappings of the psychiatrist in *Blind Alley*. Dr. Jaquith runs a clinic called Cascade, which resembles a country manor much more than an asylum and where he is right at home with his air of easy grace and authority (plate 8). He also exudes an ethereal kind of sexuality, even though the film does not allow him to focus his sexual emanations on any one character. Bette Davis (Stine 1974) has said that she believes a continuation of the incidents in *Now, Voyager* would have shown her married to Jaquith and helping him at Cascade after she realizes that she cannot marry Jerry (Paul Henreid). It would be difficult, however, to imagine Dr. Jaquith coming down to earth long enough to become romantically involved with a woman. Furthermore, when Charlotte Vale (Davis) takes over the treatment of the daughter of her married lover (Henreid), Jaquith accepts it with good humor, even though the film suggests that the girl needs mothering more than the conventional, perhaps cold treatment that Jaquith administers.

The exact nature of Dr. Jaquith's treatment is uncertain since we never really see him working with a patient. Unlike *Blind Alley* with its crude Freudianisms, *Now, Voyager* contains nothing reminiscent of psychoanalytic theory or technique. Instead, Dr. Jaquith dispenses homilies such as "independence is reliance upon one's will and judgment." He tells Charlotte that people come to him when they are "tired" or "confused," and when he first encounters Charlotte in her domineering mother's house, he tells Charlotte, "You don't need my help," and he scolds her mother. *Now, Voyager* did a great deal to domesticate and demystify the image of the psychiatrist in the United States, but it did so by shying away from any real confrontation with the technical aspects of psychiatry, even avoiding the expressionistic dream sequences of *Blind Alley*, which were rapidly becoming conventionalized in films of the 1940s. Here, as in several films we discussed in the portion of chapter 1 devoted to the "cathartic cure," mental illness is presented as overexposure to an unsympathetic parent, and the cure is a cruise on a luxury liner and a new boyfriend. Later on, when Charlotte blames herself for her mother's death and returns to Jaquith's sanitarium, the main reason is the

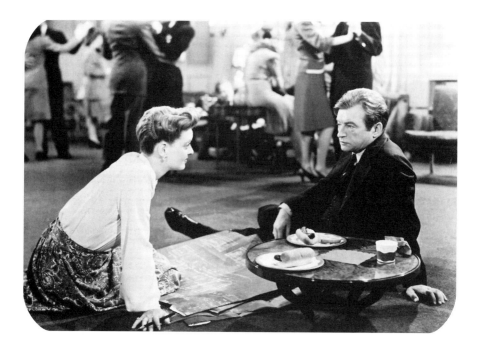

PLATE 8.   Claude Rains in *Now, Voyager* (1942) is almost godlike, but he is not above joining Bette Davis for a hot dog. Warner Brothers. The Museum of Modern Art/Film Stills Archive.

plot necessity of bringing her together with Jerry again. Other than that, she commits herself because she is a little sad.

Now, Voyager is one of several "women's films" that comfortably provide a niche for psychiatrists, involved as these films are with the problem of identity that women faced during the upheavals of the 1940s (Walsh 1984). We have already discussed *Lady in the Dark* in this context; we should also mention *Since You Went Away* (1944), *Possessed* (1947), and the English *The Seventh Veil* (1945) as films that also appropriate psychiatry as an important element in women's search for identity. Alfred Hitchcock's *Spellbound* (1945) fits into this category as well, despite the picture's more ambitious scope and the casting of a woman as a psychiatrist. Like *Now, Voyager* and *Since You Went Away*, *Spellbound* was based on a novel, still the major source for movie plots involving psychiatrists in the 1940s.

At one point in *Spellbound*, Dr. Bruloff (Michael Chekhov), the crusty old analyst who trained Constance Peterson (Ingrid Bergman), says, "Women make the best psychoanalysts until they fall in love. Then they make the best patients." Actually, at least in *Spellbound*, he is wrong. Women make mediocre analysts *until* they fall in love. Then they become superb analysts, detectives, and, of course, helpmates. Dr. Peterson, a psychoanalyst on the staff of a clinic called Green Manors, first appears as a somewhat mousy woman, hiding her beauty behind a long white coat, a cigarette holder, glasses, and an unflattering coiffure. As if to emphasize her lack of femininity, her first patient is a flamboyantly beautiful woman (Rhonda Fleming) who plays out her sexual passions by first enticing and then physically attacking the male members of the clinic's staff. Bergman accomplishes virtually nothing with the Fleming character, and their brief session together ends with the patient throwing a book at the psychoanalyst before being taken away by an orderly. A male psychiatrist on the staff of Green Manors then lectures Dr. Peterson on her icy conduct as both an analyst and a woman. He is clearly interested in forming a romantic liaison with her, but she blithely ignores his sexual overtures as well as his critique of her professional abilities. Soon, however, an amnesiac Gregory Peck arrives, and she immediately begins to demonstrate substantial competence in a variety of roles.

Dr. Peterson falls in love with the Peck character, even though he quickly reveals himself to be an extremely troubled individual. Suspected of murder, he himself is unable to recall whether or not he killed Dr. Edwardes, the new director of the clinic whose identity he has assumed. Undaunted by these uncertainties, Bergman's character flees with her lover to Dr. Bruloff. Michael Chekhov, the eminent Russian actor and nephew of the playwright Anton Chekhov, plays Bruloff with occasional moments of irascibility and clownishness but presents both these qualities as necessary components of a wise and complex personality. When Dr. Bruloff scolds the Bergman character for succumbing to female emotionalism in her seemingly irrational conviction that Peck is innocent, he speaks with great authority. Yet Constance Peterson also speaks with authority, and it is with her that the film ultimately asks us to side, as should be clear from one of the film's production stills (see plate 26, chapter 5). She tells Bruloff, "You know only science. You know his mind, but you don't know his heart." Later she adds, "The heart can see deeper. . . . I couldn't feel this pain for someone who is evil." Bruloff responds, "This is baby talk."

The scenes between Ingrid Bergman and Michael Chekhov contain the first detailed discussions of countertransference in the American cinema. As with *Private Worlds* in the thirties, the producers of *Spellbound* enlisted a practicing psychiatrist for technical assistance: the credits list May E. Romm, M.D., as "psychiatric advisor." Nevertheless, the demands of Hitchcock's film necessitate the juxtaposition of a traditional female's nurturing instinct with the professional training of an experienced male. Constance Peterson can succeed only by exchanging her psychoanalyst's background for the emotional responses of a woman in love, and she herself says so. In this sense the film endorses the emerging ideology of the postwar years and implicitly supports the biological determinism of writers such as Lundberg and Farnham (1947). On the other hand, Constance's instincts turn out to be correct: she cures the psychological afflictions of the Peck character, and she personally solves the crime for which her lover has been convicted. The film says that women are ineffective as psychoanalysts unless they are fulfilled as women, but it also suggests that the efforts of an emotionally involved woman are vastly superior to those of male psychiatrists *and* male detectives. Dr. Peterson is even vindicated in her disputes with the wise old Dr. Bruloff. In reconciling contradictory myths about female psychiatrists, *Spellbound* provides an excellent illustration for the comparison between studio bosses (such as *Spellbound*'s David O. Selznick) and "naïve anthropologists" (Ray 1985, 13).

Spellbound also contains several conventions that were already established, or soon would be, in films about psychiatrists. In addition to the psychiatrist as lover and the psychiatrist as detective, the film gives us the psychiatrist as criminal in the villain of the piece, Dr. Murchison (Leo G. Carroll). We also witness the conventional cathartic cure when Gregory Peck both regains his memory and recovers from a childhood trauma after a single skiing descent down a mountain slope. Miklos Rozsa's score for the film introduces the eerie sound of the theremin, an instrument that was part of the melodramatic trappings that accompanied several cinematic probings into the darker reaches of the human mind, although by 1948 the theremin was already being used for tongue-in-cheek purposes in *Let's Live a Little*. Although *Spellbound* is a long way from the free-flowing collection of Freudian dream images that made up the 1928 surrealist masterpiece *Un Chien andalou*, both films contain contributions from Salvador Dali. The brief montage of images appearing on the screen when Gregory Peck recounts his key dream was based on drawings by Dali and represents a further refinement in the rendering of dreams on the screen. No American film has matched the revolutionary mise-en-scène of the German expressionist classic *The Cabinet of Dr. Caligari* (1919), but *Spellbound*'s Daliesque dream sequence is a much more authentic and resonant representation of the dream work than the theatrical pageants of *Lady in the Dark* or the simple switch to negative stock in *Blind Alley*.

In addition to listing the services of a psychiatric adviser, the opening credits for *Spellbound* conclude with a truncated quotation from Shakespeare, "The fault . . . is not in our stars, but in ourselves . . . ," followed by these lines: "Our story deals with psychoanalysis, the method by which modern *science* treats the emotional problems of the sane. The analyst seeks only to induce the patient to talk about his hidden problems, to open the locked doors of his mind. Once the complexes that have been disturbing the patient are uncovered and interpreted, the *illness* and confusion disappear . . . and the *evils* of *unreason* are driven from the human *soul*" (emphasis added). This is a fascinating statement with revealing contradictions and ambiguities. Although psychoanalysis is at first named a science, it is later associated with both medicine and religion in the same sentence. But in spite of the broadly suggestive claims in its prologue, *Spellbound* does not take the practice of psychoanalysis much beyond the convention of the simple cathartic cure. When Gregory Peck arrives at the clinic, he is unaware that he is impersonating a dead man. Nevertheless, he is capable of functioning normally for the first few hours after his arrival, and he is even able to form a lasting romantic bond with the Bergman character. The film never questions the strength of a relationship initiated while one partner was not acting in an entirely rational manner. In fact, Peck's mental illness in *Spellbound* manifests itself entirely as an occasional lack of affect or as the sudden onslaught of panicky feelings. The "talking cure" suggested in the prologue appears only briefly, and ultimately "the evils of unreason" that threaten the one disturbed character in the film are exorcised by detective work rather than psychoanalysis. Hitchcock himself called *Spellbound* "just another manhunt story wrapped up in pseudo-psychoanalysis" (Truffaut 1984, 165).

Two years after *Spellbound*, the talking cure was again subordinated to criminal matters in *Nightmare Alley* (1947). In fact, the patient in this film would have been much better off if he had kept his neurosis to himself. Stanton Carlisle (Tyrone Power), a mentalist who performs in a fashionable Chicago nightclub, visits "counseling psychologist" Lilith Ritter (Helen Walker) after he is driven into panic by the odor of rubbing alcohol. During the film's earlier carnival scenes, Stan accidentally gave wood alcohol to Pete (Ian Keith), a down-and-out alcoholic mind reader. Stan's guilt over the old drunk's resulting death surfaces later when he has become a success by employing many of the techniques for phony mind-reading acts that Pete's female partner had taught him. Lilith Ritter terminates his guilt feelings in a brief therapy session, but this is not the end of Stan's problems. The psychologist enlists the mentalist into her elaborate scheme for extorting money from wealthy patients who are obsessed with deceased loved ones. Armed with religious rhetoric, the psychologist's privileged information, and his own audacity, Stan convinces one Chicago plutocrat (Taylor Holmes) that he is in touch with the girl that the wealthy man loved long ago before her death. The man even donates $150,000 for the construction of a "tabernacle," but the mentalist entrusts the money to Lilith. The psychologist's given name should have tipped Stan off, for when his project is exposed and he must flee Chicago, Lilith keeps the money for herself. When Stan threatens to expose her, she begins speaking in the patronizing tones of a therapist whose patient cannot remember the lessons of previous sessions. Just as she has done with the wealthy patients who have become her victims, Lilith has recorded Stan's confessions in their one session together, and she is prepared to use the information about Pete's death against him. The end of the film recalls its beginning, in which a young and naïve Stan had expressed disbelief at the daily routine of the carnival geek whose act consisted of biting the heads off chickens. Unable to find work after fleeing Chicago, Stan drifts into alcoholism and eventually to a traveling carnival where the job of geek seems to be awaiting him.

Nightmare Alley is still an intriguing piece of filmmaking and one of the best examples of film noir. Literally "black film" in translation from the French, films noir involve violent plots, often with a heavy dose of sexuality, and ruthless characters such as hard-boiled detectives, double-dealing women, and tough-talking criminals. Most of the films in this tradition were made just after World War II, and they reflect the less optimistic vision of American life that was emerging in this period as well as a growing fascination with psychiatry. Just as psychiatrists were out of place in Frank Capra–land, they were welcome and even necessary in the more complex world of film noir. The darker corners of the mind that create irrational behavior were widely exposed and popularized in accounts of the psychiatric treatment for returning servicemen, and Hollywood had no trouble translating this knowledge into cinematic terms. The heavy emphasis on shadows and the "visual feel" in film noir were influenced by expressionist directors and cinematographers, especially those from Germany and, to a lesser degree, France, where there was a much greater interest in psychoanalysis. Fritz Lang, who made several classic noir films in the United States, had earlier used a number of expressionist techniques in Germany for his cycle of Mabuse films about a mad psychiatrist. On the other hand, much of what we now call film noir was only obliquely related to psychiatry; much of it grew naturally out of the wide range of techniques that American filmmakers employed to render the bleak and dangerous nighttowns of many novels of this period, particularly the detective fiction, mysteries, and psychological thrillers of Raymond Chandler, Dashiell Hammett, James M. Cain, and Cornell Woolrich. *Nightmare Alley* effectively exploits the techniques of this tradition and, like many other noirist films, creates a sinister world of victims and victimizers, populated by women of threatening, often ambiguous sexuality.

Helen Walker's Lilith Ritter dresses mannishly, and, as the ultimate victimizer in *Nightmare Alley*, she provides one of the most complete examples of how film noir depicts women (E. Kaplan 1989) (plate 9). *Nightmare Alley* is another interesting example of how Hollywood has dealt with the troublesome image of a beautiful woman in an authoritative occupation. As we will demonstrate in chapter 5, female psychiatrists in the movies generally help their male patients only by falling in love with them. Lilith Ritter is an exception to test the rule. On the one hand, she does express some interest in forming a sexual relationship with Tyrone Power's character when she suggests a rendezvous in her cabin at the boat club. This overture is hardly consistent with the behavior of a sympathetic female therapist, especially since Stan (Power) is married. He refuses her offer, however, on the grounds that they cannot risk being seen together, and none of the conventional therapeutic romance we witness in *Spellbound* and many other films ever takes place. On the other hand, the psychologist's success with her patient is the work not of a competent professional but of a scheming and unscrupulous blackmailer with no "female" compassion whatever. She can help him recover from guilt feelings, but her real agenda is markedly different from that of more honest therapists. The evil female psychiatrist in *Nightmare Alley*, who operates entirely without the nurturing spirit, is the obligatory complement to the more familiar female psychiatrist who can function successfully only by making sacrifices for the man she loves. Significantly, Lilith Ritter uses the term "transference," the magic word that women therapists in the movies often use in their first feeble efforts to cope with the sexual chemistry between themselves and their patients. Coming from Lilith, however, the word is part of a speech that has been carefully prepared both to convince the hero that he is mad and to keep him in place until police arrive.

Another intriguing speech in *Nightmare Alley* takes place during the first meeting between Stan and Lilith. At this point they are still circling each other, trying to determine what scheme the other is concocting. When Stan asks about her occupation, Lilith says, "Ever been psychoanalyzed?" Stan replies, "Saw it once in a murder movie. A good mentalist could have solved the whole thing in five minutes." Although the filmmakers involved with *Nightmare Alley* probably do not agree with this statement, it does capture the attitude toward psychiatry so often adopted in crime melodramas, or to use the genre suggested by Stan, "murder movies." Psychoanalysis is regularly confused with or relegated to detective work, partially because its methodologies require gathering clues and following through on hypotheses, but also

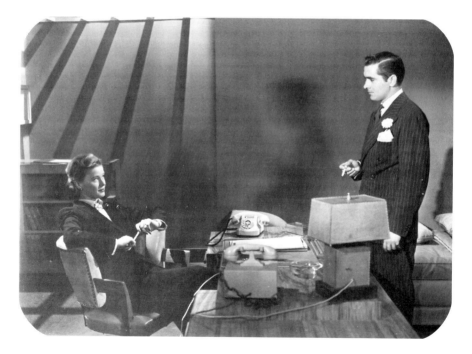

PLATE 9.   The seductive and evil Lilith Ritter (Helen Walker) with Tyrone Power in *Nightmare Alley* (1947). Twentieth Century–Fox. The Museum of Modern Art/Film Stills Archive.

because crime detection provides a neatly simplified version of psychiatry—problems can be thoroughly solved and forgotten once a culprit has been identified. This is one of the reasons why the easily identified parent is so often the cause of an individual's sufferings in psychiatrically oriented movies. Stories about people in trouble with their minds are often built upon the same foundations as stories about people in trouble with the law.

Other examples of films in which psychiatry appeared along with the conventions of film noir include Rudolph Maté's *The Dark Past* (1948), which used noirist techniques to retell the same story as *Blind Alley* of 1939, and Steve Sekely's *Hollow Triumph* (1948, later released as *The Scar*), in which Paul Henreid plays a man who kills and then replaces his psychoanalyst double with a great deal of success—at least at first. In Curtis Bernhardt's *High Wall* (1947), Audrey Totter plays a psychiatrist who, like Ingrid Bergman in *Spellbound*, falls in love with an accused man (Robert Taylor) before she identifies the man who framed him.

Robert Siodmak's *The Dark Mirror* (1946) introduced a psychiatrist to the phenomenon of the "evil twin," a cliché that has surfaced in numerous films (such as Brian De Palma's *Sisters* and Paul Henreid's *Dead Ringer*) and that, like many cinematic conventions, has moved on to entrench itself thoroughly in television melodrama (such as major network made-for-television movies in the 1980s starring Jane Seymour and Ann Jillian). One of the twins in *The Dark Mirror*, both played by Olivia de Havilland, has committed a murder. The police know that one of the twins is guilty, but since they cannot discover which one, they are unable to indict either. Eventually they enlist the help of "psychologist" Scott Elliott (Lew Ayres), M.D., Ph.D., M.S., who has done research on the pathology of twins. (Actually, Ayres's character behaves much more like a psychologist than a psychiatrist, administering tests to the twins rather than working on a talking cure.) Dr. Elliott eventually identifies the guilty one (and falls in love with the other) largely through his findings with Rorschach, free association, and lie-detector tests, work that he does with the foreboding accompaniment of Dimitri Tiomkin's dark, tense noir score.

Lew Ayres's performance as Scott Elliott in *The Dark Mirror* marks a further step in the acceptance and demystification of psychiatry in the movies of the 1940s. Although Dr. Elliott smokes a pipe, plays chess, listens to Brahms, and owns an office full of books, he also dotes on lemon drops and carries himself with the boyish charm that we expect from a clean-cut, relatively innocent leading man like Ayres (plate 10). Once again, the work of the psychiatrist is largely indistinguishable from detective work, and once again, the therapeutic relationship leads inevitably to romance, but the film also makes an effort to show how mental health professionals treat their patients. In several scenes we can compare the sharply different reactions of the twins to the same Rorschach blots and free-association series. Neither Freud nor medicine is invoked here, but in its attempts to make the mysteries of the unconscious accessible, the film suggests that by 1946 an audience that came to see a whodunnit could also appreciate the work of a psychotherapist.

The Snake Pit of 1948, also starring Olivia de Havilland, tries to present the dilemmas surrounding the treatment of mentally disturbed patients but, true to the Hollywood pattern, ultimately displaces them into melodrama. *The Snake Pit* fits most neatly into the genre of postwar social problem films best exemplified by *Gentleman's Agreement* (1947), *Crossfire* (1947), and *Pinky* (1949). The conclusion of *The Snake Pit* resembles that of *Crossfire*, a murder mystery that takes anti-Semitism as its principal theme. Although

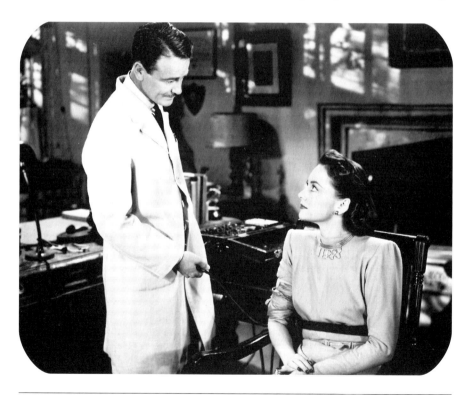

PLATE 10.   Lew Ayres probes the mind of Olivia de Havilland and her "evil twin" in *The Dark Mirror* (1946). Universal Pictures. The Museum of Modern Art/Film Stills Archive.

the ugliness of anti-Semitism is plainly demonstrated in the nearly pathological behavior of the film's villain (Robert Ryan), his discovery and death at the end suddenly seem to suggest that the much more pervasive evils of Jew-hating have been completely eliminated. Similarly, the recovery of the heroine at the end of *The Snake Pit* seems designed to make the audience forget the distress of the mental patients who are left behind.

In relation to the evolving history of psychiatry in the movies, *The Snake Pit* is important because it questions the profession's effectiveness from a more informed point of view. In films such as *Mr. Deeds Goes to Town*, psychiatrists are simply quacks, out of touch with the world in which human beings actually live. In *The Snake Pit*, on the other hand, psychiatrists can heal the sick, but our society and the institutions it builds for troubled people do not always make psychiatric work easy. *The Snake Pit*'s incipient notion that society may be at the root of people's problems would become fully developed in the 1960s.

The Snake Pit dramatizes the chaos in state mental hospitals and replaces the gracious country manors of *Now, Voyager* and *Spellbound* with a bedlam that can aid recovery only by giving the patient the desire to leave as soon as possible. The film sends Virginia Cunningham (Olivia de Havilland) back and forth between the healing efforts of her psychiatrist (Leo Genn) and the disastrous effects of conditions at the Juniper Hill state mental hospital. Virginia first arrives at the hospital after a breakdown resulting from a crisis in her marriage. She is unable to accept love from a man because of guilt feelings stemming from the death of her father as well as from the subsequent death of a boyfriend who resembled him. We know this because Virginia tells part of the story while she is under the effects of narcosynthesis, a process that also appears in *Possessed* (1947) and *Home of the Brave* (1949), perhaps the first films in which psychiatrists use any kind of drug therapy. (The same process was used in the 1946 documentary *Let There Be Light*.) We learn the rest of Virginia's story when her psychiatrist explains it to her while a portrait of Freud on the wall looms like an icon throughout the scene.

Virginia's psychiatrist in *The Snake Pit* is played by the English actor Leo Genn (plate 11), whose foreign accent is meant to be consistent with an unpronounceable last name, affectionately shortened by characters in the film to "Kik." He possesses a self-effacing but authoritative manner, and, like Claude Rains in *Now, Voyager*, he frequently taps his pipe. In spite of his good intentions and sympathetic nature, Dr. Kik is up against more than just his patients' early traumas. Leo Genn's character may be the first cinematic psychiatrist to contend with the inadequacies in state institutions, including overcrowding, arbitrarily authoritarian nurses, and incompetent administra-

tors, all of which were widely publicized in the late 1940s. Even this knowledgeable practitioner must subordinate his treatments to decisions made in
boardrooms. As a result, Dr. Kik tells Virginia's husband (Mark Stevens) that
he must take "shortcuts" because of a lack of time. We also know that Kik's
superiors have pressured him to release Virginia as soon as possible because
there are already too many patients in her ward.

As we pointed out in chapter 1, *The Snake Pit* simultaneously portrays
ECT as barbaric and as helpful. The film also expresses ambivalence toward
psychiatry in the immense difference between the analytic scenes, in which
Virginia works out her own ambivalence toward her parents, and the more
broadly played scenes involving other patients. The seriousness of her sessions with Dr. Kik could almost be part of an "educational" documentary
about psychoanalysis. The scenes in the ward, on the other hand, exploit the
horrifying as well as the farcical aspects of mental institutions. Virginia is
clearly not helped by the flamboyant antics of the other patients or by the

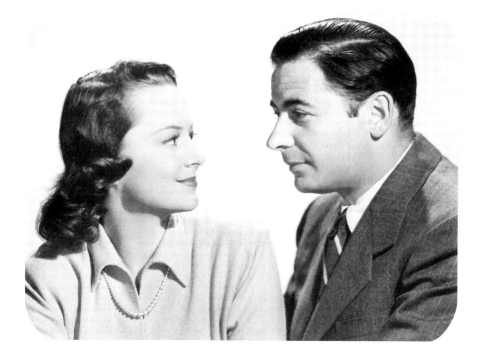

PLATE 11.   Olivia de Havilland with caring, effective psychiatrist (Leo Genn)
in *The Snake Pit* (1948). Twentieth Century–Fox. The Museum of Modern
Art/Film Stills Archive.

mindless regime enforced by the nurses. While other patients appear to be truly psychotic, Virginia's illness is almost charming, thanks especially to the affecting facial expressions and gently humorous line-readings that won de Havilland an Academy Award nomination and made *The Snake Pit* one of the five top-grossing films of 1949. At one point, the film actually invites us to sympathize with Virginia when she bites the finger of a ridiculous psychiatrist who is badgering her with questions (plate 12). Since the occasion is a hearing to decide her readiness for release, Virginia's action is certainly counterproductive. Yet within the context of the scene, her defiance seems as reasonable as it is crowd-pleasing. De Havilland's performance itself may have been as important as any of many other elements in *The Snake Pit* for fulfilling Hollywood's goal of presenting a serious problem and then deflecting it toward a single sympathetic character.

Films such as *Lady in the Dark, Spellbound, Nightmare Alley*, and *The Snake Pit* clearly appropriate psychiatry for their own specialized purposes, but they do show a more sophisticated understanding of the subject than the films of the 1930s and before. Lest we give the impression that the 1940s were entirely characterized by this new sophistication, we should mention at least a few other films. Assorted quacks played highly conventionalized roles in *My Favorite Wife* (1940), *That Uncertain Feeling* (1941), *Murder, My Sweet* (1945), *Miracle on 34th Street* (1947), and *The Gay Intruders* (1948). In 1946, *Bedlam* appeared, featuring no less than Boris Karloff as the malevolent warden of an insane asylum in eighteenth-century London. *Shock* appeared in the same year with Vincent Price as a psychiatrist who kills his wife and then endeavors to dispose of the only witness (Anabel Shaw) to his crime. As if to demonstrate the potential menace of his professional skills, the psychiatrist first attempts to drive the witness crazy and then provides her with an overdose of insulin. Bosley Crowther of the *New York Times* was more indignant than usual about what he considered socially irresponsible films like *Shock*, and his review expresses the sort of public response eventually responsible for the Golden Age of psychiatry in American film: "One is forced to challenge this picture as a social disservice at this time. Treatment of nervous disorders is being practiced today upon thousands of men who suffered shock of one sort or another in the war. A film which provokes fear of treatment, as this film plainly aims to do, is a cruel thing to put in the way of those patients or of their anxious relatives. Aubrey Schenck, who produced this picture, and Twentieth Century–Fox, which is releasing it, have evidenced here a lack of public consideration that is most deplorable" (1946, 10).

When he wrote these words, Crowther may have still been under the spell of *Let There Be Light* (1946), a documentary about the achievements of

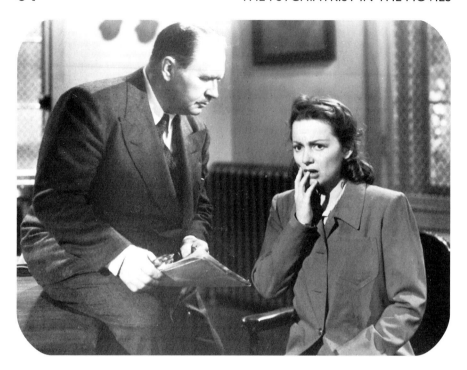

PLATE 12.   Olivia de Havilland with incompetent quack (Howard Freeman) in *The Snake Pit* (1948). Twentieth Century–Fox. The Museum of Modern Art/Film Stills Archive.

Army psychiatrists directed by John Huston long before he filmed the biography of Freud in 1962. This film may be the most impressive piece of psychiatric propaganda ever made. The cameras follow several returning servicemen through eight weeks of therapy in a hospital on Long Island. All suffer initially from serious disorders related to their experiences during the war; their symptoms are graphically presented in a series of individual interviews. Early on, psychiatrists are shown using narcosynthesis and hypnotism on four male patients and achieving immediate results. Later, these same patients are shown learning to talk and even joke about their problems in group therapy sessions. And by the end of the film, all the men are filmed laughing, singing, and playing softball, apparently restored to emotional and physical well-being. According to Huston, the Army had wanted "a film to show industry that nervous and emotional casualties were not lunatics; because at that time these men weren't getting jobs" (Kaminsky 1978, 43). However, Huston also maintains that the Army decided not to release the film, citing the lack of signed consent forms from several of the patients who appear in it. According to materials in a file on *Let There Be Light* compiled by David Culbert for the Audio Visual Division of the National Archives, Huston claims the consent forms disappeared from a bank vault in Astoria, Queens. James Agee, one of a handful of critics who had the opportunity to see the film, offered a different explanation for the film's suppression: "The War Department has mumbled a number of reasons why it has been withheld; the glaringly obvious reason has not been mentioned: that any sane human being who saw the film would join the armed services, if at all, with a straight face and a painfully maturing mind" (1958, 236). Agee may be correct, but a document in the clipping file at the National Archives quotes the legal officer of the Signal Corps as stating that the consent forms stipulated that the film could "only be used in furtherance of the war effort." He interpreted this to mean that it could be shown only to military personnel. The film was finally made available to the public in 1981. Even if allowed greater exposure at the time it was made, *Let There Be Light* would likely have done little to alter Hollywood's depiction of "the treatment of nervous disorders." With the exception of Mark Robson's *Home of the Brave* (1949), American films of that period seemed uninterested in psychiatry's efforts to heal psychological scars borne by servicemen. *Shock* was typical of Hollywood's much greater fascination with the more sensational aspects of how doctors treat the mind.

The Fifties: Prelude to the Golden Age

The American cinema continued to spin out its ambivalent mythology of psychiatry throughout most of the 1950s. While the profession was sometimes idealized, it was also shamelessly exploited in films such as *Glen or Glenda?* (1953), directed by the legendary Edward D. Wood, Jr. (best known for *Plan 9 from Outer Space*, a film that some jaded, tongue-in-cheek archivists have identified as the worst movie ever made). *Glen or Glenda?*, subtitled *I Change My Sex*, features Bela Lugosi as a sort of occult philosopher surrounded by skulls, mysterious vapors, and other typical paraphernalia of the wizard's studio. Lugosi lectures the audience on the order of nature and then introduces a pompous psychiatrist who, in turn, narrates the story of a man haunted by the desire to dress in women's clothes. The film ends happily as the transvestite's understanding fiancée hands him her angora sweater in the final moments. The directorial ineptitude of Ed Wood makes unusually clear Hollywood's desire to "have it both ways," a tradition that goes back at least to Cecil B. DeMille. In *Glen or Glenda?* the psychiatrist articulates the dominant ideology's notion of normality while he simultaneously legitimizes the voyeuristic fascination with what is forbidden.

Another semiprimitive film also reveals the complex ways that psychiatry can function in the movies. *I Was a Teenage Werewolf* (1957) touches on a number of anxieties characteristic of the 1950s. The unleashing of the destructive forces in the atom is typical of metaphors that dominated the era's science fiction and horror films (most notably Gordon Douglas's *Them!* of 1954), and psychiatry had much in common with the scientific mystification of nuclear power: both were easily characterized as modern inventions for uncovering nature's forbidden forces. Just as Americans held mixed feelings about optimistic promises of "atoms for peace," they may have harbored the unconscious concern that psychiatry derepresses powerful instinctual drives and leaves a patient in the throes of aggressive and sexual forces beyond his control. *I Was a Teenage Werewolf* expresses precisely this view. Whit Bissell plays a familiar B movie mad scientist who works in a laboratory with an assistant named Hugo and dreams of saving the world from nuclear destruction by returning mankind to its primitive origins. The film seems to have identified the doctor as a "consulting psychologist" employed at an aircraft factory for the sole purpose of engineering his meeting with the young protagonist (Michael Landon), who comes to the doctor for help with his violent temper. The psychologist finds the teenager to be the perfect subject for his experiments and with the help of drugs and hypnosis Bissell transforms him into a lycanthropic monster. As the film ends with the police shooting the werewolf, they discover that the monster has killed his doctor. One of the more theologically inclined officers observes that "it's not for man to interfere in the ways of God."

Most of the films of this decade, however, merely perpetuate well-established traditions from the 1930s and 1940s. Ineffectual or oddball psychiatrists appear in *Fourteen Hours* (1951) and *The Seven Year Itch* (1955). The beautiful but unfulfilled psychiatrist who is "cured" by a male patient appears in both *Knock on Wood* (1954) and *The Perfect Furlough* (1958). In Frederick de Cordova's *Bedtime for Bonzo* (1951), Ronald Reagan plays an amiable professor of psychology who sets out to prove the ascendancy of nurture over nature by raising a chimp in his own house. Like the equally amiable Lew Ayres in *The Dark Mirror*, the professor succeeds in his experiment and wins himself a bride. In the tradition of *Nightmare Alley*'s Lilith Ritter, *I, the Jury* (1953) offers a seductive psychoanalyst who runs a decidedly more criminal operation than her prototype. Based on Mickey Spillane's novel, both the 1953 and 1982 versions of *I, the Jury* allow Mike Hammer to make love to therapist Charlotte Manning (Peggie Castle in 1953, Barbara Carrera in 1982) before he discovers that she is the murderer of his pal. Both films end with a deadly embrace in which Charlotte hopes she can distract Hammer with her kisses while she reaches for her gun. The shot we hear, however, comes from Hammer's gun. Both films conclude with this memorable exchange:

CHARLOTTE: How could you?
HAMMER: It was easy.

Although it has little else in common with *Mr. Deeds Goes to Town*, the 1953 version of *I, the Jury* also relies on a nostalgic vision of stable individuals in stable communities to dismiss the unsettling claims that psychiatry makes for its legitimacy. Not only does the sex of the psychoanalyst in *I, the Jury* symbolize social disruption, but when Hammer first arrives outside her office and sees the shiny nameplate near the door, we hear his omniscient voice on the sound track: "'Charlotte Manning, Psychoanalysis.' Things have changed since I was a kid. Shingles were wood and carried a lot of weight. Now they were brass and could still weigh nothin'."

The vast majority of films of the fifties that included psychiatrists were still based on novels and plays. Henry Koster's *Harvey* (1950), for example, translated Mary Chase's popular stage comedy to the screen almost verbatim, including the conceit that Elwood P. Dowd (James Stewart), the good-natured drunk with the giant invisible rabbit, is less in need of help than the psychiatrists to whom his sister commits him. At one point he provides solace to the chief headshrinker, Dr. Chumley (Cecil Kellaway), whose one ambition is to escape to Akron, Ohio, where a sympathetic woman will continually say to him, "Oh, you poor thing. You poor, poor thing." Eventually, everyone comes to realize that the sanest person in the film is Elwood P. Dowd, whose vision of the world, except for the invisible rabbit, could have been borrowed from a Frank Capra film.

A few films from this period do, however, show a change in the image of psychiatry. Hollywood's drift toward a more positive view, one anchored in the unambiguous conviction that some people really do need help, is well illustrated by *The Shrike* (1955), a film based on the 1952 Pulitzer Prize–winning play by Joseph Kramm. José Ferrer was director and star of both the Broadway play and the film, but there are substantial differences between the two works. In the New York production of Kramm's play, Ferrer played Jim Downs, a failed stage director who is committed to a New York psychiatric hospital after a suicide attempt. He soon learns that he is the captive not just of the unsympathetic corps of psychiatrists who examine him but also of his estranged wife, Ann, who has convinced the doctors to release him only into her custody. The wife even succeeds in severing any possibility of contact between her husband and Charlotte, the woman Downs fell in love with shortly before abandoning his marriage. In the play's disturbing conclusion, Downs realizes that he can leave the prisonlike atmosphere of the institution only if he is willing to become the prisoner of his wife. He therefore capitulates, misrepresenting his true feelings toward her and telling the psychiatrists that he is prepared to reassume the traditional role of husband. In the play, when he finally walks out of the institution, he is a pathetically broken man.

By concentrating on the dark side of marriage, the play attacked what we have been calling "the dominant ideology." The 1955 film version of *The Shrike*, however, suggests that American movies were not yet prepared to make so drastic an appeal and that the pattern of reconciliation was still thoroughly entrenched. In the film, Jim Downs (José Ferrer) again finds himself the victim of his wife, Ann (June Allyson), and her co-conspirators in the psychiatric community, but screenwriter Ketti Frings has added a scene toward the end in which one of the psychiatrists, Dr. Bellman, uncharacteristically asks Ann if she has ever considered therapy. She reacts strongly in the negative, but at the end of the film, when Downs has been released into her custody, she reveals that she eventually went back to Dr. Bellman for treatment. Ann then tells her husband that she has seen the error of her ways and that she is prepared to let him go back to his lover, Charlotte, if he wishes. In an even more dramatic departure from the play, Downs tells his wife that he will stay with her and give their marriage another chance. The myth that any marriage can be transformed by two willing souls replaces Kramm's original vision of marriage as imprisonment. On one level, the film has simply added an upbeat "Hollywood ending" to a story that movie audiences might have found too depressing. On the other hand, *The Shrike* can be seen in the context of a gradual warming toward psychiatry in Hollywood films in the years just before the Golden Age. *The Shrike* belongs to the genre of institution films in which psychiatrists are little more than jailers, but the part of Dr. Bellman (played in both film and original New York production by Kendall Clark) has been clumsily rewritten. In the new version, Bellman suddenly becomes the oracular psychiatrist, capable of identifying and healing psychologically wounded people, that was about to become a staple of the American cinema.

Another film released in 1955, *The Cobweb*, not only echoes this tendency but presents the most elaborate treatment of the psychiatric profession in any Hollywood film to date. Produced by John Houseman and directed by Vincente Minnelli, the film employs an all-star cast and the wide-screen look of MGM CinemaScope. In fact, the film's lavish production values seem more appropriate to the musicals that Minnelli directed during the 1940s and 1950s (*The Band Wagon, Brigadoon, Kismet, Gigi,* etc.) than to a serious drama about the daily operations of a mental institution. Ultimately, the plot in *The Cobweb* revolves around a set of drapes, and the disparity between subject and treatment may have been largely responsible for the movie's failure to attract as large an audience as Minnelli's other dramatic films from the period (*The Bad and the Beautiful, Lust for Life,* and *Tea and Sympathy*), not to mention his musicals.

Based on William Gibson's novel of the same name, *The Cobweb* takes place at the "Castle House Clinic for Nervous Disorders" in Riverwood, Nebraska. The clinic and its fictional location were suggested by the Menninger Clinic of Topeka, Kansas, where Gibson lived while his wife, Margaret Brenman Gibson, was in psychoanalytic training. Like *Private Worlds* from twenty years earlier, *The Cobweb* is much more about the personal lives and interactions of the staff members than about mental illness and its treatment. Yet unlike *The Snake Pit* of just seven years before, it makes a fairly coherent attempt to connect the private lives of psychiatrists with their work. Whereas Dr. Kik (Leo Genn) in *The Snake Pit* is almost faceless, with no established family or personal problems and no apparent connection to the crazy patients and crazy nurses who surround the film's female protagonist, Dr. Stewart McIver (Richard Widmark) in *The Cobweb* has more difficulty dealing with the crises in his home than he does dealing with those of his patients. In fact, his most important clinical problem is one resulting from an action taken by his wife, Karen (Gloria Grahame). And whereas *The Snake Pit* gave us at least one godlike therapist surrounded by grotesquely disturbed patients in a chaotic institution, *The Cobweb* presents several very human psychiatrists with only mildly troubled patients in an elegantly furnished institution. Of course, we must keep in mind that these two films concern, respectively, a state institution in an urban setting and an expensive private sanitarium in the cornfields of the Midwest. Still, compared to *The Snake Pit,* *The Cobweb* suggests that psychotherapy was rapidly losing the exotic, scientifically complex associations it had once held for the American mind.

The Cobweb begins with Gloria Grahame offering a ride in her car to a pleasant young man named Stevie (John Kerr). They joke about the nearby institution, at one point saying that it is difficult to tell the doctors from the patients. Minnelli surprises us early in his film by revealing that Stevie is an inmate with free access to the area around the sanitarium and that Karen (Grahame) is the wife of the head psychiatrist (Widmark), even though we might have suspected that Karen, not Stevie, was the inmate. The interchangeability of "disturbed" and "normal" people is the central theme of the film, and a full half-hour goes by before all the doctors and staff have been distinguished from the patients.

One of the staff members is Victoria Inch (Lillian Gish), the ill-tempered business manager of the institution, who has little sympathy with Dr. McIver's (Widmark) newfangled ideas such as self-governance for the inmates. She has already picked out the drapes that she intends to put in the common room where the patients meet to discuss their problems, but at least two other parties become involved in the decision. One is Karen McIver, who has also chosen a pattern for the drapes; the second is Stevie (Kerr), whose paintings the other inmates feel should be printed onto curtains and placed in their meeting room.

The issue of the drapes creates a flare-up between Karen and Vicky Inch, which then becomes an issue between Karen and her husband. Widmark plays Dr. McIver as a no-nonsense therapist and administrator, who, despite his professional competence, is unable to devote enough time to his children and his scatterbrained wife. The film nevertheless portrays him as a loving father with equally understanding children, although his daughter claims to wish she were a patient so that she could see more of him. Because of the tension with his wife, McIver drifts into a romantic interlude with Meg Rinehart (Lauren Bacall), a sympathetic therapist at the clinic who lost her husband in the war and her only child to polio. McIver's wife is herself tempted by the institution's Don Juan, Dr. Douglas Devanal (Charles Boyer), an older analyst who turned to liquor and womanizing when his promising career became stalled. At one point he stares longingly at the faded cover of his own 1934 monograph, *The Theory and Practice of Milieu Therapy*. Presumably, he has written nothing in the twenty years since.

The most prominently featured patients in *The Cobweb* are played by Oscar Levant, John Kerr, and Susan Strasberg. Largely a comic character in the tradition of Shakespeare's Jaques, Levant enjoys his melancholy and cynicism but is often neglected by his therapist, Devanal (Boyer). Kerr and Strasberg, the juvenile and ingenue of the piece, are presented as beautiful losers who have been damaged by the outside world. Anticipating Keir Dullea and Janet Margolin in Frank and Eleanor Perry's *David and Lisa* (1962), Kerr and Strasberg's relationship becomes all the more appealing as they timidly help each other to conquer their fears. They both seem to make progress when they are able to go out together to see a movie without suffering excessive anxiety.

At the film's climax, Karen (Grahame) learns that her husband has been seeing Meg (Bacall). She decides to punish him by putting up her own drapes in the patients' meeting room, even though the group has decided to put up the set of drapes that bear Stevie's artworks. When he sees Karen's drapes in the room, Stevie flies into a violent rage and runs away from the institution. The doctors are so distracted by his disappearance that the inmates are left unsupervised. While the staff and police are busy searching for Stevie, even dragging the bottom of a nearby river, the patients quickly become involved in wild parties that just happen to take place before the clinic is to be visited by its board of directors. Dr. McIver's inspirational speech at the end convinces everyone that his unconventional methods of patient governance and freedom are working, and he is even reconciled with his wife after Stevie shows up at his house alive. The final moments of the film depict the happy home of husband, wife, and two children extended to include the much-improved Stevie, who sleeps peacefully on the couch.

The plot of *The Cobweb* is much more complex than this summary suggests, and it does afford the audience an extensive dramatization of life both inside and outside the clinic. As in *Now, Voyager*, however, there is little psychiatry practiced in the film, and its Hollywood ending is unfaithful to the novel, especially the film's suggestion that Stevie has undergone some kind of cathartic cure and is vastly improved after giving vent to his rage.

Although the film ultimately accepts the necessity of psychiatric treatment for troubled individuals, it questions the administration of that treatment as strongly as did *The Snake Pit*. It also introduces in Dr. McIver the soon-to-be-stereotyped image of the effective psychiatrist who can bring well-being to others but cannot establish harmony in his own life. (The same theme comes to the fore in Otto Preminger's *Whirlpool* [1950] as well as in the 1954 English film *The Sleeping Tiger*.) Although Charles Boyer's Dr. Devanal is more fleshed out than, say, the character played by Peter Sellers in *What's New, Pussycat?*, Boyer plays the typical philandering psychiatrist, who disguises his lust with professional jargon. What is most significant about *The Cobweb* is the humanization of psychiatrists: unlike the oracular or godlike therapists of *The Snake Pit*, *Blind Alley*, or *Now, Voyager*, Dr. McIver in *The Cobweb* is a more complete individual, with recognizable problems and responses. Like many female therapists in the movies, the Lauren Bacall character is one more woman in need of a man to bring her fulfillment, but at least the film does allow her to continue practicing therapy after she has made the difficult decision to break off her affair with McIver. Moreover, she identifies herself as someone to whom psychoanalysis has given the courage to go on living after the loss of her family, so her character provides not only a slightly more positive image of a woman psychiatrist on film but also a slightly more interesting one.

Another film from the 1950s that reflects the historical plan we have outlined is Edward Dmytryk's *The Caine Mutiny* (1954). The film was based on the novel by Herman Wouk and was produced by Stanley Kramer, who also produced five other films involving psychiatry: *Home of the Brave* (1949), *The Men* (1950), *My Six Convicts* (1952), *Pressure Point* (1962), and *A Child Is Waiting* (1963). These films all present a thoroughly positive image of psychiatry, but *The Caine Mutiny* is a little more complex in how it handles the issue. In the film, three distinctly different officers aboard the USS *Caine* during World War II become concerned about the conduct of Captain Queeg (Humphrey Bogart), whose compulsive fondling of ball bearings convinces the audience that something is wrong with him. Keefer (Fred MacMurray), a writer in civilian life, puts ideas into the head of Maryk (Van Johnson), a lifelong Navy man, who eventually agrees that Queeg's behavior is strange. The story is told primarily through the eyes of the third officer, an idealistic young student, Willie Keith (Robert Francis). When Queeg panics during a storm, Maryk submits to the urgings of Keefer and takes control of the ship. A crucial witness against the defendants in the ensuing court martial is a psychiatrist, played by the ubiquitous Whit Bissell, one of the most faceless of actors, who played at least four psychiatrists during the 1950s and 1960s. (His other films are *Invasion of the Body Snatchers*, *Third of a Man*, and *I Was a Teenage Werewolf*.) In *The Caine Mutiny*, Bissell portrays the psychiatrist as slightly pompous, and although his judgment is called into question by the defense attorney, he testifies that Queeg is sane and should not have been relieved of command. However, the defense attorney (José Ferrer) is able to win acquittal for the officers by reducing Queeg to a raving paranoid on the witness stand.

It is easy to forget that the opinions of the psychiatrist are largely vindicated in the final scene when the attorney arrives drunk at the mutineers' celebration and throws wine into the face of Keefer (MacMurray). He accuses the intellectual of sowing discord instead of supporting Queeg, holding Keefer responsible for the captain's breakdown during the storm. With drunken lucidity, he argues that regular Navy men like Queeg and Maryk would have conducted the war successfully without troublemakers like Keefer and Keith. Students and intellectuals only come into the service during war, he asserts, and they should not interfere with the men who keep the country safe in war *and* at peace. Even though the mutineers are acquitted, the film makes a strong argument in favor of Queeg, and the psychiatrist, though faceless and pompous, is shown indirectly to have been correct. Unlike the novel by Herman Wouk (1951), in which the psychiatrist is savaged, the film casts the psychiatrist and the attorney (Ferrer) as spokesmen for a society that, though it may have been unsettled by the trauma of World War II, can still preserve the values that made it great. In fact, the film's final credits go so far as to dedicate the film to the U.S. Navy. By encouraging the audience first to root for the mutineers and then to feel compassion for Queeg and pride for the military, a liberal filmmaker like Stanley Kramer could successfully negotiate the ideological minefields of the McCarthy era. Robert B. Ray sees *The Caine Mutiny* as an excellent example of how Hollywood's thematic paradigm could not hold up under postwar pressure to support the less glamorous official heroes such as Bogart's Queeg (1985, 174). The old pattern of reconciliation, which had characterized *Casablanca* and most of the films from classical Hollywood, was now breaking down, and even a psychiatrist could not conceal the absurdity in *The Caine Mutiny*'s last-minute attempts to exalt an obviously neurotic hero. In many ways, the idealization of psychiatry that was about to become entrenched in American movies can be understood as a somewhat desperate means of preserving Hollywood's consoling paradigms for an American public that was increasingly unlikely to believe in them. This was surely the case for the awkward use of psychiatry to provide reconciliation at the end of *The Shrike* as well as *The Caine Mutiny.*

Whit Bissell appears as another psychiatrist in a film that also bears the mark of McCarthyism, Don Siegel's *Invasion of the Body Snatchers* (1956). Actually two psychiatrists appear in this film: the local mind doctor in Santa Mira (Larry Gates), who turns out to be one of the "pod people," and the hospital psychiatrist (Bissell), who treats the protagonist (Kevin McCarthy) in the beginning and end of the film. Bissell's part was inserted late in production in an effort to tone down the film's disturbing conclusion. Like *The Cabinet of Dr. Caligari* (1919), the original version of the film was considered to be too unsettling for audiences, and a "frame" was added. *Invasion of the Body Snatchers* was supposed to end with Miles Bennel (McCarthy) running up and down the highway screaming "They're here!" while cars whiz by, unheeding. The final shot was to be a close-up in which he looks directly at the camera and warns the audience, "You're next!" The executives at Allied Artists overruled director Siegel's intentions and decided to add scenes at the beginning and end suggesting that the invaders may not have entirely succeeded in taking over the world. The opening scenes show Dr. Hill (Bissell) being brought in to treat the raving Miles Bennel, who tells a story that turns the original film into one long flashback. When we return to the framing device at the end of the film, the psychiatrist and another doctor (Richard Deacon) assume the man is mad. However, when they overhear another patient talking about the curious pods that fell out when a truck was overturned, they realize that McCarthy is telling the truth. Dr. Hill jumps into action and confidently orders the police to call the FBI. In chapter 12 we will discuss how the premise of *Invasion of the Body Snatchers*—that our closest friends and relatives can suddenly be transformed into enemies—plays on early infantile anxieties as effectively as it does on 1950s' anticommunist hysteria.

The first few depictions of psychiatrists in the American cinema responded primarily to highly conventionalized plots about characters such as escaped lunatics. We have suggested that the almost complete absence of mental health professionals from movies throughout the first three decades of the century is a result of their incompatibility with the earliest scenarios for silent films as well as of Hollywood's isolation from the psychoanalytic establishment. When producers began looking for scripts for the new talking pictures, they found a large library of books and plays that reflected the greater fascination with psychiatry existing in the eastern half of the country. And yet, when Hollywood made the plots of this literature their own, they recast them to accommodate the handful of cultural myths that kept Americans flocking to the cinema. Meanwhile, psychiatry was often found to be compatible with the needs of genres like the detective film, the women's film, and the screwball comedy, but only so long as the realities of the profession did not disrupt the illusions of escapist fantasy. Of course, the increasing acceptance of psychiatry as a part of American life in the 1930s, along with the profession's own willingness to give up its avant-garde image, resulted in the idealized portraits found in *Now, Voyager, Since You Went Away, Spellbound*, and *The Dark Mirror*. But even in these cases, celluloid psychiatrists rarely practiced anything resembling true psychotherapy. So long as they were little more than glorified guidance counselors, doctors of the mind could help effect the consoling resolutions that characterized nearly all Hollywood films of the classic period. At the same time, however, the complexities of the profession presented genuine problems for the movies, and throughout the thirties, forties, and fifties, a bifurcated myth of psychiatry emerged. For every idealized healer, there was a thick-accented, incompetent, and frequently malevolent quack. For every psychotherapist who spoke the culture's inherent ideology, another confirmed it by embodying an unacceptable alternative.

CHAPTER 3

The Golden Age

The Golden Age of psychiatry in the movies was over almost before it began. For a half-dozen years in the late 1950s and early 1960s, films reflected—however imperfectly—a growing conviction in American culture that psychiatrists were authoritative voices of reason, adjustment, and well-being. Before this view went on to become orthodoxy, however, the American cinema began responding heartily to the cultural upheavals of the mid-1960s, questioning the old ideas of sanity and conformity, and turning against the champions of these redefined concepts. Several historical forces played a role in making the Golden Age possible. Intrigued by successes with World War II casualties, young physicians had flocked into psychiatric residency training programs in the late 1940s, the same period during which *Life* magazine and other transmitters of popular ideology were making psychoanalysis fashionable for middle Americans. By the 1950s, Dr. Spock was advising mothers on the principles of psychoanalytically informed child rearing; psychoanalytic ideas were appropriated as cure-alls for a variety of social ills; and middle- and upper-middle-class professionals looked forward to the opportunity to lie down on The Couch.

During World War II, movie psychiatrists had been frequently idealized, especially in *Since You Went Away* (1944), a film that made a straightforward effort to contribute to the war effort by raising the morale of the women who kept the home fires burning. In the years immediately after the war, this shining image was considerably dimmed as a new disillusionment, pervasive in American society, began to set in. Film noir was one manifestation of this new malaise, but so was the inability of the social problem film to fit the old themes of reconciliation. The best example here may be the curiously ambiguous role of the psychiatrist played by Whit Bissell in *The Caine*

Mutiny (1954): audiences are asked first to reject his diagnosis and then to accept it some twenty minutes later. By the late 1950s, however, Hollywood was consistently producing idealized images of psychiatry: competent, compassionate, and lovable psychiatrists could be seen in at least twenty-five American films from 1957 through 1963.

One explanation for the new idealization of psychiatrists may lie in John Burnham's argument that the Golden Age of medicine in this country was coming to an end in the early 1950s (Burnham 1982). Perhaps the movies responded to this new disillusionment with medical doctors by shifting the sacerdotal mantle—which doctors had themselves appropriated from the clergy in the predominantly secular world of movie mythology—to increasingly demedicalized psychiatrists. In fact, some films extolled the virtues of psychiatrists at the expense of medical doctors. For example, the sexual anxiety that bedevils the two teenagers (Warren Beatty and Natalie Wood) in Elia Kazan's *Splendor in the Grass* (1961) produces shrugs and nervous laughter when Beatty asks the family physician for advice on how to deal with his desires. But when Natalie Wood's breakdown sends her into the care of an understanding and witty male psychiatrist, he is thoroughly knowledgeable about all aspects of her situation, and she emerges a wiser and healthier individual at the end of the film.

Burnham also provides a model for a more complex understanding of the Golden Age. We have already referred to his discussion of an important change in the role that analysts play in American culture. According to Burnham, the first doctors to practice psychoanalysis in the United States, such as A. A. Brill and Trigant Burrow, devoted themselves more to disseminating the revolutionary ideas of Freud than to actual practice, and as a result they were often associated with such avant-garde movements in the arts as "cubism, futurism, modernism . . . the problem play" (Burnham 1979, 128). The barrage of attacks upon Freud and his followers that were regularly published in conservative periodicals such as *Current Opinion* during the 1910s and 1920s allowed analysts like Brill, who took pleasure in shocking the sensibilities of mainstream Americans, to consider themselves in the vanguard of an intellectual revolution. In the 1930s and 1940s, however, as the emphasis in psychoanalytic circles shifted to practice, the field became one of many subspecialties in a bureaucratically organized medical establishment. Psychoanalysts could still see themselves as avant-gardists, but they just as likely might consider themselves part of a pluralistic society that could tolerate a variety of points of view. The avant-garde role had more or less disappeared by the end of World War II, and analysts were by now regularly engaged in providing "a defense of traditional civilization" (Burnham 1979, 132).

Hollywood movies of the 1930s and 1940s only vaguely absorbed the roles described by Burnham, in particular by making little distinction between psychoanalysts and other psychiatrists or mental health professionals. Films of this period seldom acknowledged the iconoclasm of psychoanalysts, unless occasional oddballs such as the jargon-spouting quacks in *Free Love* (1930) or *Murder, My Sweet* (1945) can be understood in these terms. We suggested in chapter 2 that the oracular creature played by Ralph Bellamy in *Blind Alley* (1939) may have embodied an idealized synthesis of both the avant-garde and tradition-defending roles that Burnham identifies. Within a few years, however, psychiatrists in films such as *Lady in the Dark* (1944) and *Now, Voyager* (1942) spoke exclusively as advocates for a supposedly enlightened—but in fact highly conventional—view of the world, even when the films portrayed their practice of psychotherapy simplistically or not at all. As psychiatry flourished in the postwar period, filmmaker Stanley Kramer showed this type of enlightened psychiatrist practicing a more dramatic, if not a more sophisticated, style of treatment in *Home of the Brave* (1949).

Negative stereotypes of psychiatry were still very much alive, but in the 1950s the acceptance of psychotherapists in American life finally trickled down to the highly conventionalized world of movie myths. This process was in large part facilitated by a crisis in the Hollywood cinema, an industry beset by numerous forces, not the least of which was what Ray calls "the breakdown of the homogeneous audience" (1985, 129–52). As viewers began to drift away to television and European "art films," as audiences became more politically and aesthetically sophisticated, and as the film industry coped with assaults such as communist witch hunts, desperate attempts were made to keep the old formulas alive. Ray lists the problem picture, the epic, and the "inflated genre" film as examples of this trend. "These 'serious' movies revealed very little about postwar developments or about the concerns generated by them. Instead, they limited themselves to a few domestic issues (particularly race), dealt with along the safe, official lines encouraged by a studied ideological optimism. These movies almost never portrayed the central American anxiety of the time—the fear that World War II had permanently altered the conditions of American life on which so much of the culture's mythology depended" (Ray 1985, 154). This statement is especially true of the many problem pictures that featured psychiatrists during the Golden Age. The cinema's compassionate, effective healer of troubled minds, already perfected during the war years, was readily available to assist in Hollywood's project to revive its ailing formulas.

By the late 1960s, however, therapists who embraced the wisdom of "traditional civilization" had become easy targets for the increasing number of movies that absorbed a new set of "avant-garde" ideas and questioned out-right the myths that had previously dominated American cinema. This chapter will focus primarily on American films made during a seven-year period in which psychotherapists were most often characterized as competent healers and admirable human beings. We will divide the period into three shorter ones, examining the transitional films that led into the idealized portraits of psychiatry in the high Golden Age as well as those that heralded its rather definitive fall from the pedestal in the mid-sixties.

The First Transitional Period

The 1956 version of *Invasion of the Body Snatchers*, which we addressed in the final pages of chapter 2, is one of the films anticipating the era of almost consistently positive images. The psychiatrist in the frame solves the mystery of Kevin McCarthy's story and immediately gives orders to begin the salvation of the world. Although the psychiatrist functions largely as a plot machine to set up a flashback, he anticipates the oracular character played by Simon Oakland at the end of *Psycho* (1960), who thoroughly explains the workings of Norman Bates's (Anthony Perkins) mind and then instructs the police on how Norman should be treated as well as on how they can find the bodies of three more murdered women. The 1956 version of *Invasion of the Body Snatchers* is transitional, however, because it contains the oracle (Whit Bissell), who is characteristic of the Golden Age, as well as the psychiatrist in the inner film (Larry Gates), who provides the stereotypically "rational" contrast to those who appreciate the powers of the unworldly. Much the same can be said of *The Shrike* (1955), with its good and bad asylum doctors, as well as the more complex *The Cobweb* from the same year, which offers an ambivalent view of the profession essentially by humanizing psychiatrists to the point of dwelling on their inadequacies.

Although it appeared slightly too late to fit perfectly into the transitional period before the Golden Age, Otto Preminger's *Anatomy of a Murder* (1959) may also be seen in this context. Orson Bean has a small part as the psychiatrist who testifies for the accused murderer (Ben Gazzara), defended by James Stewart. The attorney is attempting to prove that his client was temporarily insane when he committed the murder, and the psychiatrist testifies to that effect. What makes the film transitional is its self-conscious introduction of Orson Bean as a new breed of psychiatrist. When Stewart's sidekick (Arthur O'Connell) arrives at the train station to meet the psychiatrist, he apparently expects to see a Viennese gentleman with goatee and pince-nez or at least someone like Whit Bissell. He is not prepared for the youthful and friendly character played by Bean, and the psychiatrist's first speeches are aimed at countering the stereotypes of his profession. Although actors like Lew Ayres in *The Dark Mirror* (1946) and Charles Drake in *Harvey* (1950) had played youthful, good-looking psychiatrists before, in *Anatomy of a Murder* Bean seems to have been cast as a psychiatrist largely for the purpose of instructing audiences to dismiss the old stereotypes.

Anatomy of a Murder belongs more to the transitional period than to the Golden Age because the testimony of the youthful psychiatrist is under-mined by the film's conclusion: it turns out that Stewart's client (Gazzara) was sane when he committed the murder. In a sense, this conclusion repre-sents the complement to what happens at the end of *The Caine Mutiny* (1954). In *The Caine Mutiny* a rather unsympathetic psychiatrist is vindi-cated, whereas in *Anatomy of a Murder* a fresh-faced psychiatrist is discred-ited. Unlike *The Caine Mutiny*, however, which exposes Hollywood's failure to adapt the old paradigms to postwar attitudes, *Anatomy of a Murder* under-mines its psychiatrist's testimony primarily to set up a surprise ending. Much the same can be said of the 1985 mystery film *Jagged Edge*, which also at-tempts to throw audiences off the track by briefly introducing a rumpled psychiatrist to attest to the sanity of the central male character (Jeff Bridges), who is later revealed to be a psychotic killer.

A true transitional film that fits more precisely into our historical pattern is Robert Mulligan's *Fear Strikes Out* (1957). This film suggests that studio executives at Paramount were unsure whether audiences were ready to ac-cept an entirely humanized psychiatrist who can do no wrong. Lawrence Alloway (1971) has described the dilemma facing movie producers, who must spend money on a venture that may no longer be to audience taste when it is released months or even years later. As a result, movies speak to a "half known future" with images that cannot easily be dated, as can, for ex-ample, the clothes worn by women in forties' films, poised "in a strange re-gion of use, somewhere between negligee and ball gown" (Alloway 1971, 15). The tentativeness at the beginning of the Golden Age about audience accep-tance of idealized psychiatrists may explain why *Fear Strikes Out* takes a sup-posedly true story for its text and casts the faceless Adam Williams as the psychiatrist. Unlike Leo Genn's Dr. Kik in *The Snake Pit* (1948) or Richard Widmark's Dr. McIver in *The Cobweb* (1955), Williams plays a sympathetic psychiatrist working effectively in an institution where *nothing* goes wrong. As we emphasized in chapter 1, *Fear Strikes Out* even forgoes the opportu-nity to dramatize shock therapy. The treatment is portrayed as benign, with soothing music accompanying the shots of a bedridden Jimmy Piersall (An-

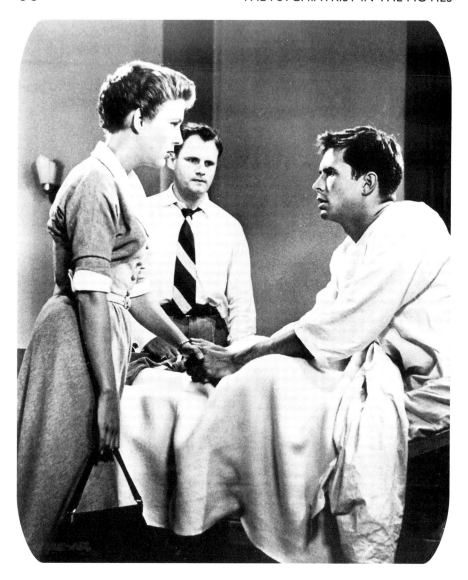

PLATE 13.   Like the audience for *Fear Strikes Out* (1957), Jimmy Piersall (Anthony Perkins) and his wife (Norma Moore) hardly notice the faceless psychiatrist (Adam Williams). Paramount Pictures. The Museum of Modern Art/Film Stills Archive.

thony Perkins) moving in and out of the door marked "electro therapy." We only see the room from the outside, and in each session Piersall's psychiatrist stands by with a compassionate expression (plate 13). The uncaricatured presence of a psychiatrist in such a film strongly suggests that the movie industry was granting new acceptance to the profession during these years.

The perfect complement of *Fear Strikes Out* is Nunnally Johnson's *The Three Faces of Eve*, which, like *Fear Strikes Out*, was released in 1957. Both were problem pictures that grossly simplified actual case histories and gave no hints that the protagonists were not completely cured as the films concluded (Piersall and Hirshberg 1955; Sizemore 1977). In fact, Jimmy Piersall, like Chris Costner Sizemore ("Eve"), continued to suffer from mental illness for many years after the film was released. Both films also painted psychiatrists as competent healers with none of the personal or professional problems that confronted many of their celluloid predecessors. However, just as the other transitional films seem tentative about presenting unabashedly positive images of psychiatry to the public, *The Three Faces of Eve* actually harks back to the apologia for psychoanalysis that began *Spellbound* in 1945. While the earlier film ran a message explaining psychoanalysis in terms inconsistent with the romance and suspense film that Hitchcock actually made, *The Three Faces of Eve* begins with an appearance by Alistair Cooke, behaving exactly as he had for several years on television's *Omnibus* and as he would later as the host of *Masterpiece Theatre*. His function in *The Three Faces of Eve* is to confirm the "truth" of what the audience is about to see, but even if he were to say that the entire film is a fabrication, his posturing legitimizes the film much more effectively than the prologues and "psychiatric advisers" of earlier films such as *Spellbound* and *Private Worlds*.

As much as anything else, *The Three Faces of Eve* is a star turn for Joanne Woodward (plate 14), who won an Academy Award for her performance. Her Eve Black expresses as much sexuality as the waning Production Code was beginning to allow in 1957. In fact, this film was one of the first to use the pathology of mental illness to step beyond the usual limitations imposed on sex in the movies. In one scene, Eve's befuddled husband Ralph (David Wayne) realizes the common male fantasy of being married to two women, one for public acceptance and one for sexual adventure. Unfortunately for Ralph, Eve Black uses her sexual allure only to entice him into buying her clothes and does not provide anything in return. Eve Black also makes eyes at the principal psychiatrist in the film, Dr. Luther (Lee J. Cobb), telling him that he is "kinda cute." As Golden Age psychiatrists were wont to do, Dr. Luther deftly parries her sexual overtures, as much from personal as from professional ethics. Cobb as Eve's psychiatrist even has some moments of gentle

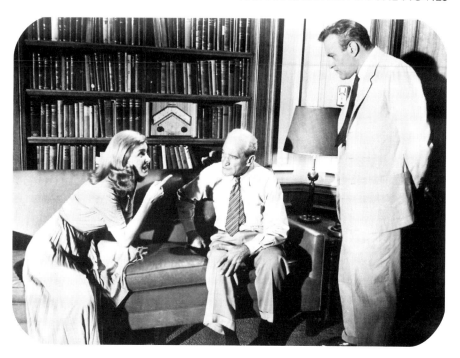

PLATE 14.   Joanne Woodward as Eve Black, one of *The Three Faces of Eve*
(1957), confuses Lee J. Cobb and Edwin Jerome. Twentieth Century–Fox. The Museum of Modern Art/Film Stills Archive.

humor, such as his attempt to explain the phenomenon of multiple personality to her husband. As Ralph stares at him blankly, Cobb slips into jargon and
then catches himself with a double take. The easy self-knowledge displayed
by Dr. Luther in this scene is definitely part of the humanizing process,
which does not begin in American films until the 1950s. It would be difficult
to imagine even Claude Rains in *Now, Voyager* or Leo Genn in *The Snake Pit*
registering anything like Cobb's double take.

   Although much less ambitious than *The Three Faces of Eve*, another transitional film is *Oh, Men! Oh, Women!* These two films make a remarkable pair
since they were both written, directed, and produced by Nunnally Johnson in
1957. (Johnson had dealt with psychiatric subjects in his screenplay for *The
Dark Mirror* in 1946.) But whereas *The Three Faces of Eve* was hailed as
something of a masterpiece, *Oh, Men! Oh, Women!* was dismissed as a mindless trifle. An English reviewer remarked: "CinemaScope discovers a solution
for the problem of filling the wide screen; the characters spend most of their
time full length on the psychoanalyst's couch" (Halliwell 1983, 602). Al-

though this may not have been exactly true, the flashy use of new technology for the rather straightforward translation of a play to the screen does not hold up well today, especially in comparison with the almost documentary feel of *The Three Faces of Eve*. (Ray [1985] would call *Oh, Men! Oh, Women!* "an inflated genre film," since it is basically a large-budget screwball comedy.) In fact, celluloid psychiatrists of the 1950s seem much more out of place in the Eastmancolor *The Cobweb* and *Oh, Men! Oh, Women!* than in the black-and-white *Freud, The Three Faces of Eve*, and *Fear Strikes Out*. This may stem from the fact that many people report that they dream in colorless images. (In *Whose Life Is It, Anyway?* Richard Dreyfuss's dreams are in black and white.) On the other hand, the illusion of grainy realism offered by black-and-white cinematography captures the ethos of the social problem film much better than the fairy-tale quality inherent in the gaudy palette of Technicolor and Eastmancolor.

Oh, Men! Oh, Women! fits squarely into the transitional period because of the script's ambivalence toward its central character, a psychoanalyst played by David Niven. The beautiful leading lady is played by Barbara Rush, whose exasperating flightiness fails to deter the analyst from asking her to marry him. Dr. Alan Coles (Niven) is shown to be an extraordinarily effective guidance counselor when it takes him a mere five minutes to put back together the marriage of two of his patients, Dan Dailey and that ubiquitous analysand Ginger Rogers (plate 15). In his dealings with his fiancée, however, Dr. Coles has trouble handling his emotions, leading her to insist that he is too intellectual and detached to be a good lover, even though she also disapproves when he deals violently with a meddling patient (Tony Randall) whose neurosis is coincidentally related to his failed relationship with her. To paraphrase Freud, it is never exactly clear what this woman wants, but by the end she has told the analyst that their engagement is off. At this point Niven is visited by the man who appears to be his training analyst, Dr. Kraus (John Wengraf). Sporting the inevitable goatee and Viennese accent, the older analyst utters the sentence, "The distance from the library to the bedroom is astronomical, but it is worth the trip." Shortly after hearing this non sequitur, the Niven character unintentionally creates a situation that convinces his fiancée that he really loves her and that he desires to take charge of their relationship in a manner acceptable to her. All is well as the movie ends. As in Golden Age films, the analyst played by Niven is a swiftly and almost casually proficient mental health professional, even if the problems of the couple he treats have little to do with intrapsychic problems. But unlike the vast majority of Golden Age films, *Oh, Men! Oh, Women!* looks into the private life of the analyst and finds the same kind of trouble that beset Richard Widmark in *The*

Cobweb: the occupational hazards of a psychiatrist get in the way of personal relationships. The image of psychiatry in *Oh, Men! Oh, Women!* is actually strongly positive—it would take a saint to endure the Barbara Rush character—but we have not yet encountered the psychiatrist who is a paragon in both professional and private life.

The Canonization

Fear Strikes Out was only one of many films from this period in which psychiatrists without personal lives were regularly portrayed as effective practitioners of healing arts. By 1958 these saintly doctors were already appearing in fictionalized stories as well as in pseudodocumentaries. In Mervyn LeRoy's *Home Before Dark* (1958), Jean Simmons barely maintains her sanity while her husband (Dan O'Herlihy), a dispassionate philosophy professor, neglects

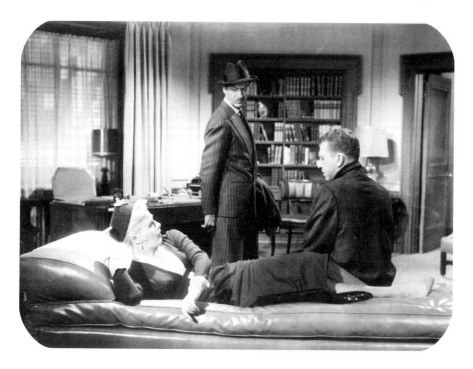

PLATE 15.   Ginger Rogers (with David Niven and Dan Dailey) in her third decade as an analysand in *Oh, Men! Oh, Women!* (1957). Twentieth Century–Fox. The Museum of Modern Art/Film Stills Archive.

her in favor of her stepsister (Rhonda Fleming). As the film begins, the Simmons character has just been released from an institution, and a faceless psychiatrist specifically instructs the husband to do everything that we later see O'Herlihy not doing. By the end, the psychiatrist's admonitions have been thoroughly verified: Simmons reacts irrationally to the not-so-benign neglect of her husband, surviving her ordeal only because her husband's sympathetic but alienated colleague (Efrem Zimbalist, Jr.) stands by her. (*Home Before Dark* probably fits best in the genre of women's film, but by identifying the character played by Zimbalist as Jewish, it also recalls the tendency of post-war problem films to confront racial issues.) When Simmons leaves her husband to join Zimbalist at the end, she vows that she will go to the big city and begin a life of her own that will include regular visits to a private psychiatrist.

We should mention a few other problem pictures from the Golden Age that present psychiatrists who are idealized but without a personal dimension. In an English/American production, Guy Green's *The Mark* (1961), Rod Steiger plays a heroic therapist who helps Stuart Whitman overcome the forces that drove him to commit sexual crimes against small children. Steiger then saves his patient again when the past comes back to haunt him. By the end, the Whitman character has established a healthy relationship with an attractive widow and her young daughter. In Joseph Cates's *Girl of the Night* (1960), Anne Francis plays a young woman who turns to prostitution because of a childhood rape trauma. She finds her way to the couch of a psychotherapist (Lloyd Nolan), who first cures her of the need to sell her body and then protects her when her pimp attempts to force her back into business. Whit Bissell appears as a psychiatrist once again in Robert Lewin's *Third of a Man* (1962), the story of how a small-town carpenter (James Drury) comes to accept his mute brother Doon (Simon Oakland), whom he has hidden away in a mental institution. The psychiatrist protects Doon from a posse after he escapes from the institution and eventually helps the Drury character to understand that people in sanitariums need love too. The film ends with the brother saying that he will visit Doon the next day. Doon then utters the first word he has spoken in years, "tomorrow."

There were other films from the early 1960s in which psychotherapists' private lives went completely unexplored. Simon Oakland appears again in Alfred Hitchcock's *Psycho* (1960), this time as a psychiatrist who is as successful a detective as he is a mind doctor. In Elia Kazan's *Splendor in the Grass* (1961), Natalie Wood's psychiatrist gracefully helps her put her life back together. Michael Callan in David Swift's *The Interns* (1962) idealizes Dr. Bonny (J. Edward McKinley), a faceless psychiatrist whose stature is so august that intern Callan is prepared to lie and cheat in order to procure a residency with him. And as we have suggested, Andrew Duggan in George Cukor's *The Chapman Report* (1962) brings the proper balance of science and humanism to his study of the sex lives of several beautiful women so that audiences can rationalize their voyeurism.

The Golden Age culminates in 1962 with, among other films, Frank Perry's *David and Lisa*. The fully integrated human being in psychiatrist's clothing emerges in this film as Dr. Swinford, played by Howard da Silva (plate 16). Significantly, da Silva was performing on the screen for the first time after twelve years on the blacklist. The politically committed character of da Silva's return to the screen complemented the film's breakthroughs in its treatment of psychiatry and in its inauguration of an American tradition of low-budget "personal films." Made outside the studio system, films such as Robert Wise's *Odds Against Tomorrow*, John Cassavetes's *Shadows*, and Perry's *David and Lisa* attempted to abandon the old Hollywood myths and seriously examine themes of the family, love, and human communication. Although *David and Lisa* appropriates psychoanalysis in the same spirit as the old classic films, "as a doctrine of self-help" (M. Wood 1975, 38), it nevertheless brought a new, less sensationalized image of mental illness to the screen. In one scene, a group of young inmates on an outing are subjected to the abuse of a local man, who tells them that they do not belong in his town. Unlike several Laingian films yet to come in the 1960s (Philippe de Broca's *King of Hearts* of 1966 is the best example), *David and Lisa* does not go so far as to say that the emotionally disturbed are superior to "normal" people, but it does confidently embrace psychiatry as the best hope for misunderstood and troubled individuals, equating the local man's hostility, in effect, with blind conformity and intolerance. Furthermore, the film establishes its credentials as "art" by undermining familiar movie myths of America as a homogeneous culture exempt from unsettling ruptures such as mental illness.

David and Lisa also overturns myths of family in several scenes that emphasize the complete alienation of David (Keir Dullea) from his insensitive mother. American films of the classic period often created tension in their treatment of the cultural mythology, and as the Editors of *Cahiers du cinéma* (1985) have written, even a filmmaker such as John Ford, who powerfully endorses the dominant ideology, contradicts that ideology through his personal style of filmmaking in *Young Mr. Lincoln* (1939). The much sharper critique of family in *David and Lisa* can be understood by comparing it with a somewhat similar situation in *Now, Voyager:* Bette Davis's alienation from her unsympathetic mother also takes place in close proximity to psychiatric discourse, suggesting that both films strain at the same cultural myths. However, although the audience is allowed to cheer Davis's rebellion against her

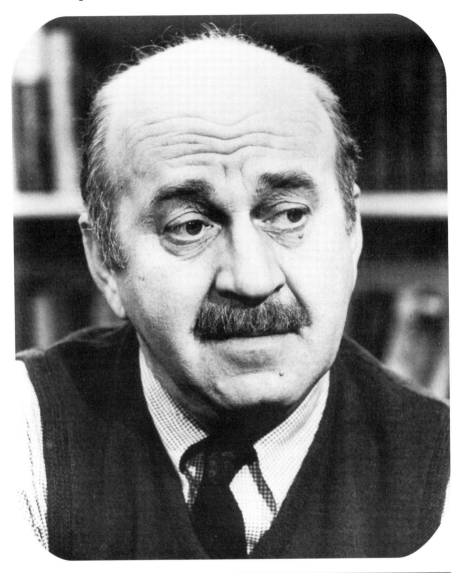

PLATE 16.   The face of compassionate competence: Howard da Silva as Dr. Swinford in *David and Lisa* (1962). Continental. The Museum of Modern Art/Film Stills Archive.

mother's repressive regime, the heroine pays dearly for this act when she feels responsible for her mother's death. The film extols values associated with family in other ways, including Paul Henreid's unwillingness to leave his wife and Davis's mothering of Henreid's daughter. *Now, Voyager*, following the Hollywood pattern of reconciliation, does not acknowledge that families can fail nearly so directly as does *David and Lisa*, in which David is effectively abandoned by his mother. Consequently, *David and Lisa* has much greater need for the healing powers of psychiatry and the parent surrogate of da Silva's Dr. Swinford. Ideologically, *David and Lisa* no longer casts psychiatry as an agent for the project of verifying American myths; instead, the psychiatrist functions as the best hope in a fallen world without the consoling promise of eternally nurturing families. Even when the doctor performs the conventional function of telling David to forgive his parents, his quietly understated performance makes the statements seem fresh and even daring. Part of the film's success lies in da Silva's ability to communicate the compassion his character has for his patients without letting the trappings of the profession impede him. Swinford seldom uses jargon, and he occasionally reveals that David's attacks affect him, even though he tries not to show it. Almost four decades after it was made, many psychiatrists still refer to *David and Lisa* as one of the most "realistic" depictions of psychotherapy.

The handling of countertransference feelings is actually the central issue in another film, Hubert Cornfield's *Pressure Point* (1962), certainly the best example of a racially oriented problem picture from the Golden Age. The film, however, has much more in common with *Home of the Brave* (1949) than with *David and Lisa*, especially since both films were produced by Stanley Kramer. Furthermore, *Home of the Brave* and *Pressure Point* substituted black characters for Jewish ones in their respective literary sources. But unlike *Home of the Brave*, *Pressure Point* makes the psychiatrist the central character and casts a black actor for the part rather than for the patient's role. Significantly, the first film appearance of a black psychiatrist takes place at the height of the Golden Age, and Sidney Poitier, the cinema's icon of the movement for black equality, endows psychiatry with his special aura during this period. (Poitier was quickly followed by Joe Adams as the good-natured black psychiatrist working with Frank Sinatra to save America from a communist takeover in *The Manchurian Candidate*.) *Pressure Point* begins when a psychiatrist in a state institution (Peter Falk) enters the office of the unnamed chief psychiatrist (Poitier) and asks to be taken off the case of a black youth who has suffered at the hands of white people and who has not responded to more than seven months of Falk's treatment. The body of the film is a flashback illustrating why Poitier believes that Falk should continue to treat the boy. Twenty years earlier, Poitier had been a prison psychiatrist treating a disturbed bigot (Bobby Darin) who had been incarcerated for wartime sedition as an advocate of Nazism (plate 17). In spite of Darin's constant taunting, Poitier eventually finds the root of his patient's problems—

his hostility toward his father. (The film uses expressionist camera work in flashbacks to Darin's childhood.) The film does not hesitate to show us that Poitier is offended by many of Darin's remarks, but it also argues that Poitier's professionalism always subsumes his personal feelings and that his only goal is to treat the young man. On several occasions, Darin tells Poitier that he is a fool to think that his white superiors will support a black man over a white man, even over a white convict who espouses Nazism. His prediction is borne out when Darin is paroled over the objections of Poitier, whose insistence that the bigot needs more treatment is interpreted by the warden as personal hostility. Poitier resigns from his job in the prison, and we learn that Darin is hanged for murder ten years after being released. Yet the black psychiatrist always believed that he could have helped the Darin character, and his insistence that Falk continue treating the black youth confirms this conviction. As in *Home of the Brave*, the real issues of racism that *Pressure Point* raises are finessed, and as in *The Caine Mutiny*, the solution of-

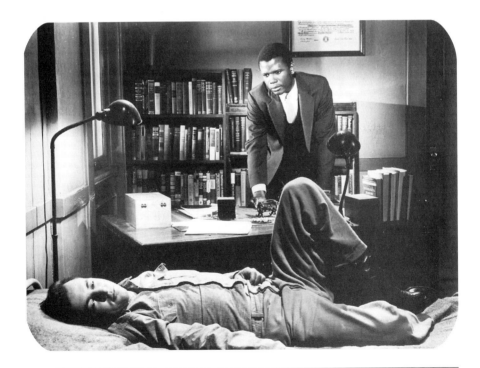

PLATE 17.   Sidney Poitier, as the movies' first black psychiatrist, overcomes the racism of Bobby Darin in *Pressure Point* (1962). United Artists. The Museum of Modern Art/Film Stills Archive.

fered at the film's conclusion does not ring true: the insuperable difficulties faced by Poitier in treating Darin contradict his optimistic belief that Falk can overcome the intractable resistance of a black patient. Obviously, the Poitier character himself should take over the case. Nevertheless, the heroism that the film finds in Poitier's struggle with himself is also invested in creating the portrait of a fully rounded, if idealized, human being whose expertise as a psychiatrist goes hand-in-hand with his nobility as a person.

One obscure film from the Golden Age is of interest primarily because of its title. Roger Kay's *The Cabinet of Caligari* (1962) hardly lives up to its name, even though its script is by Robert Bloch, who wrote the book on which Hitchcock's *Psycho* is based. In *The Cabinet of Caligari* (not the classic 1919 silent film of similar name), Jane (Glynis Johns) is trapped in a strange house where everyone is dominated and sometimes even abused by a mysterious physician named Caligari. The one sympathetic character in the group is Paul (Dan O'Herlihy), a pipe-smoking, avuncular fellow who offers advice and comfort to Jane. But Paul is ultimately revealed to be Caligari in disguise, and the heroine feels more trapped and alone than ever. Only at the end does the film make clear why it has been named after a classic of the silent German cinema: all but the final moments of the action turn out to have taken place entirely within Jane's deranged mind. Paul (O'Herlihy) is actually Jane's psychiatrist, whose attempts to reach her have transformed him into a monster in her fantasies. The film ends with the revelation that in fact Paul has cured her, and as she leaves the sanitarium we meet (much as in *The Wizard of Oz*) all the people from the sanitarium who inspired characters in her earlier dream. The expressionist mise-en-scène of the original *The Cabinet of Dr. Caligari* is suggested only vaguely in one scene, and little else connects the film with the source for its title. Nevertheless, this "remake" is typical of the Golden Age, constituting a grand apologia for psychiatry: all the tricks with which Caligari seems to torment Jane are actually valid healing techniques that only a disturbed mind would regard as threats. When O'Herlihy appears at the end, he is the avuncular character from the dream, in other words, the typical film psychiatrist of the late 1950s and early 1960s.

We should call attention in this chapter to another lower-budget film from the period, Philip Dunne's *Wild in the Country* (1961), one of the few Golden Age movies that feature a female psychiatrist. As we mentioned in chapter 1, Irene Sperry (Hope Lange) is perhaps the only female psychiatrist prominently featured in an American film who successfully treats a male patient without being transformed into his helpmate. (In 1935, when a young man thanks Claudette Colbert for curing him in *Private Worlds*, his total time on the screen is less than a minute.) Furthermore, *Wild in the Country* does not suggest at the outset that Dr. Sperry has chosen her profession because of her inadequacy as a woman. Nevertheless, she is sexually attracted to the Presley character and attempts suicide when their few chaste moments together in a hotel room are misinterpreted. This is, after all, an Elvis Presley film. On the other hand, Dr. Sperry is portrayed as a competent, compassionate therapist who transforms Presley from a juvenile delinquent into a promising young fiction writer and who at the end is capable of overcoming her feelings for him and returning to her practice. That all of this is accompanied by the obligatory fistfights and Presley's crooning should be sufficient proof that there was in fact a Golden Age of psychiatry in the American cinema.

We must also acknowledge that even during the Golden Age, women were only occasionally allowed entry into the American cinema's psychiatric pantheon. In Blake Edwards's *The Perfect Furlough* (1958), Army psychologist Janet Leigh goes through the usual process of losing her heart to her leading man after he has thoroughly manipulated her for his own purposes. Leigh is, of course, a sympathetic character, but she is no different from female psychiatrists in movies from earlier decades who found their true calling in the arms of a male lover. Irwin Allen's *Voyage to the Bottom of the Sea* (1961) reserves an even harsher fate for its female doctor of the mind: Joan Fontaine plays a seemingly competent psychiatrist who has undertaken a study of men under stress on the futuristic submarine *Seaview*, the brainchild of a scientific genius played by Walter Pidgeon. The plot presents the scientist with a fire in one of the two Van Allen radiation belts that is about to destroy the world. When Pidgeon sets out in his submarine to implement a controversial plan to extinguish the fire with a nuclear missile, Fontaine begins to spread doubts about his sanity among members of the crew. In this inflated genre picture, her function is a slight variation on that of psychiatrists in horror/science fiction films who deny the reality of supernatural forces. Rather than espousing a strictly rationalist unbelief in the supernatural, the Fontaine character in *Voyage to the Bottom of the Sea* fails to understand Pidgeon's unconventional but brilliantly effective plans. When Fontaine eventually resorts to sabotage to frustrate those plans, she receives a lethal dose of radiation for her troubles. Before she can expire from radiation sickness, however, she is eaten by a shark that another scientist (Peter Lorre) keeps aboard the submarine. Fontaine's sabotage attempts fail, and when Pidgeon finally launches his missile, he does in fact save the world. At the risk of overstating our thesis, we must point out that Fontaine, appearing in a film made during the Golden Age, is surely the least malevolent of all the negative female psychiatrists we have been able to locate in American movies. Unlike the villainesses in *Night-*

mare Alley, I, the Jury, and *Shock Treatment,* Fontaine is motivated by concern for the safety of the ship's crew rather than by simple avarice.

We should also point out that a few films from the period 1957–63 take a
skeptical view of psychiatry, even when the practitioner is male. In both *Pillow Talk* (1959) and *Lover Come Back* (1961), Tony Randall presents an unmanly contrast to Rock Hudson as Hudson pursues Doris Day. In the earlier
film, when Randall discovers that Hudson has been wooing his girlfriend
(Day), he says: "I should have listened to my psychiatrist. He told me never
to trust anyone but him." Capitalizing on the success of *Pillow Talk,* Delbert
Mann's *Lover Come Back* cast the same three actors in similar roles, this time
allowing Randall's psychiatrist (Richard Deacon) to appear briefly and to
dominate his neurotic patient as if Randall were a small child. In these two
films, as in *Oh, Men! Oh, Women!,* Randall became stereotyped as an insecure male whose dependence on his therapist is a function of his unmanli-
ness. The Rock Hudson of the movies would never be so conflicted about his
sexuality as to require psychiatric treatment (not to mention a sham marriage
demanded by the studio bosses). Twenty-five years later, revelations about
Hudson's sexual preference provided a thorough unmasking of this simplistic
notion of masculinity.

Delbert Mann again poked fun at psychiatry in still another Doris Day vehicle, *That Touch of Mink* (1962). In William Castle's *Zotz!* (1962), a psychiatrist fulfilled the conventional role of the unenlightened rationalist who
cannot appreciate the fact that the hero (Tom Poston) possesses magical
powers. However, in these light comedies, psychiatry is hardly central,
providing a few brief jokes as, for example, in *Call Me Bwana* (1963) when
Bob Hope flies past the window of a psychiatrist, who immediately lies down
on his own couch, begins talking about his childhood, and then is seen no
more.

At least one film from the Golden Age poses special problems for our historical analysis of the psychiatrist in American films. Henry King's *Tender Is
the Night* (1962), taken from the equally problematic novel of F. Scott Fitzgerald, can be seen as the straight version of a definitely post–Golden Age
film, Marshall Brickman's *Lovesick* (1983). Dick Diver (Jason Robards, Jr.) is
a handsome, well-liked, and promising young psychiatrist at a Swiss clinic
who treats a wealthy young woman, Nicole Warren (Jennifer Jones). Nicole's
mental illness gives her the same qualities possessed by Olivia de Havilland in
The Snake Pit, Susan Strasberg in *The Cobweb,* and Janet Margolin in *David
and Lisa*—a charming naïveté and vulnerability. Against the advice of his
thick-accented supervising analyst, Dr. Dohmler (Paul Lukas), Diver falls in
love with Nicole, and we hear this exchange:

DOHMLER: Love! How can a first-class brain with a brilliant fu-
　　ture fall in love so-called with a broken mind healing?
DIVER: There have been cases of good marriages between patients
　　and psychiatrists.
DOHMLER: You cannot be both lover and psychiatrist to the
　　same woman. You cannot be a guide, a doctor, a god, and a
　　husband. For when she discovers that she married a human
　　being, a fallible human being . . . crash, disaster, for one or
　　the other or for the both.

Nevertheless, Dick marries Nicole and accepts the invitation of her manipulative sister, Baby (Joan Fontaine), to devote himself full-time to showing Nicole the good life. As Nicole's guardian, Baby can and will contribute
unlimited financial resources toward her sister's happiness. But Dick and
Nicole's marriage becomes one long binge during which Nicole has regular
breakdowns. Returning to visit Dr. Dohmler some five years after leaving the
clinic, Diver finds the old analyst on his deathbed. Dohmler repeats many of
the remarks that he had made to Diver earlier, warning of the "tyranny of the
weak" and of Dick's role as a "fallible human being, not a god." When
Dohmler begins a sentence with the words, "And when the relapses end,"
Diver finishes it for him: "the love ends." Dohmler suggests, perhaps for the
only time during the Golden Age, that the profession of psychiatry may actually attract people with personal problems. He even says that Nicole would
get better without Dick and vice versa. Robards's performance suggests,
however, that Dick simply loves Nicole and wants to help her. The film also
suggests that, almost until the end of their relationship, Nicole desperately
needs Dick and that his love for her has forced him to succumb to the temp-
tations offered by Baby.

　Dick goes back to practicing psychiatry only when his little daughter becomes ill from drinking champagne, which constantly lies about in glasses
during their extended celebrations. Both Dick and Nicole, who has continued to improve, realize that they should get their lives back on track. But
Dick returns to the clinic to discover that Dohmler has died and that Franz,
the psychiatrist who has replaced him, is not fully prepared to accept Dick on
his own terms. To complicate matters, Dick is no longer as effective a therapist as he was for Nicole, and in one scene he even attacks the father of one of
his patients. During a later scene in which Dick uses terms like "anaclitic"
and "countertransference," Franz suggests that Nicole has become the stronger member of their marriage. Their relationship continues to deteriorate
until Dick decides to go back to upstate New York where he was born,

presumably to start life over. Both Nicole and Dick realize that they must separate for their own good, but the film, unlike the novel (Fitzgerald 1934), suggests that the love that they still feel for each other might eventually have saved their marriage.

Tender Is the Night does not hold up well because of its soap opera treatment of what was already an overdrawn novel. The film follows Dick's degeneration and Nicole's improvement as if she were a vampire sucking the mental health out of him. A number of reasons are offered for Dick's succumbing so easily to this process, but none of them adequately explain why the physician cannot heal himself. Old Dr. Dohmler was right to warn Diver not to fall in love with Nicole, but he speaks with a much better understanding of countertransference than the movie shows in its plot. Fitzgerald's novel is probably unfilmable, but it was especially so in 1962, the year in which the image of psychiatry had reached its apex in the American cinema. The picture of Dick Diver drowning in wasted love (Fitzgerald's onomastics are particularly bald in this story) clashes with the idealization of psychiatry that has seeped into the film from its historical context.

This idealization also comes to the movie directly from its source. *Tender Is the Night* is a largely autobiographical novel drawn from Fitzgerald's troubled marriage with the schizophrenic Zelda (Berman 1985, 60–86). Fitzgerald considered making his protagonist a film technician before deciding upon a psychiatrist. This choice was significant and not just because Fitzgerald took psychiatry to be the best available equivalent for his own work as an artist. Dick Diver in *Tender Is the Night* also stands for "the decline of the supposedly solid, turn-of-the-century American morality, the disillusionment of the so-called Lost Generation, the ultimate futility of seeking material possessions, the emptiness of a purely sensual existence" (Guthmann 1969). Fitzgerald wanted to dramatize this vision by chronicling the destructive effect of these forces upon even a character who should be most equipped to withstand them. Even more so than in the film, the Dr. Dohmler of the novel represents the lofty traditions to which Diver's generation cannot measure up. It can be argued that the film version of *Tender Is the Night* does not possess the Golden Age qualities of, say, *Pressure Point* or *David and Lisa*. On the other hand, Dr. Dohmler is the most august and sympathetic elder statesman since Michael Chekhov in *Spellbound*. As played by Jason Robards, Jr., Dick Diver is a handsome, witty man who falls in love and then tries to pick up the pieces of his life (and his practice), leaving behind the woman he loves essentially for her own good. If the film had been made before 1955, there is little doubt that the portraits of the psychiatrists would have been much less positive. After 1963, the film simply would not have been produced except as a made-for-television movie. In fact, a new version of *Tender Is the Night* appeared in 1985 as a mini-series on Showtime, a "premium" cable television service.

The 1962 version of *Tender Is the Night* did not present the only dark cloud in the golden skies of cinematic psychiatry. A curious film from this period that deserves mention is Joseph L. Mankiewicz's *Suddenly, Last Summer* (1959), based on a short play by Tennessee Williams. Three years before he was to act the part of Freud, Montgomery Clift plays a promising young brain surgeon who appears to be the only doctor in a mental institution that bears a great resemblance to the one in *The Snake Pit*. Strictly speaking, Clift does not belong in our study since his specialty in the film is surgery, not verbal therapy. Yet no brain surgeon could be more unlikely. Clift was still recovering from a disastrous 1957 automobile accident and was becoming enmeshed in an addiction to alcohol and drugs that would plague him for the rest of his career and his life. One scene in *Suddenly, Last Summer* shows his character about to perform a lobotomy, even though Clift himself is apparently unable to keep his hands from shaking. Ultimately, however, Clift plays another idealized doctor of the mind, intervening in behalf of the institutionalized heroine (Elizabeth Taylor) and finally providing her with a complete cathartic cure and more than a suggestion of love interest. What makes the film problematic is its subtext: not only is Clift barely able to walk through several of his scenes, but the portrait of institutional care for the mentally ill falls back on the bedlam conventions of the 1940s, complete with wildly aroused male patients, arbitrarily repressive keepers, and a corrupt sanitarium director (Albert Dekker) willing to lobotomize a patient in return for the donations of a wealthy patron (Katharine Hepburn). According to Vito Russo (1981), Tennessee Williams's psychiatrist had recently convinced the playwright that he should renounce his homosexuality, and so Williams earnestly responded by writing a short play that portrayed Sebastian (the son of Hepburn's character in the subsequent film) as a homosexual monster. Mankiewicz's film expands this drama into a baroque horror film, featuring cannibalism, slightly displaced incest, and a conclusion that recalls the original *Frankenstein*, in which outraged villagers chase the monster to the top of a hill before destroying him. The spectacle of a barely functional Clift— however idealized his character— only contributes to the portrait of a moral universe that is profoundly askew and far beyond the control of one benevolent therapist.

A number of films by Alfred Hitchcock present a similar ambiguity. Interestingly, many of the director's most respected films were made during our Golden Age, and many of them feature a vision of psychiatry that seems on the surface to be rather positive. But the subtexts of almost all of these films undermine the grandiose claims by and for psychiatry during this time. Unlike *Suddenly, Last Summer*, in which the subtext seemed unintentionally at odds with the film's plot, Hitchcock's work reflects a carefully articulated vision that engaged psychiatry at several levels. The later films are much more interesting from a psychoanalytic view than is *Spellbound* (1945), which features psychiatrists much more prominently in its plot.

Perhaps the bleakest film of Hitchcock's career is *The Wrong Man* (1956), a semidocumentary account of a musician (Henry Fonda) who finds himself the victim of an astonishing array of coincidences that link him to a robbery he did not commit. During the long legal process to which the protagonist is subjected, his wife (Vera Miles) suffers a breakdown and is institutionalized. In his one brief scene, the wife's psychiatrist (Werner Klemperer) appears competent and concerned. Nevertheless, the profound pessimism of the film works against the hope offered by therapy. At film's end, although the hero has been vindicated, his wife is still deeply disturbed, and there is no suggestion that his Job-like sufferings will be requited.

Much the same can be said of a film that many critics and filmmakers consider to be Hitchcock's masterpiece, *Vertigo* (1958). When Scotty (James Stewart) collapses after what he assumes to be the death of Madeleine (Kim Novak), he is treated by an articulate psychiatrist whose diagnostic formulation and treatment recommendation are perfectly reasonable. Nevertheless, when he encounters Judy, the woman who had previously posed as Madeleine, the hero's obsession leads him on a necrophilic quest in which he finds himself hallucinating Madeleine over Judy's shoulder even as he is succeeding in transforming Judy into Madeleine. In his essential essay on *Vertigo*, Robin Wood has pointed out how well the film succeeds in its psychologically complex investigation of the human tendency "to form an idealized image of the other person and substitute it for the reality" (1977, 93). By the end, Scotty has been cured of his vertigo, but without the intervention of a therapist. More importantly, "his cure has destroyed at a blow both the reality and the illusion of Judy/Madeleine, has made the *illusion* of Madeleine's death real. He is cured, but empty, desolate. Triumph and tragedy are indistinguishably fused" (Wood 1977, 95). More important than the brief appearance of the therapist in this film is a subtext that finds madness in love, betrayal in friendship, and death in the displaced sexual climax when Scotty and Judy breathlessly arrive at the top of the church tower.

Even *Psycho* (1960), which we will discuss in more detail in both chapters 4 and 7, finds means for undermining the seemingly definitive statements of its psychiatrist, Dr. Richmond (Simon Oakland). Several critics have suggested that *Psycho's* psychiatric coda is actually a Hitchcockian joke or that the glib explanations of Dr. Richmond are inadequate to dispel the profoundly disturbing issues of matricide, voyeurism, and audience complicity that lie at the core of the film (Braudy 1968; Wood 1977). Harvey Greenberg argues that Hitchcock is a much better Freudian in his creation of "*Psycho's* authentic ambience of the dream" than in the "inexact" pronouncements of the "officious" Dr. Richmond (1975, 134).

We maintain, however, that in the context of the Golden Age, in which psychiatrists were the ultimate authorities, Simon Oakland's formulation is presented by Hitchcock as a compelling explanation of the events that have unfolded in the film. The casting of Oakland, whose line readings convey a powerful sense of certainty and a persuasive credibility, speaks for itself. By contrast, in the 1998 remake by Gus van Sant, Robert Forster's portrayal comes across in an entirely different vein. The speech has been considerably cut in the remake, and Forster's befuddled look suggests that he has serious reservations about his own diagnostic understanding.

Robert Ray has identified Hitchcock's themes during this Golden Age period. "His crowning achievements, *North by Northwest* and *Psycho*, specifically dealt with money, mothers, and movement. Of all his films' great sequences, the most memorable was the crop-dusting sequence in *North by Northwest*, an image that took the very basis of the American dream, open space, and revealed its hidden capacities for danger and claustrophobia" (1985, 158). In upsetting the old formulas so thoroughly, Hitchcock was hardly interested in the pat remedies that psychiatry so frequently offered in the social problem films of the Golden Age.

In spite of these few films that tarnished the psychiatric goldenness of the late 1950s and early 1960s, our period culminated in 1962 with John Huston's *Freud*. The film is interesting if only for the role played by Jean-Paul Sartre in the genesis of its script. Huston had been planning a film about Freud ever since he had the opportunity to watch psychiatrists in action while filming *Let There Be Light* in 1946. Even though Huston refers to Sartre in his autobiography (1980) as an anti-Freudian, he says that he considered him to be the ideal writer for a script about Freud. "Sartre disagreed with Freud in a social sense rather than in a scientific sense. He regarded Freud's studies as valuable for what they discovered about the human mind, but of little social import because the role of the psychoanalyst was in fact so limited. I'm inclined to agree. Bored wives and problem children of the affluent make up the bulk of a top-ranking psychoanalyst's practice. Fees are exorbitant, and treatment is usually a matter of years. The movers and shakers have no time for it, and those who most need psychiatric counseling are precisely those who can't afford it" (Huston 1980, 294). Interestingly, the film that Huston eventually made carries none of the spirit of these remarks; in fact, it transforms Freud into a Christ figure. Huston's statements in his autobiography reflect his (and typical Hollywood) ideas of 1980 much more than they do any ideas expressed in *Freud*.

According to Huston, Sartre wrote two drafts for a script, the first of which was long enough for a five-hour movie. After meeting with Huston for several days in an effort to make the script more manageable, and after being told not to worry about censorship, Sartre then produced a second draft, which was twice as long. (Sartre's *Freud* script was published in 1986 by the University of Chicago Press.) Some time later, Huston wrote a much shorter treatment with Wolfgang Reinhardt, son of the director Max Reinhardt. (Charles Kaufman also received credit, though Huston says that his contribution was minimal.) Unlike Axel Corti's German film *Young Dr. Freud* (1977) or the six-hour miniseries made for British television in 1984, Huston's film takes a number of liberties with the chronology of events in Freud's life, and

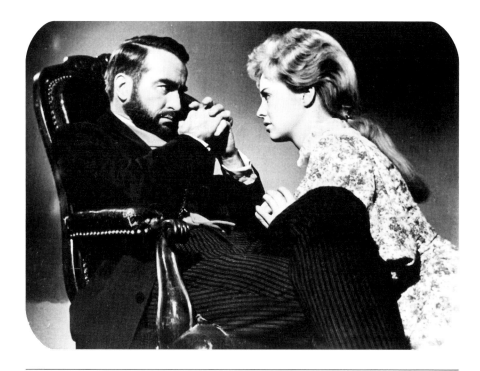

PLATE 18.   Young Sigmund Freud (Montgomery Clift) is about to come to terms with the problems of Cecily (Susannah York) as well as himself in John Huston's *Freud* (1962). Universal Pictures. The Museum of Modern Art/Film Stills Archive.

some characters, such as Susannah York's Cecily (plate 18), are composites. The script relied on Sartre's work as its "backbone," particularly its focus on Freud's early career when he was developing the theory of the Oedipus complex while confronting his own conflicts with his father. Yet Sartre denounced Huston when he eventually saw the script and demanded that his name not be associated with the film. Sartre never told Huston why he objected, even though the director felt that the $25,000 Sartre received for his screenplay entitled Huston to an answer.

Still, the film is surprisingly frank about Freud's work, in particular his theories concerning infantile sexuality. On the other hand, the film attempts to romanticize and sensationalize Freud's work at the same time that it evokes a performance from the ailing Montgomery Clift so solemn as to completely obscure Freud's famous wit. The film is also the most claustrophobic of Huston's many works, employing a larger percentage of close-ups than any of his other films, or, for that matter, the films of almost any other Hollywood director (Kaminsky 1978, 140).

The movie's opening credits tell us that not one but two technical advisers were present during filming. We then hear John Huston's overripe narration behind obscure Rorschachesque images and Jerry Goldsmith's atonal score. After comparing Freud to Copernicus and Darwin for their "blows dealt us in our vanity," Huston introduces the Christ parallel by telling us we are about to see "the story of Freud's descent into a region almost as black as hell itself—man's unconscious—and how he let in the light." (The use of the word *light* in this context also recalls Huston's *Let There Be Light*.) The music of Goldsmith, whose effective score for Ridley Scott's *Alien* will be discussed in chapter 12, often telegraphs the psychosexual importance of what happens in the film. For example, when Freud learns through hypnosis that a troubled young man (David McCallum) has attacked his father because the son believed that his father raped a "young girl," a string crescendo and then a moment of pregnant silence precede McCallum's terse identification of the young girl as "my mother." Another musical flourish marks the oedipally charged moment when Freud unintentionally breaks the family heirloom pocket watch just after his father has given it to him.

In its cinematographic depiction of dreams (plate 19) and simple cures, *Freud* is in some ways no more sophisticated than the much earlier *Blind Alley* (1939). There is even a familiar cathartic cure for Cecily, the central patient in the film, played by Susannah York (plate 18). (Both Huston and Sartre had wanted Marilyn Monroe to play the part, but according to Huston, Monroe's own analyst objected on the grounds that Anna Freud had not approved the project.) As Sartre had intended, the film unites Freud's progress

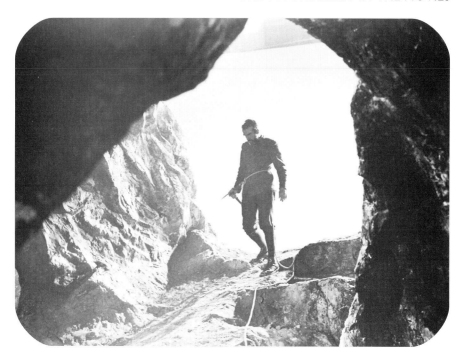

PLATE 19.   Freud's dream is also a metaphor for his perilous journey into the unexplored regions of the mind: *Freud* (1962). Universal Pictures. The Museum of Modern Art/Film Stills Archive.

toward defining the Oedipus complex through the parallel analyses of Cecily and himself, arriving simultaneously at an understanding of why he and his patient both entertained troublesome feelings toward their parents. After a nocturnal moment of self-doubt when Freud's wife attempts to encourage him by reading to him from his diary, the truth of infantile sexuality suddenly becomes clear to him. As he realizes the importance of his discovery, his wife opens the drapes and the morning light pours in symbolically, recalling Huston's opening narration. The notion that Freud's discovery came from a stray remark by his wife is a little reminiscent of the joke about Beethoven hearing the opening motif of the Fifth Symphony in his wife's laugh. Like the author of the Beethoven joke, who capsuled a complex process into a single pregnant moment, Huston and his collaborators have attempted to find a cinematic means for presenting in concentrated form a discovery that was actually a series of processes within one person's mind. A film such as *Freud* provides an excellent example of the trivializing power of cinema, especially when, ironically, it attempts to impress us with the seriousness of what it has undertaken. Most film theorists agree that movies succeed more often when they put aside pretension and turn to material that is suited to a popular medium like the cinema. This is not to say that films cannot be serious or significant, but rather that they suffer when the complexity of the material lies outside the range of what cinema can effectively dramatize.

Ernest Callenbach, the editor of *Film Quarterly*, said of *Freud*, "It is impossible, I would think, for any educated person to sit through *Freud* without bursting into laughter at least once" (Halliwell 1983, 303). This judgment may be harsh, especially of a film made during the unique moment when American films were most earnest in their romance with psychiatry, a moment that has been especially vulnerable to the changing attitudes and styles in the American cinema of the last two decades. In all fairness to Huston, we should point out that substantial portions of the film were excised under pressure from the heads of Universal-International, who nevertheless expected the film to be the studio's most important release of the year. However, like most psychiatrically inclined films from the Golden Age, *Freud* was a box-office disappointment. Psychology was never as successful in attracting audiences as the singing and dancing and biblical pageantry that often characterized box-office hits in the late 1950s and early 1960s. When *Freud* was rereleased in 1963 with the subtitle *The Secret Passion*, it was still unsuccessful. Huston is probably correct in his explanation of *Freud's* failure to attract audiences: the film seemed far more interested in education than in entertainment, while its ability to produce titillation—or moral outrage—was greatly exaggerated. "Audiences didn't give a damn whether children thought about, were influenced by or practiced sex. They were, if anything, disappointed that there wasn't more sex in the picture, especially on an adult level. But what they wanted was 'healthy' sex—the Marilyn Monroe kind of sex" (1980, 304).

The Second Transitional Period

Still, *Freud* is the ultimate example of a phenomenon toward which the American cinema had been moving since its inception: the portrayal of a sensitive human being dealing successfully with the interrelated problems of himself and others. It is no coincidence that in the single year 1962 we meet this figure not only in *Freud* but also in *Pressure Point, David and Lisa,* and, to a certain extent, *Tender Is the Night*. The Golden Age comes to an end quickly, however, and like 1957, 1963 is a transitional year in which we can see a new, negative view of the profession emerging. Golden Age myths popped up briefly in 1963 films such as Daniel Mann's *Who's Been Sleeping in My Bed?* in which Martin Balsam cures Dean Martin of compulsive woman chasing, or Norman Jewison's *The Thrill of It All*, in which James Garner wins back the attentions of his wife (Doris Day), thanks to the guidance counseling of a slightly eccentric psychiatrist. Yet both these movies are comedies, and like *Pillow Talk* and *That Touch of Mink*, they anticipate the irreverence toward psychiatry that was soon to become a regular feature of satirical comedies in the sixties and seventies.

For our purposes, the most interesting transitional film of 1963 is David Miller's *Captain Newman, M.D.* Gregory Peck plays the title role of a psychiatrist during World War II who cares deeply about his patients but who must resist the efforts of his superiors to send men back into combat before he can finish curing them. Tony Curtis and Angie Dickinson appear in the film, largely for the purpose of showing the many ways in which Newman can be human and loving as well as effective and compassionate. However, he has mixed results with the three principal patients whom we see him treating. He never really succeeds in reaching an obsessed officer (Eddie Albert) who eventually jumps to his death from a tower. On the other hand, he wins a victory in his treatment of a nearly catatonic soldier played by Robert Duvall. The most effective element in the cure of Duvall comes when the doctor encourages Duvall's dispassionate wife (Bethel Leslie) to express more affection and to dress more alluringly. When his wife takes the advice and adopts a new approach to her marriage, the Duvall character has an outburst that turns out to be another cathartic cure. The most important patient, however, is played by Bobby Darin, just one year after his well-received performance in *Pressure Point*. After encountering more difficulty with him than with anyone else, Captain Newman turns the Darin character into a healthy individual and returns him to his unit a new man. In the final minutes of the film, however, the news comes back that Darin has been killed in action. Although the film's primary message has already been clearly stated, it ends with the psychiatrist bemoaning his fate of patching up the psyches of troubled soldiers only to send them off to be slaughtered. Psychiatry works, but it is no match, unfortunately, for the problems of the world. The suggestion that the diseases of society negate or mock the efforts of psychiatrists was present in earlier films such as *The Snake Pit*, but it becomes central to the view of psychiatry throughout the 1960s and 1970s. *Captain Newman, M.D.* is a transitional film because this theme appears alongside Peck's portrayal of one of the most idealized of all movie psychiatrists. Unlike *David and Lisa*, *Captain Newman, M.D.* is the big-budget product of a Hollywood studio that at this point appears to have abandoned the project of reconciliation and consolation. However sentimentalized its ending, the film does not blink at the terrible irony of Dr. Newman's career. The introduction of the idea that the world's problems render psychiatry ineffective also signals the end of the brief Golden Age of psychiatry in the American cinema.

The abrupt and unexpected end of the Golden Age coincided with an equally abrupt and unexpected decline in governmental support of psychiatric research and education (see chapter 6). In this context, we should mention one of the last Golden Age films, Hall Bartlett's *The Caretakers* (1963), in which Robert Stack plays an innovative young psychiatrist of idealized qualities who assumes command of a clinic and then overcomes the resistance of an authoritarian head nurse, appropriately named Lucrezia (Joan Crawford), in his efforts to help patients. The film, however, also exploits the sensational aspects of ECT and titillated the audience when a dazed but attractive female patient (Polly Bergen) wanders into a ward full of men, all of whom appear to be steely-eyed rapists. *The Caretakers* was a strangely inappropriate film to ride the Golden Age wave and to garner the publicity benefits of being selected for a special preview screening before the U.S. Senate. The chairman of the Senate Committee on Labor and Public Welfare, Lister Hill, wrote to director Bartlett praising him for a film that "contributed to creating the very favorable climate and presenting the challenge that brought the victory in the passage of the Mental Health and Mental Retardation Act by an overwhelming vote" (Knight 1963). However, just as the movies were to begin projecting a much less flattering vision of psychiatry, the U.S. government was on the verge of reversing itself and cutting its expenditures for mental health. After two decades of dramatic increases, grant support from the National Institute of Mental Health for psychiatric research and education reached a peak and then began to decline in the mid-1960s (Pardes and Pincus 1983). The special attention afforded *The Caretakers* had little lasting effect on the government or, for that matter, on Hollywood itself.

The Migration of a Genre

We conclude this chapter both by departing from our exclusive concentration on theatrically released features and by pointing out that the idealized image of psychiatry does not disappear entirely from popular media after 1963. By the late 1970s, films such as *I Never Promised You a Rose Garden* (1977), *An Unmarried Woman* (1978), and *Ordinary People* (1980) depicted psychotherapists who would not have been out of place in the Golden Age. Nevertheless, the most positive images of psychiatry traveled from movie houses to television along with many other elements of the social problem film. The earnest realism of this genre quickly lost its allure for the increasingly youthful movie audiences of the 1960s, but its comforting view of souls being healed seemed ideally suited for the "cooler" medium of television. In 1962, the culminating year of the Golden Age of psychiatry, several therapeutically oriented films appeared that illustrate this point. Arthur Penn's *The Miracle Worker* from this year won Academy Awards for Patty Duke, who played the young Helen Keller, and Anne Bancroft, who played her teacher, Annie Sullivan. The story had originally appeared as an episode on television's high-art series, *Playhouse 90*, before moving on to Broadway and then to the silver screen. Significantly, when *The Miracle Worker* was remade in 1979, it was not for theatrical release but for television once again, as a run-of-the-mill "movie of the week." (Scripts for all three versions of *The Miracle Worker* were by William Gibson, who also wrote the novel on which *The Cobweb* was based.) Similarly, in 1976 *The Three Faces of Eve* was more or less remade for television as *Sybil*. The continuity between the originals and the remakes was established by casting Patty Duke as Annie Sullivan in the television version of *The Miracle Worker* and Joanne Woodward (who had played the title role in *The Three Faces of Eve*) as a psychiatrist treating a patient with multiple personality (Sally Field) in *Sybil*. In 1981, Richard Sarafian directed an almost shot-for-shot television remake of *Splendor in the Grass* with the same Golden Age vision of psychiatry that had characterized the theatrically released original in 1961. As we will see in chapter 4, reassuring stories about people overcoming their problems were practically nonexistent in the movies made for theatrical release after the Golden Age.

The issue of alcoholism offers an even better illustration of how social problems move between media. In Billy Wilder's *The Lost Weekend* (1945), Hollywood exploited alcoholism for its shock value and then tacked on a preposterous happy ending. In 1958, television's *Playhouse 90* presented a more disturbing look at the subject in *The Days of Wine and Roses*. Blake Edwards made the film version of J. P. Miller's teleplay for *Wine and Roses* in the crucial year of 1962, when audiences could also see *The Miracle Worker*, *David and Lisa*, *Pressure Point*, and *Freud*. In fact, in the film of *The Days of Wine and Roses*, Jack Klugman plays a recovered alcoholic whose selfless devotion to helping the protagonist (Jack Lemmon) would have made him the perfect example of the Golden Age psychiatrist if only the film had decided to call him "doctor" instead of leaving his occupation unstated. *The Days of Wine and Roses* purposefully explores the dangers of alcoholism and then shows that at least some of its victims—including the Lemmon character—can recover. Compared with *The Lost Weekend*, we can hardly say that the film is optimistic, but the sadder-but-wiser ending for Lemmon's character fits perfectly into an early sixties tradition that includes psychiatrically inclined films such as *Home Before Dark, Splendor in the Grass*, and *Captain Newman, M.D.* Still, this view of alcoholism soon became the almost exclusive property of undistinguished television movies. *Sarah T.—Portrait of a Teenage Alcoholic, Beatrice: Life of the Party*, and *A Sensitive, Passionate Man* are three examples of made-for-television films that treat alcoholism with deadly seriousness, and although none of them are characterized by exceptional dialogue and acting, they all emulate the tone established by *The Days of Wine and Roses*. Theatrical films, meanwhile, have taken to portraying alcoholism through the lovable high jinks of Dudley Moore in Steve Gordon's *Arthur* (1981) or the existential metaphors of John Huston's *Under the Volcano* (1984).

As for the Golden Age psychiatrist, he has been a regular feature of made-for-television movies for many years, especially since the success of a Hollywood film that might have been a television movie, *Ordinary People*. Even when American movies were most consistently harsh in their portrayal of psychiatrists, two weekly (though short-lived) television series, *The Psychiatrist* and *Matt Lincoln*, presented heroic images of them in 1970 and 1971. This is not to say that television does not occasionally cast psychiatrists in the same negative roles in which Hollywood movies have placed them, but television psychiatrists are much more likely to solve problems, such as alcoholism, multiple personality, anorexia nervosa, and the sexual abuse of children, that in the 1960s moved off the silver screen and onto the small screen. Many millions of viewers became well acquainted with a psychiatrist of Golden Age qualities during the years that Alan Arbus played Dr. Sidney Freedman on television's *M*A*S*H*. In fact, when one of the largest audiences in television history (some 50 million viewers) watched the final episode of that program in February 1983, they saw the psychiatrist restore a deeply disturbed Hawkeye (Alan Alda) to his usual level of sitcom zaniness.

By 1957, psychiatry had become a fact of life for most Americans, at least as far as the movies were concerned. Consequently, psychiatrists were regularly appropriated for effects that they had only occasionally supplied during the previous fifty years. Psychiatrists were frequently on hand to confirm optimistic myths about how easy it is for troubled people to return to well-being, or they themselves became complex heroes, confronting issues dramatically unlike the stuff of crime plots that earlier psychiatric heroes had faced in *Blind Alley* or *The Dark Mirror*. The Golden Age may represent the culmination of several decades during which real-life psychiatrists had steadily gained acceptance, partially because of their willingness to undertake what John Burnham (1979) has called the "defense of traditional civilization," a role especially accessible to cinematic myths of the late 1950s and early 1960s. The Golden Age also seems to be related to Hollywood's desperate attempt at preserving its familiar paradigm of reconciliation, an undertaking that made great demands on the healing powers of cinematic psychotherapists. Ironically, as reconcilers and defenders of tradition, psychiatrists were left wide open for the sustained attacks that movies launched as soon as the brief Golden Age came to an end and the old formulas were revised to the detriment of psychiatry.

CHAPTER 4

The Fall from Grace

F*reud*, the culminating film of the Golden Age of psychiatry in the American cinema, begins and ends with music and paintings designed to suggest the eerie world of the unconscious. At the close of the film, these sounds and images accompany words spoken off-camera by director John Huston: "'Know thyself.' Two thousand years ago these words were carved on the Temple at Delphi. 'Know thyself.' They're the beginning of wisdom. In them lies the single hope of victory over man's oldest enemy, his family. This knowledge is now within our grasp. Will we use it? Let us hope." The earnestness of this speech with its accompanying aura of the Great Unknown becomes especially ironic in light of Huston's performance twenty years later as Dudley Moore's ridiculous supervising analyst in Marshall Brickman's *Lovesick* (1983). Although this film is a comedy, and although its unlikely romantic hero (Moore) is a psychoanalyst, it is nevertheless one of the strongest attacks yet on Freud and his followers.

The swiftness and the vigor with which American movies turned against psychiatry is as remarkable as the staying power of the negative attitudes toward the profession, which have prevailed with few exceptions since the Golden Age. The success of *Ordinary People* in 1980 suggested that this tradition might be reversed after two decades of almost unrelentingly negative portrayals. However, 1980 was the same year that *Dressed to Kill* made its equally auspicious debut on the American screen. A comparison between *Dressed to Kill* and the film that most inspired it, Alfred Hitchcock's *Psycho* (1960), is a good way to introduce the striking differences between the Golden Age and what followed.

From *Psycho* to *Dressed to Kill*

Written and directed by Brian De Palma, *Dressed to Kill* is about Dr. Robert Elliott, a Manhattan psychiatrist played by Michael Caine. Throughout most of the film, he appears to be a respectable member of society, both likable as a person and thoroughly professional as a psychiatrist. He sternly reprimands an unscrupulous police detective (Dennis Franz) for referring to mental patients as "weirdos," and he steadfastly protects the confidentiality of his patients. Earlier in the film he is compassionate and wise with his patient Kate Miller (Angie Dickinson), a sexually frustrated housewife. When she asks flirtatiously if he would like to sleep with her, the psychiatrist allows himself to be drawn into his personal reasons for refusing her, but he handles the matter gently, and few in the audience would reproach him for dealing a little awkwardly with a patient's transference wishes. At the film's conclusion, however, the psychiatrist is revealed to be a psychotic killer. He has taken a razor to Kate and is prepared to do the same to any other woman who arouses him sexually. The film asks us to believe that the doctor's personality is split into male and female halves: when the male half (Robert Elliott) is attracted to a woman, the female half (Bobbie) becomes threatened and, donning a wig and a dress, destroys the woman who has enticed the male counterpart.

Like many of Brian De Palma's films, *Dressed to Kill* is clearly—and clumsily, some critics would say—modeled after a Hitchcock film. Both *Psycho* and *Dressed to Kill* lead viewers to believe that a beautiful blonde woman (Janet Leigh and Angie Dickinson, respectively) is to be the principal character in the narrative. Hitchcock builds suspense as Marion Crane (Leigh) flees across Arizona highways with stolen money. The director increases audience involvement with Marion by having a suspicious state policeman menacingly follow her through several scenes. But before the film is half over, Marion's perforated body has been dumped in a swamp, and the policeman is never seen again. Similarly, the afternoon dalliance of Kate (Dickinson) with the man she meets at the museum in *Dressed to Kill* promises to be central to the film, especially when she finds a note in her lover's desk announcing that he has venereal disease. Here, too, the assumed heroine is dispatched early, and the syphilitic lover disappears from the film. Of course, the most obvious plot similarity between *Psycho* and *Dressed to Kill* is the eventual revelation that the supposedly female murderer of each blonde woman is a man (Anthony Perkins in *Psycho*, Caine in *Dressed to Kill*), who ordinarily behaves in a fairly normal manner but who occasionally puts on women's clothes and kills people with a sharp instrument.

The plot similarities continue after the death of the woman who appeared to be the central character: in both films a young man who was close to the murdered woman comes onto the scene in search of clues. In *Psycho* John Gavin plays Marion's lover, Sam, and in *Dressed to Kill* Keith Gordon is Peter, Kate's son. The young man is aided in his search by another attractive blonde, who is in many ways the double of the murdered woman and who is nearly killed by the same murderer. In *Psycho*, Vera Miles plays Marion's sister, Lila, who not only resembles the murdered woman but appears on the verge of inheriting her lover. The sisters have the same effect on Norman Bates (Anthony Perkins), and he tries to kill both of them. In *Dressed to Kill* Liz Blake (Nancy Allen) is a whore with a heart of gold who takes the place of Kate, a woman the film goes to some lengths to characterize almost entirely in terms of her sex drive. Both women arouse the sexual passions of the killer, but both of them treat the Keith Gordon character with maternal gestures. By the end of *Dressed to Kill* Allen has taken Dickinson's place in the house, just as at the end of *Psycho* Miles appears to have replaced Leigh.

Another similarity between the two films involves the shower scene in *Psycho*, the cinematic moment when Hitchcock perversely desecrated America's shrine to personal hygiene and transformed it into a place where no one has really felt safe ever since. De Palma suggests this scene in both the beginning and end of *Dressed to Kill*. The actual slashing takes place in an elevator, but De Palma films the scene in a style that clearly recalls Hitchcock's indelible shower slashing. In addition, both films frustrate audience expectations not only with the early deaths of supposed heroines but also with early plot devices that go nowhere. For example, the $40,000 that Marion steals in the beginning of *Psycho* appears to be the Hitchcockian "MacGuffin" (Truffaut 1984, 138), which will keep the plot going until the end but actually plays only a small role after she is murdered. Similarly, in *Dressed to Kill* Kate forgets her wedding ring in the apartment of her spur-of-the-moment lover. Since she is killed before she can retrieve it, we assume that sooner or later the ring will turn up as a clue. It never does.

The comparison between *Psycho* and *Dressed to Kill* becomes most compelling, however, when we turn to the images of psychiatry that each film presents. At the close of *Psycho*, Simon Oakland plays Dr. Richmond, a psychiatrist who thoroughly clears up any confusion that any member of the cast or audience may have had about Norman Bates's behavior. The part is both written and played for maximum effect: here is a man who speaks as an oracle of knowledge and who wears his authority without reluctance. Just before his appearance, a detective can be heard saying, "If anyone can explain this, it'll be the psychiatrist." When the psychiatrist begins to explain Norman Bates's split personality, the district attorney says, "Well, now look, if you're trying to lay some psychiatric groundwork for some sort of plea that this man intends to cop . . . ." The psychiatrist interrupts him and speaks with a kind of jocular humility, "A psychiatrist doesn't lay the groundwork; he merely tries to explain it." Obviously, Dr. Richmond can do much more than that, and before he has finished, he has solved five murders besides that of the Janet Leigh character. When the sheriff asks about the location of the MacGuffin $40,000, the psychiatrist delivers his line as if an afterthought: "The swamp. These were crimes of passion, not profit." Ordinary police work is a trivial business with which a psychiatrist has little patience. The scene ends with a policeman asking his superintendent if Norman should be allowed a blanket to keep him warm. Rather than immediately answering the policeman, the superintendent defers to the psychiatrist, who nonchalantly nods his approval while lighting a cigarette. Although Hitchcock may have purposefully undermined the psychiatrist's formulation in the film's subtext (see chapters 3 and 7), his Dr. Richmond is consistent with other cinematic portrayals during the Golden Age.

Of course, the dominant image of the psychiatrist that appears in *Dressed to Kill* is the psychotic Dr. Elliott (Caine). But as in *Psycho*, a psychiatrist also appears in the police station at the end of *Dressed to Kill* to explain the mind of the murderer. Here, however, the resemblance ends. In *Psycho*, Hitchcock had Simon Oakland standing before a seated group of spectators who look up at him and hang on his every word. In *Dressed to Kill*, the psychiatrist, Dr. Levy (David Margulies), is seated during his speech; his gestures are slightly effete, and he speaks without conviction. Furthermore, his explanation of Elliott's behavior is only subsidiary to the solution of the crime. The street-wise police detective (Dennis Franz) is the scene's focal figure, paying only minimal attention to Levy and leering at the prostitute (Nancy Allen) during the psychiatrist's gratuitously graphic explanation: "Elliott's penis became erect and Bobbie took control, trying to kill anyone that made Elliott masculinely sexual." Both *Psycho* and *Dressed to Kill* present unlikely interpretations of unlikely characters in their psychiatrically informed conclusions, but the more recent *Dressed to Kill* offers the uniquely absurd proposition that the female component of a psychotic multiple personality was being favorably considered for transsexual surgery while the male side of the character was able to function competently as a psychiatrist.

In fairness to De Palma, we must point out that he knows how to make the most of familiar film genres, both as a reverent student and as an irreverent satirist. He has learned from his idol Hitchcock—with whom he has carried on a kind of dialogue in *Hi, Mom! Sisters, Obsession, Blow Out, Body Double*, and *Raising Cain* as well as *Dressed to Kill*—that mock seriousness is often the most effective means of telling a far-fetched tale. De Palma's often perverse sense of humor can best be appreciated by the more devoted film buffs who can recognize how he toys with famous and not-so-famous conventions. This explains on the one hand why his films have seldom found a large audience and on the other why his *Phantom of the Paradise* and *Carrie* have cult followings.

De Palma's handling of psychiatrists, however, is entirely consistent with that of mainstream American films, and *Dressed to Kill* may even be remembered as a culminating film after two decades of reaction against psychiatrists. The oracular character played by Simon Oakland in Hitchcock's 1960 *Psycho* fits as perfectly into the Golden Age as Michael Caine's Robert Elliott into the years of negative characterizations of psychiatrists. Completely different images emerge from two clearly similar films. Hitchcock may have subverted the psychiatrist's formulations on a subtextual level, and De Palma probably did not care how seriously his audience took the psychiatric elements in *Dressed to Kill*. But the images of psychiatry in the works of the two directors powerfully link these two films to specific moments in cinema history.

Another comparison between a Golden Age film and one from the more recent period demonstrates how the trend against psychiatry can transform the work of a single writer-director team. Frank and Eleanor Perry created the supremely sympathetic and competent Dr. Swinford (Howard da Silva) in *David and Lisa* (1962), one of the most prominent films of the Golden Age. A mere eight years later, however, they made *Diary of a Mad Housewife* (1970), in which a psychiatrist is one of several extremely unpleasant male figures inflicted upon the long-suffering heroine. Based on a novel by Sue Kaufman, *Diary of a Mad Housewife* chronicles several days in the life of Tina Balser (Carrie Snodgress), a Manhattan housewife whose egotistical, domineering husband (Richard Benjamin) has as little to offer as her violent, mean-spirited lover (Frank Langella). In addition, her children emulate all the worst aspects of their father, and she finds absolutely no compassionate souls in the domain to which she has been confined. Nevertheless, her psychiatrist, whose dour visage usually appears upside down in the frame (as she might see him from the couch but also as the film asks us to understand his upside-down values), regularly tells her that she ought to be able to fulfill herself as a wife and mother. (Tina's psychiatrist appears in the version of the film shown on television, not in the theatrical print. The psychiatrist scenes and other footage were cut from the film just before its release and then added to the television version to fill time left by the excision of several minutes of nudity and sex.) Her psychiatrist even discourages her from expressing her creative impulses through painting, urging her instead to engage in more conventionally healthful activities such as jogging and scrubbing floors. After her lover throws her bodily out of his apartment, Tina returns to her husband only to discover that he is about to lose his job, that he has squandered all their savings on a failed investment in a French vineyard, and that he is having an affair. At the film's memorable conclusion, Tina presents her story to a collection of misfits at a group therapy session and endures a chorus of loudly unsympathetic responses as the final credits roll.

After breaking ground with a "personal" film like *David and Lisa*, the Perrys may have realized that the age of earnest realism and reconciliation was over and that a more satiric, socially critical vision was appropriate for the late 1960s. It is difficult to determine if the Perrys had a change of heart about psychiatry between the time of *David and Lisa* (1962) and *Diary of a Mad Housewife* (1970) or if they merely accommodated the new wave in serious commercial filmmaking with the required character types. According to Roy Huss (1986, 111), Eleanor Perry earned a degree in psychiatric social work before becoming a writer. Regardless of motives, however, comparison of the two films suggests that the motion picture industry's reaction against psychiatry was so overwhelming that even filmmakers who once created the most sympathetic of all movie psychiatrists were caught up in it.

The psychiatrist in *Diary of a Mad Housewife* is a feminist cartoon with roots in the "you need a man to dominate you" psychiatrist of *Lady in the Dark*, but films of more recent vintage do not always present the psychiatrist-as-society's-agent only in terms of the oppression of women. In 1971, just one year after the release of *Diary of a Mad Housewife*, Lawrence Turman's *The Marriage of a Young Stockbroker* appeared, providing an interesting comparison with the Perrys' film and illustrating the extent to which psychiatry was under simultaneous assault from both sexual camps. Both films revolve around troubled marriages; both adopt myths of the 1960s about the corrupt values of the affluent professional class; in both the husband is played by Richard Benjamin; and both films suggest that a psychiatrist intervenes to change the behavior of the character who is least in need of help. Yet, whereas in the feminist *Diary of a Mad Housewife* the female spouse (Snodgress) is asked by a male psychiatrist to sacrifice her individuality, in *The Marriage of a Young Stockbroker* the husband (Benjamin) is asked by a female psychiatrist (Patricia Barry) to do the same thing. In the earlier film, Benjamin plays Tina's husband as a domineering monster who blithely makes wildly unreasonable demands of her. In *The Marriage of a Young Stockbroker*, Benjamin plays Bill, a perfectly likable young professional who takes pleasure in looking at nude or seminude women either in pornographic movies or on beaches. Falling back on the truisms of the sexual revolution, *The Marriage of a Young Stockbroker* presents these activities as the natural and completely understandable result of Bill's boring job and his difficulty in communicating with his pretty wife, Lisa (Joanna Shimkus). The villain of the piece is the wife's sister, Nan (Elizabeth Ashley), who encourages Lisa to leave Bill because of his voyeurism but who is willing and even eager for him to gaze at her own body.

The antifeminist ideology of *The Marriage of a Young Stockbroker* argues that women are prepared to give up normal sexuality for the sake of controlling men, and Nan's husband, Chester (Adam West), is a thoroughly controlled male. We learn that Chester has been brainwashed by the psychiatrist, Dr. Sadler (Barry), a friend of Nan (Ashley), whose psychobabble includes words like "insight" and "productive" but who clearly seeks to turn healthy, normal men into docile breadwinners for their domineering wives. Dr. Sadler sets to work on Bill as well, but he is immediately able to see through her manipulative and acquisitive motives; after learning that she charges $50 per half hour for her time, he pays her in cash and sends her away after ten minutes. The film ends when Bill quits his stifling job as a stockbroker and seduces Lisa in the women's locker room of a country club. As they are about to drive away in renewed connubial bliss, Nan tries to stop them by demanding that Chester "do something." Chester, however, has had enough, and he pushes his wife to the ground. Now both men have overcome the efforts of the emasculating female therapist.

Another pair of filmmakers whose portrayal of psychiatry and its practitioners appears to have changed with the times is the producer/director team of Alan J. Pakula and Robert Mulligan. In 1957 they made one of the first Golden Age films, *Fear Strikes Out*. In 1966, however, they made *Inside Daisy Clover*, the story of a 1930s' child star (Natalie Wood) reminiscent of Judy Garland who is crassly manipulated by a studio mogul (Christopher Plummer). When Daisy breaks down from the strain of being a star, a pipe-smoking psychiatrist is brought in to achieve one of two goals that Plummer offers him: either she is certifiable and the studio can collect insurance money, or she is sane and the doctor must give her a quick fix so that she can get back to work. The psychiatrist weakly demurs, but he is definitely prepared to do whatever work the money men request.

The calmly reassuring image of ECT that appears in Pakula and Mulligan's *Fear Strikes Out* provides the basis for still another contrast between Golden Age films and those that followed. As soon as the Golden Age began to wane, mental institutions were made out to be something akin to torture chambers in both Samuel Fuller's *Shock Corridor* (1963) and Denis Sanders's *Shock*

Treatment (1964). The notion that ECT is used as punishment subsequently occurs most memorably in Milos Forman's *One Flew Over the Cuckoo's Nest* (1975), but also in Michael Winner's *Death Wish II* (1982). In this grim glorification of vigilante justice, Charles Bronson masquerades as a psychologist in order to kill the man who raped and murdered his daughter. Although the film portrays the villain as simply vicious rather than "insane," he escapes prosecution because a judge consigns him to a mental hospital. When Bronson gains entry to the killer's quarters, an orderly tells him that he will meet with the patient in a room full of unused electronic equipment. The orderly says that "you guys," meaning the new breed of talking therapists to which he assumes Bronson belongs, no longer use shock treatment. "Now it's all done with kindness," he says. Appropriately, Bronson dispatches the killer by jolting him with electricity after the villain's fist misses Bronson's jaw and catches in the inner workings of the ECT apparatus.

Psychiatry in the Sixties: Politics and the Hero

The drastic changes in the representation of psychiatry after the Golden Age are undoubtedly related to the cultural revolutions of the 1960s. The swiftness of the changes may not, however, reflect correspondingly dramatic changes in American attitudes toward mental health professionals. Winick (1963) has reported data from a number of studies conducted around 1960, in the middle of psychiatry's Golden Age. One study found that only 1% of the subjects polled expressed active support for the psychiatric profession, but only 7% expressed active opposition. Another study found that although psychiatrists themselves were regarded favorably, their techniques were held in extremely low esteem.

This "softness" in American attitudes apparently provided a wide range of tolerance for the wildly inconsistent images that characterized movie psychiatrists in the early 1960s as opposed to the later part of that decade. Popular films of the 1960s continued to activate myths of freedom and the primacy of the self, somewhat revised from the patterns of classic Hollywood films but still grounded in fundamental American mythology. Just as American movies had always exploited psychiatry, American psychiatry had in some ways exploited these movie myths, largely by presenting itself as a means of removing obstacles to happiness. The French psychiatrist Henri Ellenberger (1955) visited the United States in 1952 and subsequently wrote, "In Europe, people go to the psychiatrist because of a symptom, in America because of a problem." John Burnham (1978) has demonstrated how psychiatry in the United States allowed itself to become associated with an individual's pursuit of happiness through its claims of problem-solving, especially after the therapeutic successes with veterans of World War II. Consequently, psychiatry was especially vulnerable in the sixties when disillusionment accompanied the profound questioning of postwar ideas of happiness. Although few Americans appear to have had strong feelings about psychiatrists during this period, the movies pounced upon the profession's new vulnerability.

Burnham also has stressed the ease with which the profession's focus on solving "personal problems" was appropriated by the "managers of the increasingly bureaucratic American society" as "a tactic to head off, indeed, deny, the existence of social discontent" (1978, 65). Even the teachings of Erik Erikson, one of the great post-Freudians and hardly a political or social conservative, were nevertheless "easily corrupted into the conservative assumption that any changes that needed to be made were on a one-by-one, individual basis—as in psychoanalytic psychotherapy—and in that individual, not in the culture" (1978, 65). In the climate of 1960s' social protest, psychiatry could easily be tied to the supposed conformity and repressiveness of the 1950s, and psychiatrists were regularly portrayed as part of the establishment forces perpetuating the false values of old America. An excellent example of how films used psychiatry for this purpose is Jack O'Connell's *Revolution* (1968), a crude documentary that extolled the virtues of the hippies and invited their sympathizers in the audience to ridicule pious and often hyperbolic warnings by doctors, police, and psychiatrists about the physical and mental dangers of hippie culture. In a more familiar genre film, John Guillerman's *House of Cards* (1969), Inger Stevens refers to her psychiatrist as "the man who polices my psyche."

The social problem film, which had afforded psychiatry the most amenable surroundings in the early 1960s, was as good as dead by 1965. Many of the most successful films of the 1960s adopted a more overtly irreverent and satiric vision of America and its values, especially in comparison to the dominant genres of film comedy in the late fifties. Compare, for example, *Pillow Talk* (1959) with *The Graduate* (1967). Compare also Stanley Kubrick's breakthrough masterpiece, *Dr. Strangelove, or How I Learned to Stop Worrying and Love the Bomb* (1964), and its Swiftian view of world leaders and the military, with Sidney Lumet's mirthless and didactic *Fail-Safe*, which addressed the same questions of nuclear defense in the same year as *Dr. Strangelove*. *Fail-Safe* must now be regarded as one of the final films of the 1950s while *Dr. Strangelove* is one of the first in a long series of 1960s' films that took a satirical and apocalyptic view of the world and its institutions (Cagin and Dray 1984). The gravity and solemnity with which Holly-wood had handled psychiatrists in the Golden Age made them easy targets for the youth-oriented filmmakers of the sixties, who often strove to shake up bourgeois audiences as much as to confront what the filmmakers consid-ered to be the tired old conventions of earlier movies.

As we begin a year-by-year survey of Hollywood's reaction against psychi-atry just after the Golden Age, we should point out that, as in every decade, psychiatrists were still introduced for the sake of plot mechanics but that af-ter 1964 they were knocked off their pedestals even when their functions were most trivial. A classic example of the psychiatrist–as–plot machine from 1964 is J. Lee Thompson's *What a Way to Go!* In this vehicle for Shir-ley MacLaine, a psychiatrist (Robert Cummings), whose office includes a hy-draulic couch controlled by a button on his desk, listens to the story of the heroine's several marriages so that the film can cut to flashbacks. Each of MacLaine's husbands was hugely successful at earning money but quite un-successful at remaining alive. When MacLaine tells Cummings early in the film that she wants to give her $200 million inheritance to the IRS in the form of a check, he naturally assumes that it is all part of her fantasy and set-tles back to hear her story. The film ends with the psychiatrist's secretary en-tering to announce that MacLaine's check is genuine. Cummings then falls to the floor in a faint. A Golden Age psychiatrist might have done a quick dou-ble take at this information, but even if he functioned as a mere plot expe-diter, he would not have lost consciousness. *What a Way to Go!* has little of the emerging sixties' ambience, but its irreverence toward psychiatry is por-tentous.

The year 1964 also saw the release of *Shock Treatment*, in which Lauren Bacall plays another evil female psychiatrist. She runs an institution as a front for illegal financial gain, but at the end she herself becomes psychotic. The same year marked the appearance of a low-budget exploitation film, William Castle's *Strait Jacket*. This film suggests that Joan Crawford has been cured after twenty years of confinement in an institution. Yet when her ineffectual psychiatrist comes out to check up on her, he is decapitated by an ax mur-derer. *Sex and the Single Girl* presents a lecherous male psychiatrist (Mel Ferrer) as well as an easily manipulated female therapist (Natalie Wood), and in *Lilith*, Warren Beatty plays a therapist trainee who falls in love with, and is eventually driven mad by, a seriously disturbed patient (Jean Seberg).

By 1965, the reaction is complete. Psychiatrists are thoroughly devalued in at least four films from that one year: Peter Sellers plays a libidinous Vien-nese quack named Dr. Fritz Fassbender in *What's New, Pussycat?* (plate 20); "Mrs. Koogleman" (Hermione Gingold) in *Harvey Middleman, Fireman* is a female shrink too involved with her own extramarital affairs to be of any help to the eponymous hero; an amnesiac Gregory Peck, this time with no Ingrid Bergman to save him, has to make do with a pompous and thoroughly unhelpful psychiatrist (Robert H. Harris) in *Mirage*; and the familiar female psychiatrist who is "cured" by a male patient reappears as Leslie Caron in *A Very Special Favor*.

Negative stereotypes of psychiatrists adorned even more American screens in 1966. That year introduced the "Dr. Bluebeard" (Rock Hudson) of *Blindfold*; the beautiful but unnecessary psychiatrist played by Janet Leigh in *Three on a Couch*; an easily seduced prison psychologist in *Dead Heat on a Merry-Go-Round*; Natalie Wood's mentally unbalanced analyst (Dick Shawn) in *Penelope*; a female therapist (Sarah Marshall) who is driven to hysterics by Roddy McDowall's refusal to find her Rorschach blots "dirty" in *Lord Love a Duck*; a dispassionate analyst (Arthur Hill) who so neglects his

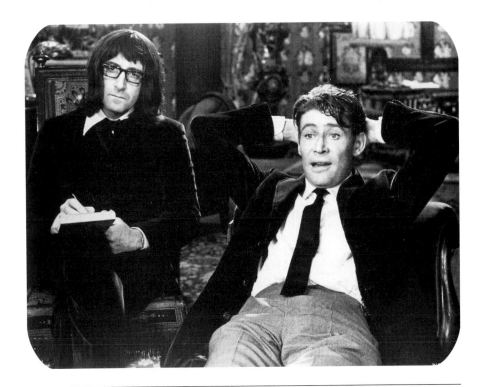

PLATE 20. Peter O'Toole details his sex life for Dr. Fritz Fassbender (Peter Sellers) in *What's New, Pussycat?* (1965). United Artists/Famous Artists. The Museum of Modern Art/Film Stills Archive.

wife (Jean Seberg) that she becomes involved in a sordid love affair in *Moment to Moment;* the willing agent of a corrupt studio boss in *Inside Daisy Clover;* and even the LSD-dispensing director of a sanitarium in a bizarre film called *Movie Star, American Style or LSD, I Hate You.* In Sidney Lumet's *The Group,* a rare distinction is made between medical psychiatry and psychoanalysis, reserving special scorn for analysis. *The Group* suggests that the inadequacies of Shirley Knight's married lover (Hal Holbrook) are a function of his dependence on his analyst. Although the film presents Knight as the solution to Holbrook's problems, he eventually drifts away, offering specious reasons supplied by his psychoanalyst. Knight finds happiness, however, when she falls in love with a hospital psychiatrist (James Broderick), outspokenly anti-Freud and anti-couch, who expresses the desire to give up his practice and devote all his efforts to "research."

The year 1966 was also the release date for Irvin Kershner's *A Fine Madness,* one of the first films that clearly cast the institution of psychiatry against the prototypical hero for the 1960s and 1970s: an eccentric but vital loner, often doomed, who rejects the obsolete values of the Establishment, even when he has not thought about them very much. Robert Ray argues that films of the 1960s and 1970s appealed to a politically bifurcated audience, generating "left and right cycles" (1985, 296–325): the mythology of classical Hollywood never died, but the 1960s marked the end of a thematic paradigm that never forced the audience to choose between an outlaw hero and an official hero. The strength of this paradigm was waning in the 1950s; the ending of *The Caine Mutiny* is incoherent because the classical formula had been strained to justify the actions of a neurotic official hero. Ray cites Howard Hawks's *Red River* (1948) as an example of a parallel phenomenon; the film's ending struggles unsuccessfully to provide the reconciliation between the official hero (Montgomery Clift) and an obviously disturbed outlaw hero (John Wayne). In the 1960s and 1970s, the official hero became the exclusive property of films of the right cycle *(Dirty Harry, Walking Tall, Death Wish),* while the outlaw hero was isolated in the left cycle *(Easy Rider, Cool Hand Luke, Little Big Man).* The choice of which hero the audience should favor was made even before the film began. In effect, Humphrey Bogart's Rick no longer played against Paul Henreid's Victor Laszlo. Although many of these films seemed radical at the time, they were still firmly rooted in American myths. Ray points out that Bobby Dupea (Jack Nicholson), the outlaw antihero of *Five Easy Pieces* (1970), is based on American heroes such as Huck Finn and Holden Caulfield. Surrounded by phonies, he impulsively decides to "light out for the Territory" at the end (1985, 297). Furthermore, Nicholson's character recalls the "roughneck classical musician" heroes of *Golden Boy* (1939) and *Humoresque* (1946).

Since the films of the right and left had abandoned the reconciliatory pattern, they no longer needed psychiatric healers. Rather, they created straw men to reinforce the validity of the hero's cause. In a right-cycle film such as *Death Wish II*, psychiatry represents a feeble, unmanly attempt to solve problems that are more effectively addressed by vigilante violence. In one scene, the ineffectual psychologist who gives directions to Bronson cannot immediately distinguish between his left and his right. The filmmakers had no such difficulty. In left films such as *One Flew Over the Cuckoo's Nest*, the power of psychiatry was more ominous than in films made for right-wing audiences. In general, the heroes of the right cycle always seemed to survive the climactic violence at the end of the film, while in left films the heroes were no match for the destructive power of the Establishment and were usually destroyed in an apocalyptic ending. This was the case in *Cool Hand Luke, Easy Rider, Bonnie and Clyde*, and even the glibly fatalistic *Butch Cassidy and the Sundance Kid*. The sixties' image of the doomed antihero was tied to perceptions of the assassination of President Kennedy and the Vietnam war, but the character type had earlier appeared in one film that deeply influenced American filmmakers of the 1960s, Jean-Luc Godard's *Breathless* (1961).

A Fine Madness, a relatively obscure film of the left cycle, finds its outlaw hero in Samson Shillitoe (Sean Connery), a brawling, womanizing New York poet who is eventually institutionalized and put at the mercy of a team of psychiatrists. The most stereotypical of the group is Dr. Menken (Clive Revill), who speaks in a thick accent about his plan to appropriate Connery for his behavioristic and dehumanizing experiments in lobotomy. A female psychiatrist, Vera Kropotkin (Colleen Dewhurst), opposes Revill's plans because, predictably, she has succumbed to the hero's sexual appeal. Although the third participant, the strict Freudian Dr. Vorbeck (Werner Peters), is broadly caricatured, he opposes Dr. Menken's lobotomy proposal on largely humanitarian grounds. The final decision must be made by the fourth psychiatrist, the no-nonsense director of the clinic, Dr. West (Patrick O'Neal), who sees through Menken's crackpot schemes. Yet when he learns that Shillitoe (Connery) has been carrying on an affair with his wife (Jean Seberg), Dr. West grimly votes to allow the lobotomy to take place. The operation turns out to be a failure, at least for the psychiatrists, and Shillitoe emerges from the experience as feisty as ever. Future victims of psychiatric intervention in left-cycle films would prove less resilient.

A Fine Madness has much in common with *One Flew Over the Cuckoo's Nest* (1975). Both are adapted from novels written in the first half of the 1960s. Elliot Baker published *A Fine Madness* in 1964, and Ken Kesey's *One*

Flew Over the Cuckoo's Nest appeared in 1962. As Jeffrey Berman (1985) has demonstrated in his thorough and psychoanalytically sophisticated study of psychiatry's image in literature, these novels were part of a literary attack upon psychoanalysis that goes back at least to 1892 with Charlotte Perkins Gilman's "The Yellow Wallpaper." Like Gilman's work, Virginia Woolf's *Mrs. Dalloway* (1925) also presents an unsympathetic psychiatrist, but negative portrayals of psychiatry became most common in the 1950s with the appearance of T. S. Eliot's *The Cocktail Party* (1950), Joseph Heller's *Catch-22* (1955), Saul Bellow's *Seize the Day* (1956), Vladimir Nabokov's *Pnin* (1957), John Barth's *End of the Road* (1958), and Iris Murdoch's *A Severed Head* (1961). All of these books present the same arguments informing the attacks on psychiatry in films after 1964: doctors of the mind are repressive, often self-deceiving egomaniacs. These novels predate the antipsychiatry movement of the 1960s, and, most interestingly, they coexisted with many of the most sympathetic treatments of psychiatrists in the movies. Their messages, however, were readily available when American films sought a new vision of psychiatry in the 1960s.

Like their literary sources, *A Fine Madness* and *One Flew Over the Cuckoo's Nest* share the more specific view of psychiatry as an emasculating activity that promotes social harmony at any cost, and both novels suggest that psychiatrists are quite willing to act out their own hang-ups to the detriment of their unsuspecting patients. *A Fine Madness* delivered this message with none of the sentimental panache of *One Flew Over the Cuckoo's Nest* and was consequently much less of a critical and commercial success. Nevertheless, *A Fine Madness* paved the way for numerous films, including *Cuckoo's Nest*, that presented psychiatry as the nemesis of those sensitive and usually victimized loners who so often emerge as the protagonists of left-cycle films. We have mentioned *Diary of a Mad Housewife* and *The Marriage of a Young Stockbroker* as films that present psychiatrists as the natural agents of a society that seeks to dehumanize its most sensitive citizens whenever they attempt to break out of the stifling lives that have been inflicted upon them. The mental health professions fill this victimizing role even in Larry Peerce's *The Bell Jar* (1979), in which the female psychiatrist played by Anne Jackson is usually caring and compassionate. But this screen adaptation of Sylvia Plath's autobiographical novel presents the soothing words of the psychiatrist as a poor anodyne for the malevolent and overpowering forces in society that drive the feminist heroine (Marilyn Hassett) to psychosis. The film makes the protagonist into still another lone antihero as it catalogs all the characters—mother, employer, fiancé, lover, friends—who would force her to become anything but her own woman. The psychiatrist must be devalued because she would prepare the heroine to accept a world that the film baldly characterizes as crazier than anyone in an institution. This conceit was taken to its most absurd extreme by "underground" director Robert Downey in his 1967 film *Chafed Elbows*. Downey's hero ignores the stern advice of his psychiatrist and fulfills his desire to marry his mother, an event that the film portrays as a joyous and fortuitous occasion for all. *Titicut Follies* and *Marat/Sade* were also released in 1967, as was Theodore J. Flicker's *The President's Analyst*, which actually turns a psychiatrist into the lone antihero.

As the credits for *The President's Analyst* roll, we see Dr. Sidney Schaefer (James Coburn) on the couch, talking presumably to his training analyst (Will Geer, made up to look like Mark Twain). We then see Dr. Schaefer in the analyst's chair while a number of different patients appear on the couch, including an attractive woman with whom he exchanges meaningful glances. Meanwhile, Don Masters (Godfrey Cambridge), wearing a curly wig and a "Dizzy Gillespie for President" sweatshirt, very professionally assassinates a suspicious man who has just accepted information from another suspicious man. The film then cuts to Dr. Schaefer sitting on the floor of his office practicing on a large Oriental gong. When his next patient enters, it is Masters (Cambridge), now dressed in a business suit. Within a few minutes, Masters has confessed to being a secret agent for a CIA-like organization as well as a killer. Assuming that the spy is there for help, Schaefer begins philosophizing about hostility, morality, society, and a paper he might write on the subject. But Masters interrupts him with the information that he has been attending the analytic sessions only because his agency is running a security check on him. Now that the check is complete, Masters invites him to proceed to a more private place since Schaefer's office might be bugged. When the doctor responds indignantly, "The sanctity of a psychiatrist's office is like a confessional," Masters replies, "Oh, really. I put this one here myself," and he picks a bugging device off the diploma on the psychiatrist's wall.

Schaefer is eventually told that he has been selected to be the analyst for the president of the United States, because, as we are told in this pre-Watergate film, the chief executive is not neurotic, just overworked and overtired. He needs to talk with someone who "does not want something from him." Honored, Schaefer takes the job and is at first fascinated with his proximity to so august a presence. Yet Schaefer soon discovers that he has become a major security risk, that he is not allowed any private life, and that he is constantly being followed by men in dark glasses. Unable to bear the strain, the hero "drops out," even joining a group of hippies for a brief journey through American subculture. The film's irreverent sixties' satire substantially increases at this point, soon careening into an exploration of political paranoia in which agents for numerous countries attempt to kidnap the psychiatrist. The film concludes with an escapist happy ending for the principals but also with the revelation that the *telephone company*, and not the various intelligence agencies of American and foreign governments, is the most powerful force in the world.

The President's Analyst has more in common with the lightweight psychedelic satire of television's *Laugh-In* than it does with *The Graduate* (the two films and the television comedy show all appeared in 1967), but it does offer an interesting synthesis of psychiatric myths since the 1930s. Like Ralph Bellamy in *Blind Alley* (1939)—our touchstone for the American cinema's idealized image of the "avant-garde" psychiatrist—Dr. Schaefer appreciates exotic cultures from the East, even having joined a presumably ancient cult of the gong sometime before he took up with hippies. The film also addresses myths of oracularity by having the psychiatrist early on engage in self-aggrandizing illusions of omniscience only to discover later that he is being controlled by a government agent. Analysands commonly fantasize that they control and manipulate their therapists rather than the other way around: Katharine Hepburn realizes this fantasy in 1938 when she outsmarts Fritz Feld in *Bringing Up Baby*. The situation becomes much more common in the 1960s, specifically in *The President's Analyst* as well as in another James Coburn vehicle, *Dead Heat on a Merry-Go-Round* (1966), in which the hero makes love to a prison psychologist (Marian Moses) only in order to win a quick parole. *The President's Analyst* is perhaps the only film in which the image of the psychiatrist as vulnerable to manipulation coexists with an attempt to cast the same psychiatrist as a lone antihero.

Of course, not all films with psychiatrists from the 1960s were characterized by irreverence and satire. Richard Fleischer's *The Boston Strangler* (1968), for instance, took the allegedly true story of Albert De Salvo seriously, even though the film indulged in some graphic violence that was very much of the later sixties. The film probably belongs more to the right cycle, but *The Boston Strangler* can be considered radical for being the first commercial film to use the potential of wide-screen projection (Panavision) for split-screen editing, offering the audience multiple views of an action on the same wide canvas. Dr. Nagy (Austin Willis), the faceless psychiatrist in this docudrama, functions somewhat like Simon Oakland in *Psycho*, a film that director Fleischer surely had in mind when he made *The Boston Strangler*. Dr. Nagy often steps forth to explain the multiple personality of Albert De Salvo (Tony Curtis), a real-life character who was charged with but never tried for the strangulation deaths of eight women in Boston during the early

1960s. As in *Psycho*, the killer has a "normal" self that has no knowledge of the murderous self. De Salvo's normal personality even lives a quiet life with his wife and children. The film reveals its right-cycle orientation when Dr. Nagy becomes involved in a professional argument with police officer Bottomley (Henry Fonda), who has been put in charge of a special task force to apprehend the strangler. The psychiatrist is convinced that De Salvo will lapse into permanent catatonia if his normal side is ever forced to confront his murderous side. Bottomley (Fonda) realizes that he will have to bring about such a confrontation if he is to get a confession, but that any confession will be useless if the strangler becomes legally insane. Eventually, the policeman decides that "cracking" De Salvo may be just as effective as a conviction. Over the objections of Dr. Nagy, Bottomley proceeds with an interrogation of the strangler that brings him to the brink of integrating the two sides of his personality. The psychiatrist tries to put De Salvo under sedation when he sees that the prisoner is about to break down. Bottomley, however, stops him.

> PSYCHIATRIST: You're looking at a sick animal.
> POLICEMAN: So were the women he strangled. I want him
> now!

In the last moments of the film, De Salvo is clearly on the verge of a complete breakdown. The final credits tell us that De Salvo has never been tried and that he is still institutionalized. We then read the following: "This film has ended, but the responsibility of society for the early recognition and treatment of the violent among us has yet to begin." The earnestness is reminiscent of the Golden Age, but the sentiment is slightly different. What is to be the "treatment" for violent people such as De Salvo if the prognosis is permanent catatonia? Unlike *Psycho*, in which psychiatry was superior to police work, *The Boston Strangler* clearly endorses the policeman's point of view over the psychiatrist's. Not only does Bottomley win the arguments with the psychiatrist, but Austin Willis (Dr. Nagy) cannot compete with Henry Fonda's star presence. As is frequently the case in Hollywood films, the casting director is as responsible as anyone for the ideology of the film.

The Artist/Analysand Comes of Age: Woody Allen and Paul Mazursky

Our year-by-year survey could be continued through the last three decades of the century with little change in the negative images of psychiatry. Nevertheless, we will abandon our chronological approach at this point and consider two directors, Woody Allen and Paul Mazursky, who deserve special attention as we move from the 1960s to the 1970s. In his own films, Woody Allen has consistently played the disenchanted analysand, a phenomenon increasingly common during this period as more and more people sought respite from the complexities of their lives on the analyst's couch. For Allen, as well as for many of his college-educated and affluent admirers, psychoanalysis is viewed as something other than a promise of bringing happiness through the elimination of "personal problems," even though the narcissistic indulgence it provides makes it hopelessly addicting. More specifically, for Manhattanites like Allen, analysis is another troublesome fact of urban life, comparable to brown tap water or pseudointellectuals who pontificate in movie waiting lines.

In *Annie Hall* (1977), Alvy Singer (Allen) delivers several one-liners about psychiatry that have been widely quoted. In the context of the critical and commercial success of *Annie Hall*, they represent the culmination of a tradition of psychoanalytic humor that goes back at least to the couch-and-notepad cartoons that first appeared in popular magazines in the 1940s (Plank 1956). Alvy/Allen says that he has been in analysis for fifteen years, but that if he has not made progress after one more year, he will go to Lourdes. Later, when Annie's family inquires about his prolonged analysis, he says, "I'm making excellent progress. Pretty soon, when I lie down on his couch, I won't have to wear the lobster bib." Alvy also delivers the following speech during a stand-up monologue before a college audience: "I was suicidal, as a matter of fact, and would have killed myself, but I was in analysis with a strict Freudian, and if you kill yourself, they make you pay for the sessions you miss."

Yet Woody Allen has brought an irony to his characterization of psychiatry that sets his films apart from the vast majority of American movies with their stereotypical psychiatrists perfunctorily fitted to generic formulas. For example, in *Stardust Memories* (1980), the filmmaker hero played by Allen is showing clips at a retrospective of his films. In a fantasy sketch from one film, "Sidney Finkelstein's hostility" is portrayed as a tall hirsute monster in the process of destroying everyone against whom Sidney bears a grudge. One of the characters who attempts to stop the beast is a man in a dark raincoat (Victor Truro) who approaches the monster and, holding up a pipe, calls out sheepishly, "Please, uh, we don't want to hurt you. We . . . we want to reason with you. I'm a psychoanalyst. This is my pipe." Allen is of course poking fun at analysis, but he is also ridiculing the B-movie idea that scientists are rationalist fools who approach violent beasts with talk instead of force. Moreover,

Allen is sending up the stale Hollywood convention of the pipe as icon of the psychiatrist's pensive intellectualism, a cliché that goes back at least as far as *Blind Alley* (1939).

In *Annie Hall*, Allen uses split-screen technique to show Annie (Diane Keaton) and Alvy (Allen) simultaneously discussing their troubled sex life with their respective psychiatrists. Each analyst asks how often Annie and Alvy have sex. Alvy says, "Hardly ever, maybe three times a week." Annie says, "Constantly, I'd say three times a week." Here Woody Allen is using psychiatry as the traditional plot device for establishing character, but the joke can be understood in several other contexts, including Alvy's Pygmalion-like attempts to transform Annie, even by paying for her analysis. Naturally, she will feel guilty if she leaves him, but any progress in her analysis would almost necessarily make her less dependent upon him and thus more likely to leave him. Psychoanalysis then becomes one of several forces making their relationship impossible, a reality that Alvy acknowledges in the joke that closes the film. A man tells a psychiatrist that his brother thinks that he is a chicken, but when asked why he does not have his brother committed, the man says, "I would, but I need the eggs." Alvy uses the joke as a focus for his feelings about relationships: they are painful and perhaps not worth the trouble, but he needs the eggs. Much the same can be said for his feelings about his analyst. Like the split-screen presentation of parallel analytic sessions, this juxtaposition of borscht belt humor with the troubling complexities of romantic love is one of several "modernist" devices Allen uses in *Annie Hall*, both to comment on earlier romantic comedies and to separate his film from this tradition (Schatz 1982). Although the psychiatrists in Allen's films often appear ineffectual or pompous, his purpose is not simply to condemn them or to exploit them for conventional generic purposes. If anything, Allen is more interested in poking fun at their *patients*. Allen also uses psychiatry, along with a wide range of cinematic techniques, to explore the ambivalences in human relationships.

Since his 1977 breakthrough with *Annie Hall*, Allen has continued to find new ways of integrating his eccentric humor, as well as his fascination with diverse traditions of filmmaking, with affecting observations about complex relationships. In *Hannah and Her Sisters* (1986) he created one of the most artistically successful syntheses of his many obsessions. Once again, Allen appropriated psychiatry as an important element in the lives of the witty, beautiful, and delicately flawed characters who interact in the film. Playing Mickey Sachs—Hannah's ex-husband and an almost peripheral character—Allen has an introspective monologue just after he discovers that he does not have the fatal brain tumor he thought was about to end his life. Reflecting on the inadequacy of philosophers such as Socrates or Nietzsche to make sense of life's absurdities, Allen's character then expresses his disillusionment with Freud: "I was in analysis for years. Nothing happened. My analyst got so frustrated, the poor guy, that he put in a salad bar." As usual, this is not the only time that the issue of psychiatry is raised. Later on, we see Elliot (Michael Caine), Hannah's husband, talking through his midlife crisis with a psychotherapist. Elliot is unsure whether to leave his well-adjusted and supportive wife (Mia Farrow) for her heartbreakingly beautiful sister Lee (Barbara Hershey). Although the briefly glimpsed therapist never speaks, Elliot eventually overcomes his infatuation with Lee and by the end appears to have reestablished a strong loving relationship with Hannah. Meanwhile, Mickey Sachs (Allen) has found the reason for living while watching the Marx Brothers in *Duck Soup*. Allen has never been a propagandist for psychiatry, and he is much too subtle a filmmaker to suggest a direct relationship between therapy and "cure." But in *Hannah and Her Sisters*, at least one character appears to have benefited from treatment.

After seeing *Hannah and Her Sisters*, a therapist might assume that Allen's own psychoanalysis was working and that he might be more upbeat about the therapeutic potential of psychoanalytic treatment. This perspective was given further credence in 1988 when *Another Woman* appeared. Gena Rowlands plays the protagonist, who listens with envy to the treatment process in the poorly insulated office next door. A perfectly reasonable analyst, whom Allen refrains from lampooning in any way whatsoever, seems to be helping a troubled woman sort out her feelings. Indeed, in *Crimes and Misdemeanors*, released the next year, Allen even cast a renowned New York psychoanalyst, Martin Bergmann, as an elderly sage much revered by Allen's character, who is devastated when the sage ultimately takes his own life.

But there is no question that Allen's view of analysis has darkened in the 1990s. In 1992, Ron Rifkin appears in *Husbands and Wives* as a psychiatrist obsessed with a patient young enough to be his daughter (Juliette Lewis), with whom he has been sexually involved. Then in *Manhattan Murder Mystery* (1993) Allen's disenchantment with the outcome of psychotherapy is evident when the Diane Keaton character suggests that she might need to go back into therapy. Allen's character discourages her from doing so, arguing that "you don't have anything that can't be cured by Prozac and a polo mallet." In 1997, with the release of *Deconstructing Harry*, Allen showed the darkest side yet of his persona, a side that resists any and all attempts at healing. The protagonist Harry Block (played by Allen himself) is seen in therapy or analysis with a series of analysts, and he ultimately marries one of them. This character, played by the outspokenly anti-psychiatry Scientologist

Kirstie Alley, suggests that they should terminate the analysis and begin seeing each other "after a suitable interval," providing a superficial gesture in the
direction of ethical concerns. Later, however, when Harry begins a sexual relationship with one of her female patients, she explodes in the presence of
one of her analytic patients, unleashing a string of obscenities in the shrillest
possible tones while her patient lies on the couch terrified.

In a December 11, 1997, article, Alley told a *USA Today* interviewer:

> I don't like psychiatry. And I don't believe it works. And I believe psychiatrists
> are neurotic or psychotic, for the most part. I wanted to play her that way, and
> Woody just totally let me do it. I said, "I want to be taking Prozac or drugs dur-
> ing the session with her patient." I wanted to show that this woman is so
> twerked out that she has to take drugs, too. She takes her own medicine. So he
> said, "Yeah! That's a good idea." (quoted in Grinfeld 1998)

In *Deconstructing Harry*, the protagonist tells one of his therapists that he
has seen six different analysts and nothing has changed. This comment has a
chilling ring in light of Allen's apparent obliviousness to the quasi-incestuous
quality of his relationship with Soon-Yi Previn. Could it be that after his
many years of analysis, there has been no deepening of his self-under-
standing, no insight into the psychodynamics of his relationships? *New York
Times* film critic Stephen Holden noted that *Deconstructing Harry* "may be
the first Allen film set in New York that isn't in some way an ode to
well-heeled Manhattan urbanity" (1998, B12). By the end of the film it is
clear that one symbol of that culture, the psychoanalyst, has been replaced by
a black prostitute, who appears to be much more useful to Harry than any of
his analysts ever were. Similarly, in Allen's 1998 film *Celebrity*, the Judy Davis character visits a prostitute (Bebe Neuwirth) to receive instructions on
how to please a man sexually. When the prostitute suggests that she may actually need a therapist, the Davis character insists that that she does not want
to get "too clinical." We will have more to say about Woody Allen in chapters
10 and 11.

Paul Mazursky's films also use psychiatry to deal with the inevitability of
ambivalence in human relationships, but his work is particularly interesting
because he has regularly cast real-life psychiatrists in his films. Donald F.
Muhich, for many years a Beverly Hills psychiatrist, has appeared in four of
Mazursky's films and has advised the director on virtually every film he has
made since 1969. Muhich gives low-key performances as a psychotherapist in
both *Bob and Carol and Ted and Alice* (1969) and *Blume in Love* (1973). He
also appears briefly in *Willie and Phil* (1980) and *Down and Out in Beverly*

Hills (1986). In *Down and Out*, the most recent (and most broadly satirical) of these four films, Muhich plays a solemnly earnest psychiatrist for a wealthy family's dog, at one point announcing that the pet suffers from "nipple envy."

On one level, the character played by Muhich in *Bob and Carol and Ted and Alice* fits into the historical pattern of reaction against the profession that in 1969 was still powerfully active in American films. For example, when Muhich is consulted by Alice (Dyan Cannon), the more traditional of the film's two eponymous women, Alice is appalled to learn that the analyst encourages his young daughter to refer to the female genitals as "vagina." Alice's befuddlement is handled comically, but so is the studiously detached pose of the psychiatrist: Mazursky's camera presents both Cannon and Muhich in uncomfortably tight close-ups and invites us to laugh at the therapist's habit of idly tugging at his cheek, a mannerism that Muhich himself created in order to achieve "the fine line between realism and satire" on which most of Mazursky's films take place (Muhich, personal communication, 1985). The session nevertheless begins to bring Alice to a better understanding of her situation; but just as she seems to be on the verge of a major insight, the analyst informs her that her time is up. Even though she protests that she needs more time, he steadfastly refuses to continue. The analyst may be acting professionally, but the audience is not asked to applaud his behavior.

In a certain sense, the psychiatrist in *Bob and Carol and Ted and Alice* is equated with the range of alternative therapies, such as encounter groups, which are sampled by the "hip" couple played by Robert Culp and Natalie Wood; neither psychoanalysis nor the more contemporary experiences offered by the human potential movement seem to be of any real help to the characters. (The most popular among the alternative therapies of the 1970s was probably est, an institution subjected to devastating parody in both *Semi-Tough* [1977] and *The Big Fix* [1978].) Mazursky's film begins with Bob and Carol (Culp and Wood) visiting "the institute," where participants in a twenty-four-hour marathon are invited to wallow in their problems ad nauseam; Muhich's arbitrarily terminated session with Alice (Cannon) may be intended as representative of the opposite extreme. On the other hand, the exchange between Alice and the therapist has some relevance to the inner lives of the four protagonists, whose failure to follow their convictions into group sex is never fully explained. The film ends with the two couples strolling out of their Las Vegas hotel room and into the world to the tune of Burt Bachrach's "What the World Needs Now (Is Love, Sweet Love)." It is unclear what kind of love the song is meant to endorse in the long dialogue-free conclusion to the film, but it is unlikely that the film's huge audience believed that the song referred to the love that, according to psychoanalysis, is inevitably tempered by unconscious hatred and aggression. Yet these forces clearly play a part in the loving relationships cultivated by the couples. Mazursky is one of several directors such as Martin Scorsese, Francis Coppola, and, to a certain extent, Robert Altman who attempted in the 1970s to strike a balance between commercialism and social criticism. Consequently, an unstable irony in *Bob and Carol and Ted and Alice* allows some viewers to identify with the couples' leisure-time explorations of cultural revolutions at the same time that it allows others to condemn their superficiality. Mazursky has not made clear just who is making the highly generalized call for love at the end of the film and how it should be interpreted. The plea for love could come from the film, from the couples, or from the crowds that they walk past, and the audience can accept the plea as genuine or satirical. Similarly, the audience is offered a number of alternatives for evaluating the experience of Alice with the psychiatrist played by Muhich. This kind of complexity has led Schneider to refer to the scene in the psychiatrist's office as "the best and most realistic therapy session ever portrayed on film" (1977, 618).

In Mazursky's *Blume in Love*, Dr. Muhich plays the psychiatrist for both Blume (George Segal) and his wife, Nina (Susan Anspach). Like Bob and Carol and Ted and Alice, Blume and his wife are upwardly mobile adults trying to cope with the new sexual/cultural mores, which they may not be young enough to manage successfully. Nina has caught Blume in the midst of a peccadillo with his secretary and has taken up with a docile drifter named Elmo (Kris Kristofferson), after which Blume drifts into an unsatisfying affair with Arlene (Marsha Mason). Blume, however, is still in love with his wife, and like Proust's Swann in a story with a similar title, he frequently stands outside Nina's quarters and stares into her windows with longing and jealousy. In a session with his psychiatrist (Muhich), Blume speaks of his spells of impotence just after he sees his wife with Elmo. The therapist, wearing an extremely wide and garish tie, inquires innocently—but to the great surprise of Blume—if he has been engaging in "sport-fucking." Although the psychiatrist insists that he is not recommending the activity as a cure for impotence or depression, the next scene shows Blume with a sexually adventurous young woman whom he has met in a bar but who does little to cheer him up. In a subsequent scene, Blume questions the effectiveness of his analytic hours:

> BLUME: Sometimes I think this is a waste of time. That it doesn't really do any good.

ANALYST: Sometimes it doesn't.
BLUME: Then why do you do it?
ANALYST: Sometimes it does. And until we find something
    better, what else is there to do?

Immediately after this scene, Blume goes home and rapes his wife.

In another crucial scene, *Blume in Love* flashes back to an earlier time when Blume and Nina were still living together and Nina was working for the California Department of Welfare. Coming home from her yoga meditation class, Nina starts to cry but cannot say why she is unhappy.

BLUME: Maybe you should go back to the shrink.
NINA *(after a pause to compose herself)*: A woman came into my
    office today . . . to talk to me about her son. He's a junkie;
    she's already on welfare; and she wants more money. Do you
    know why?
BLUME: So the son can buy dope.
NINA: It's getting very depressing there.

Not only does the film imply that an analyst is of little help to Blume and Nina, but in her deflection of Blume's suggestion that she return to therapy, Nina expresses a sixties' and early seventies' notion that reverses the vulgarized ego psychology of the 1950s identified by John Burnham (1978). Rather than locating the cause of problems in the individual and not in society, Nina implies that the real problems are in the culture as a whole and that psychiatry can do little to help. This kind of glib social criticism is typical of most of the films of this era, but like Woody Allen, Mazursky is usually less inclined to oversimplifications of this sort. As in *Bob and Carol and Ted and Alice*, the irony in *Blume in Love* is difficult to locate precisely. When Nina refuses to return to her psychiatrist by complaining that her job is "depressing," are we being asked to agree that psychotherapy can be of no help, or are we to suppose that Nina is unwilling to face her own problems? Similarly, the scene in which Blume forces his estranged wife to have sex can be interpreted in a variety of ways. Rape is not something that a filmmaker as sensitive as Mazursky is likely to endorse, but on the other hand, Nina appears to be sharing Blume's passion during the scene, and the couple *is* reunited by the end of the film. Also, the fact that Blume has committed rape just after a frustrating session with his analyst cannot be blamed entirely on the analyst. Muhich articulates most completely the unpleasant realities that Blume faces, yet it is Blume himself who ultimately must decide how he will respond to the new sexual roles for which he is not prepared. He must make this decision, just as he must decide whether to continue courting his wife and whether to continue therapy. Until recently, few American films offered their protagonists such ambiguous choices.

Blume in Love does have a Hollywood happy ending of sorts, although we should point out that the dramatic reunion of Blume and Nina in Venice to strains of Wagner could be Blume's fantasy. But if it does not take place in the hero's imagination, the film's conclusion can be understood as the fortuitous result of Blume and Nina's coming to terms with problems that were at least identified in therapy. The analyst's wide tie and his salty language can be regarded as a function of his humanity (and of the film's wry humor) as much as they can be seen as evidence of ineffectuality. Since Mazursky has used a real-life psychiatrist, chances are that his intentions toward psychiatry are at least somewhat honorable, even if he does not return to the myths of the Golden Age. In fact, Mazursky and Woody Allen have expressed an ambivalence toward psychiatry that may nevertheless represent a new and sophisticated appropriation of the profession for gently humorous explorations of complexity in loving relationships. The Golden Age psychiatrist of heroic stature never appears in Mazursky's films, but neither do the grotesque shrinks from the years immediately following the Golden Age. Furthermore, Mazursky rejects the sixties' and seventies' mystique of the lone antihero. James Monaco's statement is relevant here: "Almost alone among his contemporaries, Mazursky takes it for granted that the natural state is marriage, and that single people are anomalies" (1979, 380). He is not as likely, then, to be hostile to psychiatrists when they fulfill their usual cinematic function of reconciling patients to their social roles.

In this sense, Mazursky's *An Unmarried Woman* (1978) is similar to his earlier work. The film stars Jill Clayburgh as Erica, the unmarried woman attempting to find herself after her husband, Martin (Michael Murphy), announces that he has fallen in love with a woman he has met in Bloomingdale's. Like most of Mazursky's characters, Erica and Martin inhabit the world of sophisticated, affluent professionals who are just close enough to the audience (and Mazursky) to win affection and understanding in spite of the satirical treatment to which they are often subjected. Mazursky, who also wrote the script for *An Unmarried Woman*, had projected a scene in which Erica seeks help from a therapist who is a short, fortyish woman with a European accent. However, at the suggestion of director Claudia Weill (who later used Clayburgh in her 1980 film *It's My Turn*), Mazursky cast the six-foot-two-inch, sixtyish American psychologist Penelope Russianoff as Erica's therapist. In fact, Russianoff is the real-life author of the book *Why*

Do I Think I'm Nothing without a Man? which addresses many of the same problems Erica faces in the film. According to Russianoff (personal communication, 1984), Mazursky did several takes of the scene between Erica and her therapist in which Clayburgh read lines that Mazursky had scripted while Russianoff ad-libbed a number of different responses. The take that Mazursky eventually used presents one of the most sympathetic images of psychotherapy in American film since 1963 and clearly anticipates the return of the Golden Age psychiatrist in *Ordinary People*, a film released two years after *An Unmarried Woman*. Nevertheless, Erica later encounters the therapist at a party, and the film raises the question of the doctor's sexual orientation when she introduces Erica to her female companion. Mazursky had filmed a subsequent scene in the therapist's office in which Erica confronts her about her sexuality. Russianoff, a married heterosexual in real life, explains in the scene that she is bisexual and that Erica must accept the fact that sexual fulfillment can be found in a variety of contexts. Erica is so upset by this revelation, however, that she decides to break off therapy. After an emotional confrontation, patient and therapist embrace. According to Dr. Russianoff (personal communication, 1984), Mazursky says that he cut this scene from the final print because it made the therapist too important a character and deflected the film's focus from Erica.

Of course, the issue of the therapist's lesbianism is still present in *An Unmarried Woman*, especially in Erica's facial expression when the doctor introduces her female friend. For even after excising the discussion of bisexuality, Mazursky has introduced one of his favorite themes into the film: the fact that Erica receives good advice from a practicing homosexual underlines the morally and culturally ambiguous sphere in which she must operate now that she, like Blume, is deprived of the clearly defined role that married life offers. The doctor's unconventional sexuality may also be the same kind of offbeat humanizing touch Mazursky gave to the analyst played by Muhich in *Blume in Love*.

Mazursky's ambivalence toward psychotherapists and psychoanalysts, however, ultimately appears to follow the same course as Allen's—that is, it deteriorates into outright contempt. This transformation begins with Muhich's portrayal of the dog psychiatrist in *Down and Out in Beverly Hills*. It is difficult for the audience to view this character as anything other than a buffoon. Similarly, in his 1991 film *Scenes from a Mall*, Mazursky initially introduces Bette Midler as a famous and prospering psychologist-author. Her special expertise is in helping couples stay married. As the movie progresses, however, the Midler character unravels into a basket case as her own marriage collapses.

In his 1996 film *Faithful*, Mazursky himself appears as the therapist of a hit man named Tony (Chazz Palminteri, who also wrote the screenplay). Cher plays a bored but rich housewife whose husband (Ryan O'Neal) has hired Tony to kill her. Tony has misgivings about bumping off a woman, so he consults with his therapist over the phone periodically throughout the film. Mazursky's therapist is shown to be an unmitigated disaster. He is a compulsive gambler who does not charge Tony a fee in exchange for access to Tony's cousin, who happens to be a bookie, an arrangement that Tony refers to as "barter." The therapist tells Tony to read *The Road Less Traveled*. When his patient refuses, he prescribes, in desperation, *The Celestine Prophecy*. At one point he explains that the mind is like a toilet that fills up with "shit" and needs to be flushed out. He describes himself as "the plumber." As the convoluted plot grinds toward a resolution, Mazursky's therapist is clearly irrelevant to the process. Although *Faithful* does little to glorify the image of psychiatry, Mazursky's decision to cast himself as a therapist represents a culmination of sorts for the director. However disillusioning therapy may have been for Mazursky, his desire to assign to himself the controlling, pedagogical, and purgative aspects of the profession suggests that he has become even more obsessed with and envious of a practice that has for so long been at the center of his films. Like Hollywood in general, Mazursky cannot let go of psychiatry even if it means manically demeaning it.

Mazursky and Woody Allen, perhaps the two directors most associated with the depiction of psychotherapy and psychoanalysis in cinema history, end up in the same consulting room, so to speak, in the 1998 film *Antz*. As the animated feature begins, we hear the voice of Woody Allen emerging from an ant lying on an analyst's couch. The analyst's chair is inhabited by another animated ant with Mazursky's voice. Although both men perform brilliantly as voice actors, there can no longer be any doubt that Mazursky and Allen have been instrumental in reducing movie analysis to a cartoon caricature.

Psychiatry in the Seventies: McMurphy and Nurse Ratched

A real-life psychiatrist also appears in Milos Forman's *One Flew Over the Cuckoo's Nest* (1975), but there the similarity between Mazursky's and Forman's films ends. Dr. Dean Brooks appears as Dr. Spivey, the director of the institution to which McMurphy (Jack Nicholson) has been confined, but he seems to be little more than an administrator. The most potent figure in the film—and the one who seems most active in seeking psychiatric solutions to the problem that McMurphy presents—is Nurse Ratched (Louise Fletcher). We have already mentioned how *One Flew Over the Cuckoo's Nest* presents psychiatry as the accomplice of a culture that does not hesitate to use electroshock and lobotomy to punish its transgressors. In addition, we have identified the film's protagonist (Nicholson) as another of the era's inspirational but doomed outlaw heroes. At this point, we should also call attention to how the film transforms the treatment of mental illness into a metaphor for emasculation (plate 21). The great majority of the inmates in the institution with McMurphy are not really crazy. They are simply weak. Most have voluntarily committed themselves and are unwilling to face the real world. They are, however, content to submit to Nurse Ratched's fantasies of omnipotence. Only when McMurphy arrives in their midst do any of them begin behaving like "real men." He shows them that sitting about like women and discussing their personal feelings is not nearly so fulfilling as more mascu-

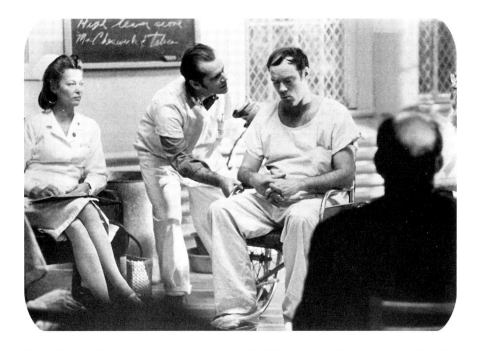

PLATE 21.   McMurphy (Jack Nicholson) looks for help in his efforts to overcome the regime of Nurse Ratched (Louise Fletcher) in *One Flew Over the Cuckoo's Nest* (1975). United Artists. The Museum of Modern Art/Film Stills Archive.

line and competitive activities such as poker, fishing, and basketball.

The sexual politics of *One Flew Over the Cuckoo's Nest* separates women into two groups: emasculating martinets like Nurse Ratched and submissive floozies like McMurphy's girlfriends. The inmates seem to prefer emasculators to hookers, even allowing themselves to be fed saltpeter tablets to repress their sexual appetites. McMurphy, who would be their sexual liberator, is especially committed to masculinizing Billy Bibbit (Brad Dourif), a stuttering mama's boy who nevertheless develops a special affinity for McMurphy. Because Billy has expressed what the film suggests is a healthy interest in McMurphy's girlfriend, the hero is readily willing to carry out his program of men's liberation by loaning her to Billy for the night. When Nurse Ratched arrives the next morning, she confronts Billy with his transgression, but now that he has partaken of the right kind of woman, Billy can talk back to the nurse, even with a marked reduction in his stuttering. He has not reckoned on all the weapons in Nurse Ratched's arsenal, however, and he loses his confidence when she threatens to report his behavior to his mother. In his panic, Billy takes his own life, and in a play upon the film's sexual themes, McMurphy dives on top of the nurse in an attempt to strangle her.

At the conclusion of *One Flew Over the Cuckoo's Nest*, lobotomy is portrayed as psychiatric vengeance against an almost Christlike savior, whose inspirational force is confirmed in Chief Bromden's eventual escape. Still, in terms of the film's sexual metaphors, the lobotomy inflicted on McMurphy is an upward displacement of the castration performed on those who would express their masculinity. The misogynist ideology of *One Flew Over the Cuckoo's Nest* did not prevent the film from garnering four major Academy Awards. The film also confirmed Nicholson's status as a superstar and established director Forman, who would later win his second Oscar for *Amadeus*, as a filmmaker to be reckoned with. Nevertheless, its casting of psychiatry in the role of assistant to the repressors was nothing new.

A few films from the 1970s deserve special attention for the extent to which they have extended this formula of psychiatrist-as-repressive-agent-of-society. In Hal Ashby's *Harold and Maude* (1971), Harold (Bud Cort) is a quietly appealing young man whose wealthy mother (Vivian Pickles) refuses to acknowledge his fascination with death and suicide, a trait that the film presents as a healthy alternative to any other activities available to him. When he decides to marry Maude (Ruth Gordon), an exceedingly eccentric and elderly woman who is, again, vastly preferable to any available alternative in the film, director Ashby sets up three complementary scenes in which representatives of establishment authority voice their opposition. In each scene a man sitting behind a desk speaks directly into the camera, presumably to the unseen Harold, while a single photograph is visible on the wall behind him. In the first scene, Harold's uncle, a hawkish Army general, expresses befuddlement, while an official portrait of Richard Nixon looks on. In the third scene, a sexually obsessed priest gives vent to his disgust beneath a picture of the pope. The middle scene places Harold's pompous and transparently foolish shrink (G. Wood) beneath a photograph of Freud as he exposes his inability to understand the boy, even with the help of psychoanalytic clichés: "A very common neurosis, particularly in this society, whereby the male child wishes to sleep with his mother. Of course, what puzzles me, Harold, is that you want to sleep with your grandmother." Sandwiched between Nixon and Pope Paul VI, Freud has become another icon for a system that demands blind conformity to a sterile and obsolete set of norms.

The idea that psychiatry colludes in society's efforts to destroy its vital but unconventional individuals is spelled out by a psychiatrist himself in Sidney Lumet's 1977 film of Peter Shaffer's play *Equus*. The audience here is asked to believe that the competent therapist Dysart (Richard Burton) envies young Alan Strang (Peter Firth), a psychotic teenager whose only passion is an occasional night ride during which he masturbates on the back of a horse. Eventually this activity issues in Alan's blinding of several horses with a metal spike. However, since Alan's relationship with horses has a strong religious component, and since Dysart sees himself as the sterile practitioner of a science that robs people of worship, the psychiatrist regrets that he must be the one to prepare Alan to lead a "normal" life. Critics and audiences shunned the movie largely because of its inability to translate the striking theatricality of the play into film, but the overstated portrayal of a psychiatrist's despair at his own success was seldom questioned. Dysart ends the film with a long speech about the damage he has done to Alan as well as to himself: "I'll heal the rash on his body. I'll erase the welts cut into his mind by flying manes. And when that's done, I'll set him on a metal scooter and send him puttering off into the concrete world, and he'll never touch hide again. Hopefully, he'll feel nothing at his fork but approved flesh. I doubt, however, with much passion. Passion, you see, can be destroyed by a doctor. It cannot be created. You won't gallop anymore, Alan. Horses will be quite safe. . . . You will, however, be without pain, almost completely without pain. But now, for me, it never stops, the voice of Equus, out of the cave. Why me?"

For the most part, the seventies continued to offer the same stereotypes of psychiatry that were introduced or refined in the late 1960s. In contrast to the heroic black psychiatrist from the Golden Age's *Pressure Point*, James Earl Jones in Aram Avakian's *End of the Road* (1970) runs a clinic in which patients are encouraged to have sex with chickens, a particularly grotesque variation on the "avant-gardist" psychiatrist played by James Coburn in *The President's Analyst*. Like many out-of-touch shrinks in the sixties, a young psychologist in Jack Lemmon's *Kotch* (1971) is entirely incapable of appreciating the problems of the elderly widower played by Walter Matthau. Joanne Woodward plays another neurotic psychiatrist who is cured by a male patient in Anthony Harvey's *They Might Be Giants* (1971), and Patricia Barry attempts to emasculate Richard Benjamin in Lawrence Turman's *The Marriage of a Young Stockbroker* (1971). Ernest Lehman's *Portnoy's Complaint* (1972) sends its characters to analysts who are completely wordless, even depriving the protagonist's psychiatrist of the one sentence that is the "punch line" in Philip Roth's novel, "So. Now vee may perhaps to begin. Yes?" In a tepidly feminist film, Bryan Forbes's *The Stepford Wives* (1975), a female psychiatrist appears to be part of a plot to replace the wives of wealthy suburbanites with automatons. A pompous psychologist in Richard Donner's *The Omen* (1976) is the conventional rationalist who has plausible but completely wrong explanations for the "fantasies" of Lee Remick, who is correct in believing that her son is the Devil. Similarly the female psychiatrists in John Boorman's *Exorcist II: The Heretic* (1977) and Jack Gold's *The Medusa Touch* (1978) are powerless in the face of supernatural forces. An Army psychiatrist asks inane and insensitive questions of a deeply troubled Christopher Walken in Michael Cimino's *The Deer Hunter* (1978); Richard Benjamin indulges in the grossest kind of countertransference as the analyst for his girlfriend in Stan Dragoti's *Love at First Bite* (1979); and in Blake Edwards's *10* (1980), Dudley Moore, in the midst of a midlife crisis, is about to call his dour black psychiatrist but thinks better of it and hangs up.

Dozens of post–Golden Age films have not been mentioned in this chapter, although the interested reader can find them listed in the filmography. If only because the negative portrayal of psychiatrists may have become overly familiar, a few films began to appear in the midseventies that were less hostile to the profession. We have already mentioned *I Never Promised You a Rose Garden* (1977) (plate 22), *An Unmarried Woman* (1978), and *Starting Over* (1979), all of which take a much more sympathetic view of therapists. We also should point out that Alan Arkin played a somewhat idealized version of Sigmund Freud in Herbert Ross's *The Seven-Per-Cent Solution* (1976), a portrait that was all the more remarkable since it coexisted with a deromanticized revision of the Sherlock Holmes myth.

Still, the most successful film to reverse the antipsychiatrist tradition, and in a sense to bring back the old pattern of reconciliation, was the Academy Award–winning *Ordinary People* of 1980. Hollywood almost always attempts to follow up on its successes, and in the next few years even more

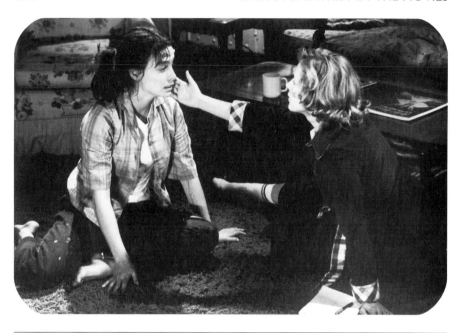

PLATE 22. Bibi Andersson heals Kathleen Quinlan in *I Never Promised You a Rose Garden* (1977). New World Pictures. The Museum of Modern Art/Film Stills Archive.

films appeared that were much less aggressive in their attacks upon psychiatry. Jack Hofsiss's *I'm Dancing as Fast as I Can* (1982) begins with the revelation that a faceless male psychiatrist (Joseph Maher) and a violent, jealous lover (Nicol Williamson) have turned filmmaker Barbara Gordon (Jill Clayburgh) into a Valium addict. Yet the second half of the film introduces the therapist Julie (Dianne Wiest), a fully rounded human being in the tradition of *David and Lisa*'s Dr. Swinford (Howard da Silva), who swallows her pain at Barbara's transference attacks and stays with the case until her patient has thrown off her addiction. Although the psychiatrist played by Kathryn Harrold in *The Sender* (1982) is the typical rationalist foil for superior supernatural powers, she is nevertheless portrayed as concerned and devoted to her possessed patient. In Bryan Forbes's *The Naked Face* (1984), Roger Moore was cast against type as a pensive, nonviolent analyst pursued by both the Mafia and a vindictive police lieutenant (Rod Steiger). The chain-smoking psychiatrist played by Jane Fonda in Norman Jewison's *Agnes of God* (1985) is similar to Harrold's character in *The Sender;* she strives mightily to help her patient (Meg Tilly), but she is completely unwilling to entertain the possibility—suggested by the film with leaden ambiguity—that

Agnes (Tilly) has been impregnated by an angel. Dr. Sam Rice (Roy Scheider) in Robert Benton's *Still of the Night* (1982) is another intrepid detective in the mold of Ingrid Bergman's Constance Peterson in *Spellbound*, and Dudley Moore is the supposedly lovable analyst hero in Marshall Brickman's *Lovesick* (1983). However, both Scheider and Moore play characters who are carried away by countertransference to an alarming extent. Even though they function according to the demands of the genre, their credibility as analysts is undermined.

Lovesick has a certain air of sophistication. After Saul Benjamin (Moore) falls madly in love with his new patient Chloe (Elizabeth McGovern) (plate 23), the ghost of Sigmund Freud himself (played by Alec Guinness) appears to admonish him that he is not in control of his countertransference and that he should refer the patient to another therapist. The analyst proceeds to go to bed with his patient anyway, but he does seek help from his mentor (John Huston), who appears to be his former training analyst. However, when Saul

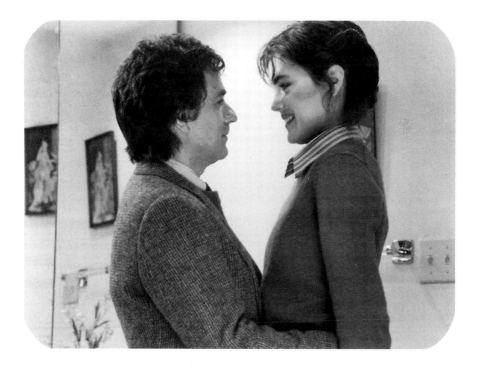

PLATE 23.   Saul Benjamin (Dudley Moore) succumbs to the spell of his patient (Elizabeth McGovern) in *Lovesick* (1983). Warner Brothers. Museum of Modern Art/Film Stills Archive.

gets on the couch and starts to talk about his countertransference love, his former training analyst proceeds to fall asleep. At a later meeting of the psychoanalytic institute's ethics committee, Saul protests that he is experiencing "real feelings" rather than countertransference (we thought countertransference feelings *were* real), and he rejects his colleagues and the profession as he strolls off hand in hand with Chloe in the moonlight. The ethical concerns of his colleagues are viewed as old-fashioned, restrictive, and irrelevant to the passions of "true love." Although *Lovesick* was not a success at the box office, *Newsweek* critic David Ansen called it "as airy and charming a movie as is likely to be made about countertransference" (1983).

As the 1980s lumbered on, the promise of more reasonable portrayals of psychotherapists offered by *Ordinary People* soon faded. For the most part, the familiar stereotypes returned. In Robert Altman's *Beyond Therapy* (1987), two therapists (Tom Conti and Glenda Jackson) are clearly much more disturbed than their patients. In Howard Zieff's *The Dream Team* (1989) and Michael Ritchie's *The Couch Trip* (1987), pompous and controlling psychiatrists end up in the patient role. In John Schlesinger's *Dead Bang* (1989), a police psychologist spins out of control when Don Johnson's hard-boiled cop tells him that he looks like Woody Allen.

Evil, corrupt, and incompetent psychiatrists abound in the movies of the eighties. At times they are comic, such as John Waters's behaviorist who shocks his patients with a cattle prod in *Hairspray* (1988). In other films the psychiatrist is more complicated, such as the character portrayed by Lindsay Crouse in David Mamet's *House of Games*. Mamet rounds up the usual assortment of con artists and sleazeballs, only to throw a psychiatrist in their midst. The narrative of the film suggests that she is ultimately corrupted by her contact with these shady psychopaths but was perhaps corrupt to begin with since psychiatry is viewed as simply one more variant of a con game. Others are more conventionally seedy, such as Michael Higgins in Alan Parker's *Angel Heart* (1987), who falsifies medical records when paid a sufficient fee.

After *Ordinary People* in 1980, few other movies in that decade portray psychotherapy as a treatment modality that may be helpful. One exception occurs at the end of the decade in Blake Edwards's *Skin Deep* (1989). John Ritter portrays the typical Edwards protagonist, a narcissistic womanizer seeking some sort of ill-defined redemption in the face of midlife woes. Numerous scenes involve the Ritter character with his analyst, played by Michael Kidd. Although the analyst is a bit unconventional in his interventions, it is clear as the film progresses that his patient's philandering ways are cured through visits to the analyst. The pivotal intervention seems to occur when the analyst compares womanizing to alcoholism. He tells his patient that when he treats an alcoholic, he gives him a simple message: "First, stop drinking." The Ritter character then stops womanizing, and after several months of celibacy, he appears ready to live happily ever after with his former wife.

This mode of therapeutic action departs from the usual cathartic cure we expect to see from Hollywood. However, the technique depicted is equally simplistic and similarly naïve about therapeutic change. The method of cure is straightforward: whatever it is you are doing, stop it. (This approach would undoubtedly be endorsed by managed care companies, who might argue that such advice could be offered in one session.)

The 1990s reveal no diminution in the appearance of psychiatrists and other therapists in American films, and no significant variations take place in the familiar cinematic mythologies about what psychotherapists are and do. Unfulfilled women therapists cannot seem to keep themselves from falling in love with their handsome male patients. Examples include Barbra Streisand in *The Prince of Tides* (1991), Lena Olin in *Mr. Jones* (1993), Madeleine Stowe in *12 Monkeys* (1995), and René Russo in *Tin Cup* (1996), to name a few. We will deal with this phenomenon in much greater detail in chapter 5.

The unbearable, pompous buffoon returns in Richard Dreyfuss's portrayal in *What About Bob?* (1991) and George Plimpton's cameo in *Good Will Hunting* (1997). Ineffectual psychiatrists are ubiquitous, as in *Groundhog Day* (1993), *Problem Child* (1990), *Primal Fear* (1996), and *Fearless* (1993). The psychiatrist who envies his patient's unfettered imagination, typified by Dr. Dysart in *Equus*, is re-created by Marlon Brando's portrayal in *Don Juan DeMarco* (1995).

Evil psychiatrists predictably surface throughout the decade. Patrick Stewart plays a corrupt CIA psychiatrist in *Conspiracy Theory* (1997). Mel Gibson, who plays a lovable cab driver, has been his guinea pig in a series of *Manchurian Candidate*–like experiments in mind control. In the Academy Award–winning Jonathan Demme film *The Silence of the Lambs* (1991), Anthony Hopkins portrays the notorious Hannibal Lecter (plate 24), who murders his patients and then eats them for dinner. While murdering and eating patients are not specifically prohibited in the ethics code of the American Psychiatric Association, these activities *are* illegal, so poor Dr. Lecter is confined to a maximum security cell where he is studied by a pompous, buffoonish psychiatrist portrayed by Anthony Heald. Rivaling Dr. Lecter in his malevolence is a psychiatrist portrayed by John Lithgow in Brian De Palma's *Raising Cain* (1992), which appeared a year later. Once again borrowing heavily from Hitchcock, not to mention his own 1980 film *Dressed to Kill*, De Palma depicts this psychiatrist as an abusive father who tortures his

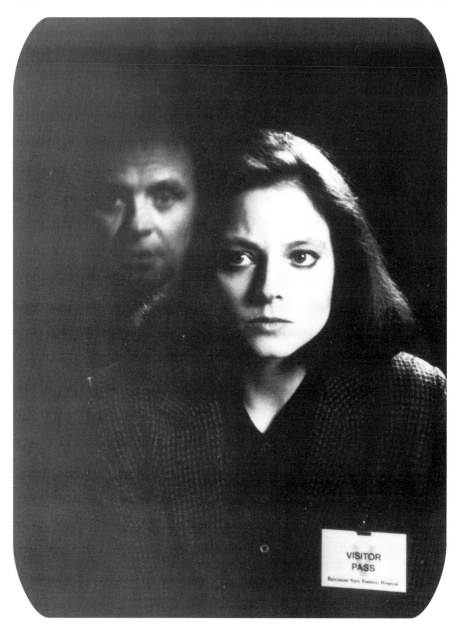

PLATE 24.   Dr. Hannibal Lecter (Anthony Hopkins) is interviewed by Clarice Starling (Jodie Foster) in *The Silence of the Lambs* (1991). Orion Pictures Company. Museum of Modern Art/Film Stills Archive.

son in an effort to create multiple personality disorder. He succeeds.

While no striking variations occur among the cinematic psychiatrists in the nineties, several lesser variations deserve mention. In what has to be one of the most hilarious depictions of countertransference ever to appear on the screen, Alan Arkin plays a jittery therapist treating a hit man (John Cusack) in *Grosse Pointe Blank* (1997). He explains to his patient that he is afraid for his life, which makes it difficult for him to be as therapeutic as he would like. When Arkin was first asked to play the therapist, he demanded a total rewrite. He felt the original version showed the therapist acting much more calmly than was reasonable. He said he wanted to have his character "pretend he's in charge, when he's really a victim screaming for help" (Appelo 1996, 63). Director George Armitage noted that Arkin insisted on having the office redesigned as an authentic replica of Freud's office in Vienna. Armitage felt that it turned out to be the best scene in the picture. We agree.

The general tendency to view psychiatrists with contempt continues throughout the nineties. An occasional exception appears, such as a sympathetic black female psychiatrist who treats Mary Stuart Masterson's schizophrenia in *Benny and Joon* (1993). A particularly interesting cameo occurs in James Brooks's *As Good as It Gets* (1997). Writer-director Lawrence Kasdan appears briefly as Jack Nicholson's psychiatrist. In the film, Nicholson plays an exaggerated version of a patient with obsessive-compulsive disorder who also happens to be a mean-spirited bigot. He bursts in on his psychiatrist asking to be seen immediately. Kasdan's psychiatrist acts in an entirely professional way and makes it clear to Nicholson's character that he will have to schedule an appointment like everyone else. What is unique about *As Good as It Gets*, however, is that it is perhaps the only example of a theatrically released American film that shows psychotropic medication as having therapeutic value for the patient. The methods of psychiatry in the American cinema have almost always involved psychotherapeutic approaches, even though the last two decades have been marked by impressive advances in the neurosciences and an extraordinary expansion of psychopharmacologic agents for the psychiatrically disturbed patient. This change in real-world psychiatry is almost completely absent from the screen.

In any case, Nicholson's character is being tortured by obsessive-compulsive disorder until he finds himself falling in love with a waitress played by Helen Hunt. At one point he tells her that meeting her and getting to know her has made him want to be a better man, so he decided to take the medication that had been prescribed for his disorder. As the film progresses, he finds himself much less concerned about stepping on cracks in the sidewalk and contracting germs, but the film is ambiguous regarding whether it is

Helen Hunt's love for him or the psychotropic medication (or perhaps both) that serves as the therapeutic agent in his obvious improvement.

The year 1997 also saw the box-office hit *Good Will Hunting*, which won an Academy Award for best screenplay. Probably no film since *Ordinary People*, which appeared seventeen years earlier, has portrayed psychotherapy in such a positive light. Matt Damon portrays Will Hunting, a young man with impulse control problems who is ordered by the court to see a therapist. He also happens to be a mathematical genius working as a janitor at MIT. A mathematics professor who recognizes his potential arranges for him to see a therapist played by Robin Williams. Much of the narrative hinges on the psychotherapeutic relationship between Williams's therapist and Damon's bad boy, who is far from a cooperative patient. Even though the movie suggests that psychotherapy is helpful, if not curative, for Will, the treatment depicted is pure Hollywood fiction. In the first session, for example, when Will indirectly casts aspersions on his therapist's deceased wife, the therapist grabs him by the throat, pushes him against the wall, and threatens him. The therapist also frequently ends the sessions by telling his patient to "get the fuck out of here." (In everyday practice, "Your time is up" or "We have to stop" is more typical.)

The mode of therapeutic action in *Good Will Hunting* owes much to Sàndor Ferenczi's experiments in mutual analysis. Ferenczi describes in his diary (DuPont 1988) an experiment in which he analyzed his patient for an hour and then switched places and allowed the patient to analyze him for an hour. Ferenczi ultimately abandoned this odd experiment because he realized that if he free-associated on the couch he would reveal confidential information about his other patients. Williams's therapist appears to have bypassed Ferenczi in his studies and proceeds to self-disclose personal details about his life to the point where the audience might begin to wonder who is the patient. This confusion of roles is exacerbated by Williams's decision to quit his psychotherapy practice at the end of the film and move on to brighter horizons, almost as though he has been "cured" by the experience of treating Will Hunting. Moreover, Will's "cure" seems to be based in part on an identification with his therapist. Rather than face the difficult and painful task of figuring out who he is, he simply decides to follow in his therapist's footsteps.

The movie also features a standard cathartic scene in which Williams repeatedly states, "It's not your fault," moving one step closer to Will with each utterance. Will, who has apparently been harboring extraordinary self-blame and guilt, although nothing in the screenplay has suggested such feelings, eventually breaks down and sobs as he recognizes that his abusive childhood

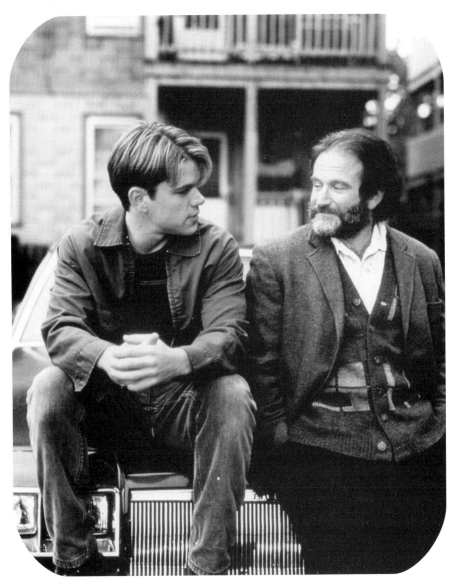

PLATE 25. Matt Damon engages in unconventional therapy with Robin Williams in *Good Will Hunting* (1997). Miramax.

experiences as an orphan were not of his own doing. This scene certainly resonates with the climactic moment of the psychotherapy in *Ordinary People*, where Judd Hirsch's kindly therapist convinces Timothy Hutton's tormented teenager that he is suffering because he held on to the boat while his brother drowned.

Barry Levinson's *Sphere* (1998) expresses the familiar ambivalence about the role of mental health professionals as pseudoscientists who lack the expertise of "hard scientists." In the film, Dustin Hoffman plays a clinical psychologist who is invited to join a team comprising an astrophysicist, a biochemist, and a mathematician in the investigation of an alien life form on the bottom of the ocean. Hoffman's character specializes in posttraumatic disorders arising from airplane accidents, but he has been brought in on this particular investigation because he wrote a report during the Bush administration on what to do if aliens ever land on Earth. He admits in the film that he has plagiarized half the report from Isaac Asimov, Rod Serling, and others. The biochemist on the team (Sharon Stone) is a former patient with whom he was sexually involved. When Hoffman announces that he is a psychologist, the mathematician (Samuel L. Jackson) quips that aliens must now be requesting their hosts to "take me to your therapist." Despite the obvious corruption in his background, Hoffman nevertheless uses his knowledge to figure out that the alien intelligence is allowing the members of the investigative team to manifest their unconscious fears in the real world. He also realizes that the sphere of the title is reflecting every image in the room except the investigative team, while all the "real" scientists miss this observation.

The portrayal in *Sphere*, which is based on the novel of the same name by Michael Crichton, is ambivalent in the sense that psychologists seem to have some knowledge and expertise worth having, even though they are basically corrupt and unethical losers. In some respects this ambivalence is an undercurrent of many of the recent portrayals of psychiatrists in the movies. Even Hannibal Lecter in *The Silence of the Lambs*, while the embodiment of evil, is also an extraordinarily astute clinician who can diagnose Jodie Foster's psychological conflicts by identifying her perfume and assessing her shoes and clothing with Sherlock Holmesian accuracy.

As the twentieth century comes to a close, psychiatry as a subject continues to fascinate filmmakers and audiences. No decline has occurred in the numbers of therapists appearing on the screen, and myths established in the 1960s and 1970s persist with few revisions. We might point out, however, that the ubiquity of psychiatric drama in the 1990s represents some degree of acceptance for therapists among the denzions of Hollywood. In the 1998 Academy Awards gala, Oscars for best actor and best supporting actor went to a psychiatric patient (Jack Nicholson) and a therapist (Robin Williams).

CHAPTER 5

The Female
Psychotherapist in
the Movies

"Women make the best psychoanalysts until they fall in love. Then they make the best patients."—Dr. Bruloff (Michael Chekhov) to Constance Peterson (Ingrid Bergman) in *Spellbound* (1945)

Since the 1930s, Hollywood has released more than one hundred films that feature a female mental health professional. Some are predatory villains as in *Nightmare Alley* (1947) and in both versions of Mickey Spillane's novel *I, the Jury* (1953, 1982). In *The Medusa Touch* (1978), *The Sender* (1982), and *The Serpent and the Rainbow* (1988), female analysts fill another conventional role that male analysts could just as easily have filled: the rationalist foil, a familiar convention of science fiction and horror films. In these genres the psychiatrist expresses a rational, psychologically plausible explanation for obviously supernatural events, thus demonstrating the impotence of science in the face of mysterious or satanic forces.

At least one stereotype, however, departs from the traditional depictions of male psychiatrists and appears to belong exclusively to the female practitioner—that is, the therapist who is "cured" by the patient. As several film historians have observed, Hollywood movies consistently tell women that they cannot have it all (Basinger 1993; Doane 1986; Haskell 1987). Career and marriage belong to an either/or equation. Women are reminded repeatedly that they have a biological function related to their role as women and that marriage and motherhood are their correct choices. However, movies frequently depict women as making the mistake of doing something else as a way of confirming the wisdom of traditional sexual stereotypes. As Basinger (1993) notes, "These movies don't say that women can't do these things, only that if they do, they'll be tripped up by love" (452). They are shown wielding power, savoring freedom, operating outside rules and conventions, having children out of wedlock, dodging bullets, settling the frontier, and entering the corporate boardroom. Stereotypes are presented, undermined, and then reinforced. The pattern in films involving female psychoanalysts is remarkably consistent, even in movies produced during the three decades following the sixties. While attempting to cure a male, and occasionally a female, patient, the female analyst is relieved of her need to practice an "unwomanly" profession. More often than not, the analyst finds her true nature when she succumbs to the romantic lure of a male patient or when she can nurture a younger female patient.

To a large extent, the depiction of women analysts in Hollywood cinema is simply an extension of the way that women in general are depicted in films. Laura Mulvey (1975) noted that the movies gratify a primitive wish for sexualized looking in the patriarchal order that characterizes mainstream cinema. According to Mulvey, the male gains pleasure from looking, while the female is the exhibitionistic object of display. Throughout the history of film, Mulvey argues, the woman has primarily been punished or fetishized in order to soothe the castration anxiety of the male spectator. Male characters advance the plot of the movie, while female characters serve as a spectacle that stops the action of the plot for brief moments of erotic contemplation.

Although Mulvey's work has been seriously questioned over the last two decades (see chapter 7 for a detailed discussion), much of what she described can be applied to the female psychotherapist in the movies. That therapist is often a woman of physical beauty who is displayed as a sex object for the visual pleasure of the male patient as well as the male audience. Moreover, the tension in the story line generally deals more with the male patient's sexual conquest of the therapist than with the technique of her treatment. Even when a woman psychotherapist treats a female patient, she is presented as an unfulfilled "spinster" or divorcée. These depictions, relatively uninfluenced by feminism, have been consistent over six decades of American cinema.

Six Decades of Countertransference Love

Perhaps the most famous celluloid analyst to fall for a male patient is Dr. Constance Peterson in Alfred Hitchcock's *Spellbound* (1945). At least at first,

Ingrid Bergman plays her as a sexually repressed automaton who focuses entirely on her work. But later, when her training analyst, Dr. Bruloff (Michael Chekhov), tells her that a woman in love makes a better patient than psychoanalyst, he is wrong. Women are mediocre analysts *until* they fall in love. Then they become superb analysts, detectives, and, of course, helpmates. Dr. Peterson, a psychoanalyst on the staff of a clinic called Green Manors, first appears as a somewhat mousey woman, hiding her beauty behind a long white coat, a cigarette holder, glasses, and an unflattering coiffure. By contrast her first patient is a flamboyantly beautiful woman (Rhonda Fleming) who plays out her sexual passions by first enticing and then physically attacking the male members of the clinic's staff. Bergman accomplishes virtually nothing with the Fleming character, and their brief session together ends when the patient throws a book at the psychoanalyst before being taken away by an orderly. On the one hand, the Fleming character highlights the lack of conventional femininity in Dr. Peterson. On the other hand, by showing femininity at its most unhinged, she provides a contrast with the woman that Dr. Peterson is about to become when she uses her feminine impulses for salvific, even heroic, ends.

After the Fleming character has made her histrionic exit, a male psychiatrist on the staff of Green Manors lectures Dr. Peterson on her icy conduct as both an analyst and a woman. He is clearly interested in forming a romantic liaison with her, but she blithely ignores his sexual overtures as well as his critique of her professional abilities. Soon, however, an amnesiac Gregory Peck arrives, and she immediately demonstrates substantial competence in a variety of roles. Dr. Peterson falls in love with the Peck character, even though he soon reveals himself to be extremely troubled. Suspected of murder, he is unable to recall whether or not he killed Dr. Edwardes, the new director of the clinic whose identity he has assumed. Undaunted by these uncertainties, Bergman's character flees with her lover to Dr. Bruloff, her training analyst. Michael Chekhov, the eminent Russian actor and nephew of the writer and playwright Anton Chekhov, plays Bruloff with occasional moments of irascibility and clownishness but presents both these qualities as necessary components of a wise and complex personality. When Dr. Bruloff scolds Dr. Peterson for succumbing to female emotionalism in her seemingly irrational conviction that Peck is innocent, he speaks with great authority. Yet Constance Peterson possesses a more compelling brand of authority, and it is with her that the film ultimately asks us to side, as should be clear from one of the film's production stills (plate 26). She tells Bruloff, "You know only science. You know his mind, but you don't know his heart." Later she adds, "The heart can see deeper. . . . I couldn't feel this pain for someone who is

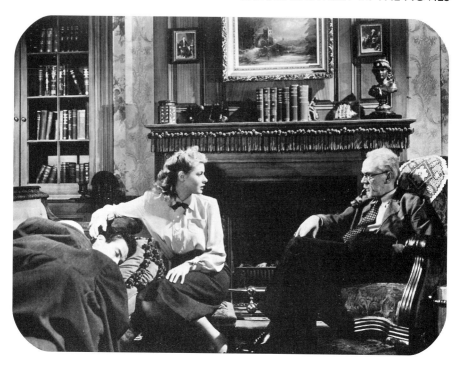

PLATE 26.   Ingrid Bergman nurtures Gregory Peck while her ex–training analyst (Michael Chekhov) looks on in *Spellbound* (1945). Selznick International Pictures. Museum of Modern Art/Film Stills Archive.

evil." Bruloff responds, "This is baby talk." Clinicians might also notice the amount of physical contact between the two analysts in this scene, suggesting that a good deal of erotic transference and countertransference may have been left unanalyzed when the treatment terminated.

Nine years after *Spellbound*, another Swedish actress, Mai Zetterling, played a psychoanalyst in a film from a totally different genre. Norman Panama and Melvin Frank's *Knock on Wood* (1954) is a combination of spy melodrama, musical comedy, and Freudian romance. Danny Kaye stars as Jerry, a ventriloquist whose breakups and disavowed feeling toward his girlfriends are spoken only by his dummy. He consequently has trouble staying engaged to women, who take issue with his dummy's statements. Eventually his case is turned over to the beautiful Ilse Nordstrom (Zetterling), who quickly determines through hypnosis that Jerry associates marriage with the constant fighting he witnessed between his parents. The session is barely over before the ventriloquist has learned, through Dr. Nordstrom's didactic, unanalytical presentation, that all marriages need not involve the same kind of strife that his parents endured. Jerry has already told his doctor that he finds her attractive, and in a second session Dr. Nordstrom acts out a scene that occurs repeatedly in movies whenever beautiful psychiatrists treat leading men: she explains to him about transference. Jerry, however, has found in her office a picture of a man in uniform whom he soon discovers to be the doctor's fiancé, killed in the war while she was a nurse. The film has nothing else to say about Dr. Nordstrom's progress from nurse to psychiatrist, a good example of how movies make little distinction between psychiatry and less technical helping professions. Jerry immediately jumps to the conclusion that she has responded to her fiancé's death by withdrawing from life and becoming a psychiatrist. The ventriloquist then makes advances, telling her that there is more wrong with her than with him. The doctor loses her professional composure and desperately suggests that Jerry see another psychiatrist. That night, Jerry sits up reading Freud (the camera reveals that he has acquired a volume of *A General Introduction to Psycho-Analysis*); the next morning he assaults Dr. Nordstrom with a jargon-laden speech, insisting that she has a "guilt complex" because her man died and not her. She has denied herself fulfillment as a woman by becoming a psychiatrist.

> JERRY: It's like punishing yourself because you didn't die too. Don't you see that? It's true, isn't it?
> ILSE (*looking down pensively and nodding as music swells*): I just didn't think it showed.
> JERRY: Maybe you'll feel better if you talk about it.

Knock on Wood illustrates a common pattern in these films, namely, role reversal. After a cursory reading of Freud, Jerry is able to diagnose the therapist, thus recasting her in the role of patient. The analyst is defined completely by her relationships with men. The Danny Kaye character immediately diagnoses her career as a doctor as an aberration, and he demands to know about her social life and her personal relationships, obviously searching for an explanation for her peculiar choice of a career over a man. Basinger (1993) points out that in the classic women's films, whenever a woman is doing a man's job, the film provides an explanation of some sort that answers the question, "What is this woman doing here?" The explanation in this film suggests that the Mai Zetterling character has become a psychiatrist as a pathological grief response to losing her fiancé. The cure for her aberration is to fall in love with Jerry.

Knock on Wood is one of many films from the postwar period that reveal the discomfort audiences must have felt at the idea of a female psychiatrist. Barbara Melosh (1983) has tied fictional portraits of aggressive nurses, specifically "Hot Lips" Hoolihan in *M*A*S*H* and "Big Nurse" Ratched in *One Flew Over the Cuckoo's Nest*, to the greater visibility of professional nurses in hospitals during the postwar years. Middle-class patients, once treated almost exclusively by male doctors and student nurses, were unsettled when more authoritative female nurses began regularly to appear at their bedsides. After World War II, fictional stereotypes of docile and devoted nurses began to give way to the officious, threatening images represented by Hot Lips and Nurse Ratched. Although the movies have seldom dealt with female medical doctors, films like *Knock on Wood* could acknowledge the significant number of women who had for a long time practiced psychiatric specialties, largely because psychiatry was not perceived as medicine. The film, however, also obscures the implicit threat of female professionalism by exposing it as a neurotic denial of feminine domesticity.

Still another beautiful female analyst with a European accent appears in Michael Gordon's *A Very Special Favor* (1965), in this case the French actress Leslie Caron. Lauren (Caron) is at first engaged to her hairdresser, played with exaggerated effeminacy by Dick Shawn. When Lauren's disapproving father, a traditional Old World male played by Charles Boyer, enlists Paul (Rock Hudson) to make his daughter a "real woman," Hudson first appears in her office with a story about how he has been unable to resist the constant attentions of women ever since an affair ended tragically. He then takes her out to dinner, where he discovers that he can easily manipulate her by appealing to her vanity and jealousy and also that she cannot hold her liquor. Paul takes Lauren home to his apartment after she has become intoxicated at the restaurant and spends the next morning attempting to convince her that she had made advances to him the night before. When his initial plans for seducing Lauren fail, Paul eventually succeeds by pretending to have homosexual tendencies. (As many have pointed out, Rock Hudson's real-life homosexuality was not entirely hidden in his various film roles.) He even goes so far as to arrange a meeting with a young man (actually his female secretary in drag), a meeting that Lauren breaks up by rushing in and eventually collapsing in Paul's arms. This shot dissolves into the final scene, showing the former psychiatrist in a maternity ward holding a baby. The camera then pulls back to reveal Paul and, apparently, five more of their children looking in from the other side of the glass. Caron's face suggests that the psychiatrist has given up psychiatry for the more fulfilling occupation of motherhood. Once she meets the right man, the formerly repressed therapist becomes not just feminine but ultrafeminine.

In Richard Quine's *Sex and the Single Girl* (1964), Natalie Wood plays
Helen Gurley Brown as an American without a foreign accent. Brown is "a research psychologist" attempting to treat Tony Curtis, an editor for a super-
market tabloid intent on exposing the details of her sex life in the wake of her
highly successful book, also called *Sex and the Single Girl* (plate 27). Posing
as a sexually inadequate patient, Curtis sweeps Brown off her feet. Wood is
able, however, to muster enough professionalism to lecture Curtis on transference, even though her formulation is presented as a joke. In fact, her analytic technique consists of hand-holding, effusions of sympathy, and other
behaviors that are more seductive than therapeutic. Nevertheless, the introduction of a didactic discussion of transference is a convention that is present
in several of these films, including not just *Knock on Wood*, but also Philip
Dunne's *Wild in the Country* (1961), in which Hope Lange begins to fall for
Elvis Presley.

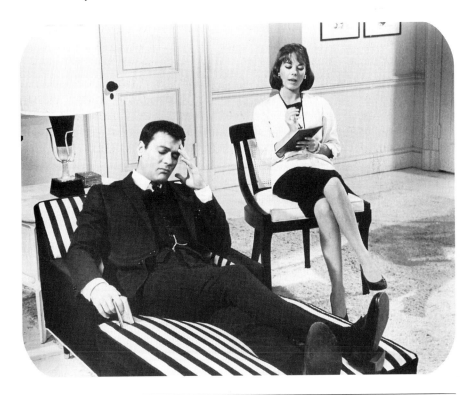

PLATE 27.   Muckraking journalist Tony Curtis about to expose Natalie Wood,
before falling in love with her, in *Sex and the Single Girl* (1964). Warner Brothers.
Museum of Modern Art/Film Stills Archive.

Perhaps the only sympathetic female clinician in a period when Hollywood films were populated with pipe-smoking saints, Hope Lange in *Wild in
the Country* plays another nonmedical therapist. Employed by the state parole board, Lange is assigned to the case of a sensitive but rebellious young
man (Presley) recently released from prison. She deals effectively with his
hostility and later encourages his talent for writing fiction before she becomes emotionally involved with him. Lange plays a widow who has been
dating at least one other man (John Ireland) since her husband's death, and
the film never suggests that she is sexually inadequate, even if it observes the
entrenched tradition of depicting female therapists exclusively as spinsters or
widows. Perhaps because the screenplay for *Wild in the Country* is by no less
a playwright than Clifford Odets, the film lacks much of the anti-
intellectualism and good-ol'-boy mystique that characterize most of Presley's
films. There is even a likable English professor (Alan Napier), who invites
Presley to come study with him at the state university. Consistent with other
films of the period, Lange's character is meant to be as sympathetic as possible, and she behaves in a relatively professional manner as she attempts to de-
flect Presley's first expressions of love with her discussion of transference.
Presley, however, dismisses her statements as "book talk" and proceeds to romance her. Before the film is over, she has saved his life by attempting suicide, thus setting off a chain of events that results in manslaughter charges
against him being dropped. At the end of the film, she puts Presley on a train
and sends him off to college. She will presumably go back to a satisfying
career as something akin to a caseworker, helping more young men like Presley, even if she has to take the kind of risks that she barely survived with him.

The sexual contact between female therapist and male patient in *Wild in
the Country* consists of a few chaste kisses, but it is clear that both characters
must exercise considerable restraint to prevent their strong feelings for each
other from leading to a sexual affair (plate 28). The Production Code, after
all, was still in effect in 1961. In addition, the film dwells on the intense feelings that Presley felt for his mother before her death. In the film, the woman
therapist, who is supposed to be about ten years older than the Presley character, performs a maternal, nurturing role. Lest by some fluke there are psychologically sophisticated individuals in Presley's audience, the film allays
any suspicions about his sexual preferences by offering both Millie Perkins
and Tuesday Weld for more traditional love interest. *Wild in the Country* is
remarkable, however, for avoiding the more familiar stereotype of the unfulfilled woman who renounces her career when the right man comes along.
Nevertheless, the positive effects that Lange has on Presley are not really the
result of professional efforts but largely the issue of a loving relationship,

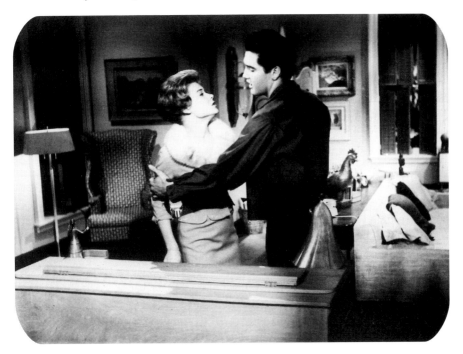

PLATE 28.   Hope Lange copes with Elvis Presley's transference in *Wild in the Country* (1961). Twentieth Century–Fox. Museum of Modern Art/Film Stills Archive.

even though the relationship is never allowed to become sexual.

In the history of female therapists in the movies, however, the seductiveness of Natalie Wood in *Sex and the Single Girl* is much more typical. Although always unfulfilled, and always in need of a man, the female analyst may be more or less aggressive in the pursuit of her man, even though he is a patient. While Mai Zetterling in *Knock on Wood* fends off the advances of Danny Kaye in her office before falling under his spell, in Irvin Kershner's *A Fine Madness* (1966), Colleen Dewhurst gives her patient (Sean Connery) a back rub as she attempts to seduce him into less sublimated forms of sexual relations. Ultimately, Dewhurst vindictively votes to have Connery lobotomized when he appears more interested in an affair with Jean Seberg.

The first time the audience sees Joanne Woodward in Anthony Harvey's *They Might Be Giants* (1971), she is treating a psychotic and mute patient in her office. However, it is she who is lying on the couch. Enter George C. Scott as a judge suffering from paranoia manifested by a delusion that he is Sherlock Holmes. Brought to Woodward for evaluation, he immediately demonstrates that he is far more competent in diagnosis and treatment than she is. In a matter of minutes he restores the power of speech to the mute patient who has consistently defied her efforts to make him talk. When he tires of her tedious questions, he turns on Woodward with diagnostic ability worthy of Sherlock Holmes: "You tint your hair and have a vitamin deficiency. You were a tomboy and an only child. Your adolescence was a nightmare, and you didn't lose your acne until your middle twenties. You can neither cook nor sew, and your apartment needs a thorough cleaning. You suffer from insomnia and sometimes drink yourself to sleep. You think you're homely, and you're glad you're growing old. You bite your nails; you're frightened that you're a failure; but you're lost without your work. . . . You've never been engaged. No one you've loved has ever loved you back." As if this were not sufficient, Woodward vividly confirms his assertions, at least about her inability to cook, by making a botch of a meal after she has invited him to her apartment for dinner. By the end of the film she has put on a prom dress and fallen for the pseudo-Holmes as well as for his view of reality, and as the film concludes, the two face the imagined appearance of Holmes's archnemesis Moriarity with equal conviction. The Woodward character, by the way, is named Dr. Watson, fated by name to be Holmes's intellectually inferior companion.

These films suggest a pattern of growing resistance to the notion that women can or should help male patients. Each film imposes progressively greater humiliations upon the female psychiatrist as the price of her desire to practice her craft. Like other heroines of the 1940s, such as Katharine Hepburn and Rosalind Russell, Ingrid Bergman in *Spellbound* retains both her dignity and her femininity before and during her love affair with Gregory Peck. Mai Zetterling in the fifties' film *Knock on Wood* is much more the cool Swede than Bergman, but she is also more the passive object of her lover's attentions. Janet Leigh, portraying an Army psychologist romanced by Tony Curtis in *The Perfect Furlough* (1958), keeps her cool except when she is dumped gracelessly into a vat of wine. By the sixties, Leslie Caron in *A Very Special Favor* is subjected to outright ridicule, as is Natalie Wood in *Sex and the Single Girl*. Neither Wood nor Caron, however, endures anything like the constant humiliations suffered by Woodward in *They Might Be Giants*. Although the women in all these films are returned to the submissive roles demanded by the dominant ideology, the movies become increasingly more aggressive in the methods they use to effect this return.

In her study of the "woman's film" of the 1940s, Mary Ann Doane (1986) observed that neuroses and even psychoses in women are frequently characterized by the woman's failure to attend to her physical appearance. In films such as *Now, Voyager* (1942), *The Snake Pit* (1948), and *Johnny Belinda* (1948), the doctor/hero's cure of these women is presented as essentially a beautification of the women's body and face. *They Might Be Giants* illustrates the same convention, although the roles are reversed. It is the analyst whose lack of narcissistic concern for her appearance is symptomatic of her emotional disturbance. Her patient is the male figure capable of transforming her and curing her of her disorder.

The women's movement of the 1970s appears to have had at least a temporary effect on the portrayal of female analysts. After *They Might Be Giants* in 1971, no women in love appear in cinematic portrayals of the mental health professions until 1983. Feminists may have made the industry gun-shy on this issue for a total of twelve years, but the industry's reticence was short-lived. In Blake Edwards's *The Man Who Loved Women* (1983), a remake of François Truffaut's *L'Homme Qui Aimait les Femmes* (1977), Burt Reynolds plays a narcissistically disturbed womanizer who goes to Julie Andrews for psychiatric help. Despite Reynolds's dubious charms, Andrews, who is depicted as alarmingly naïve, falls for him, even though he is developing the same contempt for her in the transference that he has for other women. In a scene reminiscent of the earlier scene from *Spellbound*, the Andrews character seeks out her former training analyst for consultation. She confides to him that she wants to be held in her patient's arms and to tell him that she is not the "Rock of Gibraltar." Her former analyst advises her that falling in love with a patient might be a problem, so she may want to refer him to another analyst if she wishes to become his lover. The film portrays this as a perfectly sensible decision to be made.

The Man Who Loved Women is not an isolated example from the eighties. In *Bedroom Eyes* (1986), Dayle Haddon portrays a beautiful therapist who, after initially fending off her male patient's invitation to dinner, ultimately asks *him* to dinner. In *From Beyond* (1986), Barbara Crampton plays a brilliant and beautiful woman who is a sympathetic and concerned psychiatrist. After a series of preposterous experiments involving the pineal gland, she becomes obsessed with sadomasochistic sexual activity and dresses up in the obligatory leather and chains. Also in 1987, *Hunk* features a female therapist who falls for her male patient in a recycling of the Faust story. Woody Allen's *Zelig* (1983) provides yet another example of a female psychiatrist falling for her male patient, although Allen, who often treats movie conventions with a good deal of irony, hints that the love cure results in less than enduring improvement.

The trend continues well into the 1990s. In *My Blue Heaven* (1990), FBI agent Rick Moranis is dumped by his wife, a "sports psychotherapist," who decides to run off with a baseball player who is her patient. In *The Prince of Tides* (1991), Barbra Streisand's initial professionalism is undermined when she falls in love with Nick Nolte during his cathartic recall of traumatic memories. The Streisand character is married to a man who is not a former patient, which makes her different from just about every other female analyst in American cinema. But, in *The Prince of Tides*, she turns out to be married to a philandering violinist who humiliates her with his indiscreet liaisons. Hence, she is just as unfulfilled as her predecessors, and like other celluloid women therapists, she needs a male patient to rescue her from her misery. Indeed, the audience is led to believe that the Streisand character is transformed into a "real woman" by her love affair with a "real man," not a European-accented, effeminate violinist, but a macho football coach from the South.

The 1991 film *Hot Shots* suggests that romance between a female therapist and male patient has become sufficiently commonplace in the movies to be the subject of parody. Valeria Golino, playing a military psychiatrist who

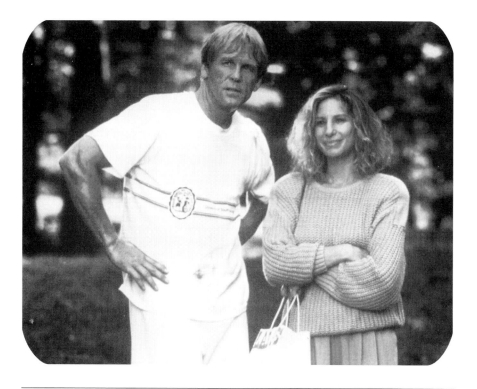

PLATE 29.   Barbra Streisand basks in the glow of Nick Nolte in *The Prince of Tides* (1991). Columbia Pictures.

doubles as a nightclub singer, seduces a patient played by Charlie Sheen. In a moment that also parodies the culinary love scenes in *9½ Weeks* (1986), Sheen cooks bacon on Golino's naturally hot belly. But *Basic Instinct* (1992) restored a new earnestness to films with female therapists. Jeanne Tripplehorn sleeps with her patient, Michael Douglas, and then endures a session of rough sex after she has ended the treatment. By the end, her bisexual past has been uncovered, and she has become the prime suspect in the brutal murder of several men. After the tremendous popularity of *Basic Instinct*, an entire genre of erotic thrillers emerged, usually with sexy, possibly murderous female psychiatrists. (Most of these films went direct to cable television and starred a woman named Shannon.) Director William Friedkin contributed to the genre with *Jade* (1995), in which a sultry therapist played by Linda Fiorentino moonlights as a prostitute and may or may not have committed a series of grisly murders.

Other films from the 1990s return to familiar paradigms in their representations of female therapists. In *12 Monkeys* (1995), Madeleine Stowe is first the rationalist foil and then the helpmate of time traveler Bruce Willis (plate 30); Diane Keaton's husband in *The First Wives' Club* (1996) has an affair with their marriage counselor; and in *Tin Cup* (1996) Kevin Costner liberates René Russo from a neurotic relationship with Don Johnson. Woody Allen takes a slightly different view of the familiar conventions in *Deconstructing Harry* (1997), first by showing Kirstie Alley terminating her treatment of Harry (Woody Allen) in order to begin a relationship with him and then by dramatizing the disasters of the resulting marriage, including Harry's seduction of his therapist wife's patients and her repetition of her boundary violation with another male patient. Falling in love with a male patient is clearly not a solution to her problems.

In *Mr. Jones* (1993), Lena Olin plays a female analyst who falls in love with her manic-depressive patient, played by Richard Gere. In many respects, the film's narrative is utterly predictable and indistinguishable from its predecessors. The Olin character is portrayed as a woman with serious problems in her personal relationships. Early in the film, we see her husband moving his things out of her house as he embarks on an affair with another woman. Just as Barbra Streisand is portrayed as an unstable woman who throws an ashtray at Nick Nolte in *The Prince of Tides*, Olin loses her temper with Gere and, at the top of her lungs, tells him to shut up. A significant difference between *Mr. Jones* and other female analyst movies is a screenplay that acknowledges the ethical violations in a sexual relationship between a patient and his therapist. The Olin character is confronted by an outraged male colleague who threatens to report her if she does not bring the relation-

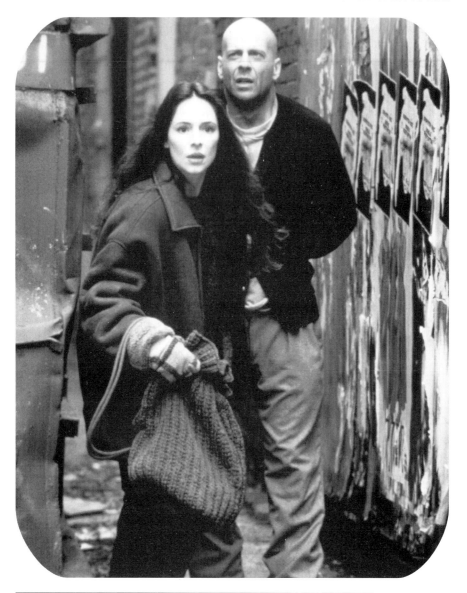

PLATE 30.   Madeleine Stowe and Bruce Willis in *12 Monkeys* (1995). Universal.

ship to an immediate end. She maintains, however, that she has already gone too far and that she cannot stop it. The audience clearly is meant to sympathize with the star-crossed lovers.

Mr. Jones ends with Olin and Gere on a dangerously steep rooftop after the patient has narrowly avoided committing suicide. The film strongly suggests that the patient has finally had a breakthrough facilitated by the therapist's love. Hospital treatment, lithium carbonate, and psychotherapy have all proved useless. Only the therapist's love has worked. Hence, although the Olin character challenges conventional ethical codes, she is nevertheless trapped in a familiar gender role as she unprofessionally succumbs to an irresistible man. The love transforms *her* at the same time that it transforms the patient. Love conquers all as the wildly manic patient loosens up the rigid therapist and helps her become free. One of the few new developments in the portrayal of psychiatrists in the 1990s may be the idea that a *male* psychiatrist can be similarly cured by a *male* patient in the critically acclaimed melodrama *Good Will Hunting* (1997). (See chapter 4 for a more detailed discussion.)

In all, we have been able to locate at least twenty-nine American films in which a woman therapist becomes romantically or sexually involved with a male patient (see table 2). By contrast, there seem to be fewer than twenty American movies in which a male therapist is similarly involved with a female patient (see table 3). This lopsided state of affairs is striking in view of the fact that actual surveys of therapists indicate that when it comes to sex with patients, male offenders outnumber female offenders 3 to 1 (G. Gabbard 1989).

Another gender comparison is equally revealing. Virtually every female analyst is portrayed as lacking a stable relationship with a male: she is either a divorcée, a widow, a "spinster," or, like Janet Leigh in *Three on a Couch* (1966), married to a former patient. In those rare instances in which a female therapist is portrayed as married, such as *Mr. Jones* or *The Prince of Tides*, the therapist is usually in the process of being dumped by her husband. *The Demon Seed* (1977) begins as Julie Christie's husband is walking out on her; she is subsequently raped by her computer. By contrast, wives or lovers of male psychiatrists appear in dozens of films.

We have been able to locate only two American films in which a female psychiatrist effectively treats a male patient without falling in love with him. *Private Worlds* (1935) and *The Last Embrace* (1979) portray such successful treatments, but in both films they are relatively insignificant and peripheral to the central action: in both films, as well, treatment involves hospitalization for a "breakdown" rather than analysis or therapy. Male therapists have much better success treating female patients (see table 4).

So long as American culture in general and Hollywood film culture in particular are invested in fantasies of "naturally" nourishing women, the narrative of the female analyst cured by the love of a male patient seems

TABLE 2. Gender Comparisons of Romantic Sexual Involvement
Between Therapist and Patient, I

Films in which a female therapist falls for a male patient:

The Flame Within (1935)	*The Man Who Loved Women* (1983)
Spellbound (1945)	*Zelig* (1983)
She Wouldn't Say Yes (1946)	*Bedroom Eyes* (1986)
High Wall (1947)	*From Beyond* (1986)
Let's Live a Little (1948)	*Hunk* (1987)
Shadow on the Wall (1950)	*The Hero and the Terror* (1988)
Knock on Wood (1954)	*My Blue Heaven* (1990)
The Perfect Furlough (1958)	*Hot Shots* (1991)
Wild in the Country (1961)	*The Prince of Tides* (1991)
Sex and the Single Girl (1964)	*Basic Instinct* (1992)
A Very Special Favor (1965)	*Mr. Jones* (1993)
Dead Heat on a Merry-Go-Round (1966)	*12 Monkeys* (1995)
	The First Wives' Club (1996)
A Fine Madness (1966)	*Tin Cup* (1996)
They Might Be Giants (1971)	*Deconstructing Harry* (1997)

TABLE 3. Gender Comparisons of Romantic Sexual Involvement
Between Therapist and Patient, II

Films in which a male therapist falls for a female patient:

Carefree (1938)	*Beyond Therapy* (1987)
Condemned Women (1938)	*Bad Dreams* (1988)
The Dark Mirror (1946)	*Husbands and Wives* (1992)
Tender Is the Night (1962)	*The Net* (1995)
Lilith (1964)	*The Evening Star* (1996)
What's New, Pussycat? (1965)	*Bliss* (1997)
Love at First Bite (1979)	*That Old Feeling* (1997)
Lovesick (1983)	*Sphere* (1998)
Duet for One (1986)	

inevitable. If the movies are any indication, audiences cannot imagine a
deeply personal conversation between a man and a woman that does not develop into a romance. The films reassure audiences that women do *not*, in
fact, hold back their affections when men reveal themselves. After the fe-

TABLE 4.   Films in Which a Male Therapist Effectively Treats a Female Patient

Reunion in Vienna (1933)	*Oh, Men! Oh, Women!* (1957)
Carefree (1938)	*The Three Faces of Eve* (1957)
Condemned Women (1938)	*Home Before Dark* (1958)
Lady in a Jam (1942)	*Suddenly, Last Summer* (1959)
Now, Voyager (1942)	*Butterfield 8* (1960)
Dark Waters (1944)	*Girl of the Night* (1960)
Since You Went Away (1944)	*Splendor in the Grass* (1961)
Bewitched (1945)	*The Cabinet of Caligari* (1962)
The Locket (1946)	*David and Lisa* (1962)
The Bachelor and the Bobby Soxer (1947)	*Freud* (1962)
Dark Delusion (1947)	*Tender Is the Night* (1962)
Dishonored Lady (1947)	*On a Clear Day You Can See Forever* (1970)
Possessed (1947)	*The Seven-Per-Cent Solution* (1976)
The Snake Pit (1948)	*Schizoid* (1980)
So Young, So Bad (1950)	*Zelig* (1983)
The Shrike (1955)	*The Stepfather* (1987)

male therapist surrenders to countertransference love, she develops insight into her denial of her domestic role. She becomes more dependent on men and accepts a subordinate role to the man in her life. She starts attending to her physical appearance. She accepts and integrates the emotional and sexual aspects of herself. Finally, she also may decide that she no longer needs her work since she has found fulfillment in a man. Occasional exceptions to this pattern occur, such as *House of Games* (1987) and *Whispers in the Dark* (1992), but even these films show the female therapist involved in serious boundary transgressions. In *House of Games*, the female psychiatrist is conned by a patient's associate into corrupt activity, eventually shooting him dead, and in *Whispers in the Dark*, the female therapist becomes romantically involved with her female patient's male lover but does not give up her practice at the end of the film.

Perhaps the most impressive exception is the 1996 independent film *Walking and Talking*, written and directed by Nicole Holofcener. Anne Heche plays a therapist-in-training who is shown doing psychotherapy in several vignettes. With one particular male patient, only once seen in the entire film, she imagines herself kissing him passionately and caressing his chest and face. The film cuts immediately to a conversation with her best friend (Catherine Keener), in which the Heche character proclaims, "I'm a bad therapist. Do you hear me? A bad therapist. . . . I'm making these people worse. . . . I've got a crush on one of my patients." Her friend responds, "What? What do you mean?" The therapist clarifies her initial statement: "I mean—this is not funny!—I mean, like a crush, like I want to fuck one of them." This scene may be the only one in American cinema where a female therapist identifies her erotic countertransference and avoids acting on it. As the audience does not see the male patient again, we have no idea whether the patient ultimately benefits from the therapy or not.

The Female Psychiatrist and the Female Patient

The most sympathetic portraits of female therapists occur in movies in which the therapist is treating a female patient. *I Never Promised You a Rose Garden* (1977) is often cited as an example of effective psychoanalytic psychotherapy with a psychotic patient. Based on the pseudonymous Joanne Greenberg's experience in treatment with Frieda Fromm-Reichmann at Chestnut Lodge, the movie shows the evolution of a positive and successful psychotherapeutic relationship in scene after scene, culminating in a cure. However, one particular scene reveals that the analyst (played by Bibi Andersson) suffers from the same affliction as her colleagues who treat men. Given the opportunity to temporarily examine her therapist, the patient (Kathleen Quinlan) discovers that her doctor is childless and unmarried. The Andersson character then implies that her nurturing energies have been invested obsessively in the treatment of child surrogates such as the young female protagonist. Throughout the history of Hollywood cinema, few films have suggested that a woman's successful analytic career and a satisfying personal life might coexist. (An exception may be the low-budget *Vampire's Kiss* [1989], in which Elizabeth Ashley is actually seen with a sexy male lover who is not a patient or former patient.)

The patient's discovery of her analyst's childlessness in *I Never Promised You a Rose Garden* is duplicated almost exactly in *Agnes of God* (1985) when Meg Tilly questions Jane Fonda. While not identified as an analyst, Dr. Martha Livingston (Fonda) is appointed by the court to do a forensic evaluation of a young nun in a convent, but she ends up doing quasi-psychotherapeutic work to solve the mystery of the dead baby found in the convent. The film strongly suggests that since Dr. Livingston is beyond childbearing age, the

Tilly character satisfies some frustrated maternal instinct, allowing her to become highly dedicated to, if not excessively involved with, her patient.

According to cinematic convention, female analysts can be competent, but only when they treat patients of their own sex. In *An Unmarried Woman* (1978), director Paul Mazursky cast real-life psychologist Dr. Penelope Russianoff as Jill Clayburgh's effective, if unconventional and certainly nonanalytic, therapist. Late in the film, the doctor appears at a social event holding hands with a female lover, indicating that she too lacks a stable male relationship. According to Russianoff, scenes were edited out of the film in which the therapist explicitly declares herself to be bisexual. Nevertheless, the film implies that Russianoff has helped Clayburgh become her own woman after a traumatic divorce. In *I'm Dancing as Fast as I Can* (1982), Clayburgh again appears as a woman in a bad marriage who is saved by her therapist (Dianne Wiest) after she has become addicted to the Valium that her previous (male) psychiatrist had prescribed.

Understanding a Stereotype

Since the beginning of the century when psychiatry was considered one of the "softer" medical specialties, women have been more likely to practice this specialty than surgery or obstetrics. Thus, on the one hand, the significant presence of women among the ranks of psychiatrists has been accurately represented by the Hollywood cinema. On the other hand, countertransference acting-out of a sexual nature by female therapists is relatively uncommon in real life, even though Hollywood's representation of the practice is deeply entrenched and seems unresponsive to cultural and historical changes. The most simple explanation is that many Americans simply cannot or choose not to believe that the close, confessional aspects of the therapeutic situation, often involving discussion of the patient's love life, do not invariably lead to sex.

Another way to understand the female analyst in the movies is to see her simply as a product of certain movie conventions and genres in which boy meets girl, boy falls in love with girl, boy and girl live happily ever after—even when the girl is treating the boy in a professional relationship. On the other hand, a pattern so consistent and so unresponsive to cultural and historical changes suggests a more fundamental explanation.

To find a more satisfying solution, it is useful for us to keep in mind the mythopoietic function of Hollywood films, specifically, Lévi-Strauss's (1975) notion that myths are transformations of fundamental conflicts or contradictions that in reality cannot be resolved. Dreams function as wish fulfillments; films provide wish-fulfilling solutions to often unsolvable human dilemmas. What we are proposing here is that these films depict a fundamental problem, particularly for the male spectator, that requires a solution that follows a consistent mythic narrative.

A woman in the role of analyst is an image that may strike terror right to the core of the male psyche. She threatens to restore the early mother-child dependent relationship and to reactivate primitive concerns that the man has fought most of his life to overcome. We would like to offer some reflections on what several of these concerns may be. One is that a powerful wish for a cure by love will emerge, a reflection of earlier yearnings that if mother only would have loved him differently or more intensely, he would now be fulfilled. The child is born without a sense of the mother as a separate and autonomous person (Benjamin 1998). A man's love for a woman always has a regressive component of searching for a perfect union with a figure whose otherness is denied. Of course, the fulfillment of this original desire is impossible. The lost paradise cannot be found because it was never there. The fantasy of fulfillment depends, paradoxically, on the inaccessibility of the object. So why not a woman analyst? This wish is closely related to the longing for symbiotic merger in the male child about which Stoller (1975) wrote so eloquently. The narrative of these films solves this problem handily by reversing the playing field. It is now the *woman* who needs the love cure. The man obliges by sweeping her off her feet and curing her with his magic wand, otherwise known as the penis. Here we find that filmmakers shade into another deeply ingrained area of cultural mythology—namely, that the cure for an unhappy woman is sex with the right man.

Freud (1914) recalled receiving a referral from the Viennese gynecology professor Rudolf Chrobak. A hysterical patient resistant to treatment had gotten the best of Chrobak, and in exasperation he told his colleague Freud that the optimal prescription for her was *"penis normalis dosum repitatur."* Freud, for all his shortcomings, had the wisdom in this case to suggest that Chrobak's treatment plan might be less than optimal. Yet cinematic mythology continues to be imbued with this particular male fantasy. Even in a feminist film like Ridley Scott's *Thelma and Louise*, we see the same mythic narrative at work. Thelma (Geena Davis) is an unhappy housewife with a Cro-Magnon for a husband. Finally, when she picks up hitchhiker Brad Pitt and goes to bed with him, she emerges the next morning with a beatific grin. At the coffee shop with her friend Louise (Susan Sarandon), she explains that she now knows what it is all about. Clearly, all an unhappy housewife requires is sex with the right man. Even a *female* screenwriter like Callie Khouri found this mythology irresistible. By devaluing female analysts as pathetic and incomplete women who need the right man to make them whole, male filmmakers and audience members reassure themselves that the patriarchal order is not disturbed.

Anxieties of a darker nature are also at work in these portrayals, which may defend against fantasies that a woman analyst might use her power to tame men into submission and render them helpless and dependent. A handful of films, such as *The Marriage of a Young Stockbroker* (1971) and *Nightmare Alley* (1947), bring that very fantasy to life.

Lerner (1974) has linked the pervasive devaluation of women in our society to envy connected with the infant's earliest experiences. The newborn is at the mercy of its mother, an all-powerful figure who is the source of life-giving nurturance and who has total control over the child. To avoid envying these maternal qualities, men may need to devalue the mother in particular and women in general as a defensive maneuver. As men grow up and become acculturated, they attempt to reverse the early mother-infant situation by placing themselves in dominant roles vis-à-vis women. "According to most cultural stereotypes, the desirable 'feminine' woman is one who embodies all aspects of the good mother (e.g., cleaning, feeding, providing emotional understanding, comfort, softness, warmth), but who possesses no elements of power, dominance, and control that are also factors within the imago of the omnipotent, envied mother" (Lerner 1974, 543).

Jessica Benjamin (1988) has pointed out that as children develop, dominance and submission soon become linked to gender—dominance to males, submission to females. Specifically she noted that for males there is "the tendency of erotic love to become erotic domination" (76). Gender prejudices are, of course, ubiquitous and effectively encoded within cinematic myths. Hollywood's attempts at having it both ways may account for why stereotypes are challenged by depicting psychoanalysts as females only to be reinforced by demonstrating that the love of a good man is what these women truly need to find happiness. Audiences can then leave the theater reassured that traditional sex-role stereotypes have not been unduly undermined. Clinical reports from female analysts who have treated male patients shed further light on these early anxieties. A man treated by a woman will very likely have to deal with his transference fear of the analyst as the phallic mother (Karme 1979). The "penetrating" insights of the female analyst may create concerns in the male patient that he will be taken over by a malevolent and omnipotent *magna mater*. She will invade him, will control him, and will know every corner of his psyche. He will then be at her mercy. She has become more phallic and more potent than he, leading to a variant of the negative Oedipus complex and to cross-gender analyses of this type. The male patient must, in essence, "castrate" his female analyst by proving himself more therapeutically potent, which is a consistent narrative development in all of these films. Females in the cinema may represent castration to some male viewers, as Mulvey (1975) has suggested, but when the woman is an analyst, the fantasy that she may *not* be castrated is often responsible for a more fundamental fear.

An examination of wayward *women* analysts on the silver screen leads ironically to a revealing glimpse of the cinematic mythology about masculinity. The Hollywood version of the "real man" does not talk to a woman about his feelings so that he can better understand himself. Consider the 1996 film *Mulholland Falls*. Four hypermasculine Los Angeles cops distinguish themselves by pushing around anyone who invades their literal and figurative territory. Surprisingly, and a bit comically, one of the four men talks throughout the movie about his experience in therapy with a female therapist. The other three cops respond to him with contempt and ridicule every time he brings up what he has learned from his therapist. He is seen as far too talkative for a "real man," and his encouragement of the star of the film, Nick Nolte, to express his feelings is regarded as totally useless. Nolte's response to his suggestion is that each man needs to "carry his own water." Women ask for help and express their feelings. Men do not. The screenwriter has given the character who sees the therapist, played by Chazz Palminteri, a woman's name, Hillary. At one point he is told by the Nolte character, "That psychiatrist of yours has made you into a piano teacher." In other words, if a man allows himself to be helped by a female therapist, he has effectively lost his male standing. Hence, we have a partial explanation of why so few films can depict a male patient being helped by a female analyst. The price, emasculation, is too great to submit to the cure.

Benjamin (1998) has suggested that part of the oedipal transformation in males is to projectively disavow the passive experience of being a helpless and overstimulated child. The mother's activity is negated as the concept of "feminine passivity" is solidified. Similarly, in these films the female analyst's activity is transformed into feminine passivity by the male patient's "cure." One further observation is that these films are truly Freudian in a specific sense—namely, they share Freud's view that women are basically unprincipled and lacking in integrity. We are, of course, referring to Freud's gaffe in his 1925 paper "Some Psychical Consequences of the Anatomical Distinction Between the Sexes," in which he comments that "for women the level of what is ethically normal is different from what it is in men. Their superego is never so inexorable, so impersonal, so independent of its emotional origins as we require it to be in men" (1925b, 257). Clearly, female analysts created by the Hollywood cinema confirm Freud's observation, even though in day-to-day practice ethical transgressions are much more common among male analysts.

We may conclude, then, that the Hollywood "dream factory" may borrow certain principles from the dream work of the unconscious. When a movie analyst succumbs to the charms of her male patient, we may be witnessing the fulfillment of an unconscious wish on the part of the screenwriters and directors, most of whom are men, as well as male audience members. The sexual conquest of a female analyst may be experienced as a triumph over anxiety stemming from the potential restoration of some of the more disturbing elements of the early mother-infant dyad. One can only speculate on the ways in which movie portrayals of female analysts have affected prospective male patients in search of treatment. What mitigates strongly against purely negative results—and accounts for the survival of many women as successful practitioners—is the much more consistently positive view of analysts, male and female, presented in other media such as print journalism and television. Advice columnists in newspapers routinely recommend that their distressed correspondents visit a therapist, just as family doctors, school counselors, priests, ministers, and rabbis are still likely to assure people that mental health professionals can help them. On television, female therapists are likely to cure their patients in soap operas, dramatic series, and the various made-for-TV movies that appear on major networks as well as on cable channels such as Lifetime. In addition, Judith Kuriansky, Joyce Brothers, and many other attractive, articulate female therapists regularly show up as talking heads on daytime television, dispensing wisdom that is much more soothing than anything in the Freudian canon. Television is, after all, much more in the business of telling audiences that everything is all right, and that therapists, like lawyers, doctors, and police officers, are in fact competent professionals. The movies, however, continue to exploit decidedly different fantasies of the therapist. No better example of the separate missions of television and cinema may be found than their strikingly different portrayals and appropriations of female therapists.

CHAPTER 6

Clinical Implications

$\mathbf{A}$s our survey of female psychiatrists in the cinema in chapter 5 suggests, the siren song of countertransference desire is far too compelling for the wayward women analysts of celluloid to resist. Audiences viewing these films might well begin to assume that female therapists have little control over their countertransference feelings and are likely to succumb to temptation.

The narrative of the female analyst, however, is only one example of a series of cinematic images that depict psychiatrists as completely incapable of managing countertransference feelings. In Graeme Clifford's 1982 film *Frances*, Jessica Lange stars in a biographical account of the tragic life of movie actress Frances Farmer. Halfway through the film, Frances is taken to see Dr. Symington (Lane Smith) at a nearby asylum. He informs her with a smile that he has followed her career and finds her to be a "fascinating case." He tells her that he looks forward to "solving her predicament." Frances is uncooperative and contemptuous of his efforts to help her. She avows that she will not tell him anything about her personal life and does not want to talk with him about her "predicament." However, Dr. Symington seems incapable of handling this negative transference reaction, and we see beads of sweat develop on his upper lip, which he seeks to hide with his hands. An increasingly menacing look appears on the doctor's face as Frances continues to devalue him and his attempt to help her. He is portrayed as so narcissistically wounded and humiliated at her refusal to be assisted that he becomes punitive. She leaves his office, and the film cuts to a scene in which Farmer is being administered insulin shock, inducing a grand mal seizure.

Perhaps the most outrageous example of countertransference enactment can be found in J. Lee Thompson's *St. Ives* (1975), in which Dr. John Consta-

ble (Maximillian Schell) is the live-in psychiatrist for millionaire Abner
Procane (played with understatement unusual for John Houseman). Although Schell plays the psychiatrist as obsequious, he eventually reveals that
he has been scheming to deprive Procane of his fortune. When Dr. Constable
produces a gun and prepares to shoot Procane, he delivers the following
speech:

> DR. CONSTABLE: What have I been paid all these years to listen
>   to your mewling little troubles? Your mewling little troubles
>   drove me mad! For nights, for hours. And what did you pay
>   me? Compared to the millions you stack in your Swiss bank
>   accounts, I have been paid in pennies.
> PROCANE (*innocently*): I had no idea. I . . . thought, John, I really
>   believed . . .
> DR. CONSTABLE: That we were friends? It was a Freudian rev-
>   elation, Abner. God knows I loved you, but God knows I
>   hate you now.

With these words, the psychiatrist shoots and kills his patient. This perversely
sophisticated exploitation of psychiatry may represent a point at which the
motion picture industry's reservations about the profession became self-
conscious to the point of parody. At any rate, it provides one of the most extreme examples of countertransference in the movies, crystallizing the worst
fears a patient may harbor.

Mental health professionals sitting through these agonizing cinematic moments are left to ponder a number of questions that are not easy to answer.
What is the relevance of these images for the clinical practice of psychiatry
and psychotherapy? Are patients or potential patients significantly influenced by these depictions? Can we assume that audiences are sufficiently
discriminating to know the difference between the celluloid image and what
they actually encounter in therapy? Do screen portrayals adversely affect patients by causing them either to overidealize or to distrust their psychiatrists?
Do the depictions of movie psychiatrists affect psychiatrists themselves and
the ways in which they practice their art? Finally, could the treatment of psychiatry in the movies be, at least in part, a cause for the decline in the public
image of psychiatry, or, conversely, is it the *result* of that decline?

Psychiatric movies are not irrelevant either to the interactions of doctors
and patients or to the public's understanding of psychiatry. The cinema is the
great storehouse for the intrapsychic images of our time, and movies touch
on fundamental human psychological processes with which both patients and

therapists identify. Film serves many of the same functions for modern audiences that tragedy served for fifth-century B.C. Greeks. In addition to providing catharsis and *anagnorisis*, the mythological (i.e., political, ideological, and spiritual) dimensions of film unite audiences with their culture as profoundly as the Aeschylean and Sophoclean visions of man in the universe were a major part of the civic and religious life of every citizen of Athens.

Perhaps the consideration of these questions should begin with another: are the screen portrayals of psychiatrists accurate? In our historical overview we attempted to avoid judgments on whether or not a particular portrayal was "realistic." Clearly, such judgments are made according to some notion of what normally goes on in the consulting room of the competent, well-trained professional. Through our experience with numerous workshops for mental health professionals and symposia at national psychiatric meetings, however, we have come to realize that the characterization of typical mental health practice is highly subjective. Repeatedly, we have been impressed at how often therapists disagree about whether or not a particular movie realistically depicts how a therapist functions. For example, while some mental health professionals feel that *Ordinary People* provided a realistic glimpse of what a human, compassionate, and effective adolescent psychiatrist is like, others laughed heartily at the idea that Dr. Berger would come out to his office in the middle of the night to see Conrad under the circumstances depicted in the movie.

It is just these kinds of disagreements that have contributed to the public skepticism about the scientific status of psychiatry (Fink 1983). When millions of Americans read news reports of sensationalized trials, they are privy to "expert" psychiatric testimony that presents diametrically opposed arguments for the sanity or the insanity of the defendant. Expert psychiatric witnesses on each side claim that because of their training, experience, and knowledge, their diagnosis and formulation are accurate, while the psychiatric experts on the opposite side are thoroughly confused and inaccurate in their appraisal.

The problem of establishing whether or not screen portrayals are realistic is even more difficult for films portraying psychiatric abuses. *Frances*, after all, is based on a true story, one might argue, and reports of psychotherapists having affairs with patients as in *Lovesick* are not at all uncommon (Davidson 1976; G. Gabbard 1989; Gabbard and Lester 1995). Horror stories about the abuses of psychotropic medications, electroconvulsive therapy, and psychosurgery in state hospitals around the country regularly surface. Are these distortions? Yes and no. On the one hand, there really are psychiatrists who are sadistic and punitive toward their patients; there really are psychoanalysts who act on their erotic feelings toward their patients; and there probably are even instances of psychiatrists who have murdered their own patients. On the other hand, these portrayals are distortions in the sense that they misrepresent typical, average, well-intentioned clinicians who attempt to understand and harness their countertransference feelings in the service of what is ethical and best for their patients. To the uninformed audience member, who may or may not have contact with a psychiatrist outside a movie theater, the movies may not be portraying just one particular psychiatrist, but rather *the* psychiatrist, just as many moviegoers regard James Bond as *the* secret agent or Vito Corleone as *the* Mafioso. Without knowing what the customary and modal behavior of a psychiatrist is, the audience has no standard by which to judge the appropriateness and the frequency of what it witnesses on the screen. Returning to the comparison of the American public's reaction to movies with that of the ancient Greeks to Sophocles and Aeschylus, audiences may perceive characters and situations as archetypes. Just as Oedipus is Man, and Thebes is the Polis, Americans may regard a particular character as representative of an entire profession, conveying its core characteristics. Hence, the psychiatrist in the cinema is a psychiatric Everyman, who is likely to make audience members think to themselves, "So that is what psychiatrists are like."

For both filmmakers and audiences, the movie psychiatrist is a transference object. Charles Brenner (1982) notes that transference is pervasive—the only difference between transference in the analytic situation and transference in life outside the consulting room being that it is analyzed in the clinical setting. In other words, at an unconscious level throughout the course of our personal and professional lives every day, we all are transforming those around us into various objects from our past. Conceptualizing the film psychiatrist as a transference object may be more valuable than quibbling about which movie psychiatrist comes closest to an accurate portrayal of his or her real-life counterpart. If it is true that transference is pervasive in all human relationships, it is also true that every relationship is a mixture of real qualities and transference distortions. Perhaps the psychiatrist, whether in movies or in real life, is particularly subject to transference distortions. As Paul Fink has pointed out: "While all physicians have their roots in the priesthood and in the rites of the society, they do not retain the mantle of magic incantation as do psychiatrists. Aesculapian authority has evolved in a nonverbal direction. Psychiatry is often called upon to deal with mental pain such as guilt (which is more akin to priestly authority than Aesculapian authority)" (1983, 673). After all, translated directly from its etymological origins, psychiatrist means "doctor of the soul." Perhaps psychiatrists are more prone to significant transferential distortions because they can so easily be regarded as supramedical mind readers who understand the dark workings of the human psyche in a way inaccessible to others. Hannibal Lecter, for example, in *The Silence of the Lambs* (1991), is virtually a mind reader despite his evil core. As Fink points out, such powers are frightening, and people may devalue or ridicule them in order to deal with their anxiety over these perceived super-human powers .

While the attribution of magical powers to psychiatrists is certainly a distortion, mental health professionals must acknowledge their own contribution to fostering such distortions. The similarities between the mystique of psychoanalytic institutes and that surrounding secret societies are the object of many humorous comments. The reluctance among psychoanalysts and other psychotherapists to make themselves accountable for what they do may encourage the belief that the therapeutic process is intuitive and magical rather than rational and empirical. Historically, psychiatry may have contributed to its own idealization and mystification by affecting omniscience and by promising remedies for highly complex social problems that were well beyond its purview (Fink 1983). The growth of psychiatry following World War II was partly related to its ability to explain behavior, such as malingering among soldiers, in a psychodynamic manner. Hence, what was previously condemned as immoral or evil behavior was now understood as psychopathological. This phenomenon provided psychiatrists, as Fink puts it, with "the external superego power of absolution usually reserved for priests" (1983, 677). Psychiatrists have thus been blamed, and not entirely without just cause, for being harbingers of an era of situational ethics and self-proclaimed experts on social issues beyond the scope of the consulting room. In 1960, Stephen Sondheim's lyrics in *West Side Story* took note of this trend in the unforgettable song "Officer Krupke," in which juvenile delinquents urge a policeman to go easy on them since they are "misunderstood" and "psychologically disturbed" rather than criminal or antisocial.

Another area in which satirical portrayals of psychiatrists are disconcertingly close to reality is psychiatrists' use of obfuscating jargon. As early as 1931, the alienist in Lewis Milestone's *The Front Page* utters the phrase "dementia praecox," even as he is collapsing to the floor with a bullet wound in his leg. Unfortunately, psychiatrists must plead nolo contendere to the charge that they have enhanced the trend toward mystification by talking and writing in a tongue that to most outsiders is as unfamiliar as a foreign language. Another frequent fantasy, that therapists are always analyzing those around them, even in social situations, is neatly captured in the scene from Claudia Weill's *It's My Turn* (1980) in which a psychiatrist condescendingly refers to another man's beard as "a classic case of compensatory displacement." While therapists would like to view this behavior as only a movie stereotype, anyone who travels in analytic circles is familiar with individuals who offer free and wild analyses of persons who are not their patients in an effort to impress their friends over cocktails. Hence, the psychiatrist in *It's My Turn* is certainly a stereotype and a figure laden with transference distortions, but he is nevertheless based on a kernel of truth.

In the final analysis, of course, art owes no debt to reality. Filmmakers and screenwriters are in no way obligated to present portraits of psychiatrists that are acceptable to the psychiatric profession. And as we have attempted to demonstrate throughout this study, the question of "realism" may even be a red herring in the study of cinema, a medium that seems to communicate almost entirely through myths and conventions. Furthermore, while surely some relationship exists between cinematic art and its sociohistorical moment, too many other factors complicate the specific issue addressed in this study— the image of psychiatry. While filmmakers are free to portray psychiatrists in any way they wish, the graver question is to what extent they influence patients' or potential patients' inclinations to seek or accept psychiatric help.

The Reaction of Patients

We have known mental health professionals who are highly skeptical when we suggest that cinematic images of psychiatrists may seriously influence a person's attitude toward his or her current or future therapist. Any intelligent person, the argument goes, can discriminate between the celluloid image and the real thing. We strongly disagree with this argument, which paints the moviegoer as a sophisticated and rational thinker who is beyond the influence of unconscious forces. We would submit that media images work on us unconsciously throughout our lives, even if we consciously reject the film stereotypes that we see. The cumulative effect of viewing film after film is the creation of a mental warehouse full of internal stereotypes stored in preconscious and unconscious memory banks. The laconic cowboy, the mad scientist, the whore with a heart of gold, and the socially inept intellectual are all examples of such internal stereotypes. Madison Avenue has long been aware of the power of these subliminally perceived and stored images, and its manipulators have used them to sell everything from toothpaste to political candidates. It would be naïve to think that audience members are so discriminating that they can easily distinguish what is depicted on the screen from what happens in real life. Indeed, when the Tom Cruise megahit *Top Gun* came out in 1986, enlistments in the Navy's pilot program dramatically increased, even though what appeared in the film was pure fantasy.

While we would argue that the *average* person may not be adept at distinguishing the reality of a particular occupation from its distorted image in the media, it is intuitively obvious that the ability of emotionally disturbed individuals, who may already experience compromised reality testing, is even more impaired. We have seen numerous clinical examples of this phenomenon. After viewing *One Flew Over the Cuckoo's Nest*, a patient in a psychiatric hospital revoked his previously given consent for electroconvulsive therapy (ECT) treatments. He explained that after seeing ECT administered in the film, he wanted no part of such treatment, thus depriving himself of a badly needed and clearly indicated intervention. Another hospitalized patient walked out of *Frances* after a scene in which patients are raped by a series of sailors who have been smuggled into the hospital by a psychiatric aide. The patient, who reported that the film made her feel "like the whole world was out to get me," said she had previously felt her own hospital unit to be a safe place but that the movie made her question both the motives of mental health professionals and their worthiness of her trust. We are also familiar with a case in which the family of a hospitalized patient refused to consent to ECT because of its depiction in *Cuckoo's Nest*.

Psychiatric patients come to the consulting room with expectations of how a psychiatrist should behave based on what they see in movies. After witnessing Elizabeth McGovern's forbidden wish acted out with Dudley Moore in *Lovesick*, one female analytic patient told her analyst that she was haunted by the thought that the boundaries of the psychoanalytic situation might not be as clear as she had thought. She commented that if she developed erotic feelings in the transference, she might not be so willing to talk about them. These thoughts came from a patient who was relatively sophisticated in terms of her knowledge of psychoanalytic ethics. One can only speculate on the impact of such a movie on prospective patients who have never seen a therapist or who do not know one. A male patient in psychotherapy with a female therapist had spent more than two years working through a highly sexualized transference. Near the end of his psychotherapy, he also saw *Lovesick* and reported that it was deeply disturbing to him. He said that if he had seen it when he first came to treatment, he would have been much less likely to discuss his feelings so openly with this therapist. He told his therapist that the movie left him with the impression that different therapists apply different ethical standards to their relations with their patients.

Just as portrayals of negatively tinged stereotypes may lead patients to expect that their psychiatrists will somehow violate them, more positive portrayals may similarly result in a patient's developing unrealistic expectations of an idealized sort. A young female college student who had seen *Ordinary People*, for example, came to psychotherapy for a variety of interpersonal difficulties. After several weeks of therapy, the patient, who carried a diagnosis of borderline personality disorder, was growing increasingly frustrated with her therapist. She insisted that he should behave more like Judd Hirsch in *Ordinary People*. She wanted him to be less formal, and, more specifically, she wanted him to hug her, just as Hirsch had embraced Timothy Hutton. The therapist explained why hugging her would not be in her best interests. The patient was not satisfied with his explanation and demanded, "If Judd Hirsch can do it, why can't you?" Her therapist maintained his position, and a split transference developed early in the psychotherapy, with Hirsch's Dr. Berger representing the idealized, all-good object and the actual therapist representing the devalued, all-bad object. Judd Hirsch's behavior was continually referred to as a standard that the therapist was failing to live up to.

This vignette demonstrates how even positive portrayals of psychiatrists in films may have adverse clinical implications because they may lead to false and overidealized expectations of what a psychiatrist can and will do for a patient. Patients who have seen dramatic results from the cinematic version of the cathartic cure often expect similar results in their own psychotherapy. Numerous patients come to psychotherapy fully expecting to immerse themselves in detective work, collaborating with their therapists to uncover the single repressed traumatic memory that has created all their symptoms. These patients may beg their therapists to hypnotize them so that they can delve into the dark recesses of their minds to locate the missing link between etiology and cure. The belief that the derepression of a buried traumatic memory will lead to cure can serve as a powerful resistance to therapeutic or analytic progress if patients repeatedly take flight from the here-and-now transference situation in search of dark secrets in their past. Patients near the end of lengthy psychoanalytic treatments often express some disappointment that they have almost completed their treatments without a blinding flash of insight, accompanied by the uncontrolled affective storm depicted in the movies.

In the case of the college student's infatuation with the Judd Hirsch character in *Ordinary People*, her therapist eventually felt that he must see the movie so that he could understand more of what she was talking about. After viewing the film, he felt much better equipped to deal with the patient's demands and to understand her expectations of him. One clinical implication of movie depictions of psychiatrists is that therapists ought to be relatively familiar with their screen images so that they are in tune with the meanings of these images to patients. A knowledge of relevant films can be a significant benefit in one's work with patients. One striking example of this benefit occurred when a young professional woman, in her third year of analysis, brought the following dream to her analyst: "I was standing naked in a bedroom drying myself off after a shower. A menacing sort of man was in the room with me. At first I was embarrassed; then I was not. I sat on his lap, and he had some sort of mask on his face so that I could not see who he was. I became increasingly frightened as he sat down on the bed with me. He leaned his head back on my breasts, and his mask fell off, revealing the face of Michael Caine. I woke up in a state of panic." The analyst asked for the patient's associations to the dream as he would any other dream. The patient's associations were not particularly productive in deepening the material or in shedding light on the meaning of the dream. The analyst, remembering that she had mentioned having seen *Dressed to Kill* not long before, wondered if Michael Caine's appearance in the dream could be understood as a way of symbolizing her analyst in disguised form. This interpretation resulted in a breakthrough in the patient's associations. She expressed intense anxiety that, just as in *Dressed to Kill*, destructive consequences would occur if she revealed her sexual feelings toward her analyst. She worried that her father had physically abused her because she had been seductive toward him, and she was terrified that the same situation would be repeated in the transference, even though she rationally knew that her analyst would not actually be violent toward her. Hence, the movie image of Michael Caine as a psychotic and violent psychiatrist had been appropriated by her unconscious to represent a not yet conscious transference fantasy about her analyst. Her analyst's knowledge of that film enabled him to be in better touch with her unconscious and to make an appropriate intervention that led to a deepening of her associations. While it is certainly not realistic to think that all therapists should keep up with current cinematic releases, this dream beautifully demonstrates how screen images come to inhabit the unconscious minds of moviegoers and potentially may surface in the consulting room.

Few movies since *Ordinary People* have generated as much discussion in psychotherapy sessions as the 1997 film *Good Will Hunting*. As we noted in chapter 4, despite the fairly preposterous behavior of the therapist portrayed by Robin Williams, the message of the film is unequivocal in its support for psychotherapy as a helpful process for Will Hunting, played by Matt Damon. Patients seeing the film made comparisons between their own therapists and the fictional therapist created by Williams. After seeing the film, a young male patient came into a session with his male therapist and asked him,

"Have you seen *Good Will Hunting?*" When the therapist replied that he had not, the patient pronounced, "That's how therapy should be. It's like there was a real bond between them."

Although this patient had been in therapy for well over a year, he steadfastly kept his distance from the therapist. He rarely spoke of any transference feelings and denied any curiosity about the therapist. He said that he regarded his therapist like a dentist or an accountant who was performing a service for him. In short, he kept his therapist at arm's length. When the therapist was absent for meetings or holidays, the patient would never bring up any feelings about missing the therapist. When pressed by the therapist about this significant omission, the patient would acknowledge that he occasionally "missed the process, but not the person." As the patient continued to talk about the film, he said, "I know it was just a comedy, but the two were so close. At the end of the therapy, they hugged each other, and the patient asked if the hug was a boundary violation. The therapist said, 'Only if you grab my ass.'" Both patient and therapist laughed heartily as the patient recounted this moment in the film.

His curiosity piqued, the therapist asked what else the patient liked about it. The patient responded that the Robin Williams character shared his own problems with the patient and allowed the patient to help him. The therapist asked the patient if he wanted more therapist self-disclosure in *his* therapy. The patient affirmed that he did. At this point the therapist commented, "I wonder if you'd think it was a good use of your money if I told you about my problems." After reflecting for a moment, the patient replied, "Probably not. I don't think I'd really want to hear about your problems. They might worry me. But I guess I *am* curious about you." The therapist then speculated that the movie may have activated a longing for closeness that was deeply conflictual for the patient. The patient blushed and said, "I'd like to be closer to you, but I'm afraid of that. What if you don't reciprocate like Robin Williams did?"

This little fragment of a psychotherapy process reflects how useful it may be to discuss certain cinematic depictions of psychotherapy in an actual treatment process. The film may serve as a "once-removed" analogue that allows the patient to express transference longings that are difficult to verbalize.

The same patient also saw *As Good as It Gets* within the same month. As we observed in chapter 4, in a brief vignette a psychiatrist appears and deals with Jack Nicholson's wish to have an immediate appointment by setting appropriate boundaries and insisting that his patient adhere to the regularly scheduled appointments. Although the psychiatrist is shown as being entirely professional and appropriate, this particular patient saw him as cold and uncaring. Movie audiences prefer their therapists to be touchy-feely and self-disclosing, even though the prospect of one's actual therapist behaving in that way may be highly disconcerting to the patient. As we have stressed throughout the book, psychotherapy in the movies operates on an entirely different set of principles than real-life treatment.

The power of the cinema is especially in evidence when a patient in treatment reports feeling "cured" by a film depicting psychotherapy. Some members of the audience identify so powerfully with the characters in the film that they may experience the therapy as if it were happening to them.

A twenty-three-year-old graduate student in the humanities came to psychotherapy for chronic feelings of depression, worthlessness, and occasional suicidal ideation. In the first three months of therapy he recounted horrific instances of childhood abuse at the hands of his father. Over time he had attributed blame to himself, which served a defensive function to maintain father as essentially a loving figure in his life. In other words, the only reason father would strike him is that he was a bad child and deserved it. In this formulation father was acting with good intentions by punishing an unruly son.

After about three months of psychotherapy, the young man saw the film *Good Will Hunting*, and he came to his session the next day and asked his therapist if she had seen the film as well. She told him she had not. The patient then started crying and said through his tears, "It was me." The therapist asked him to elaborate. He clarified that just like Will Hunting, he had always blamed his abusive past on himself, and he also said that the therapist played by Robin Williams reminded him a great deal of his mentor in graduate school. He said he was deeply moved when the therapist repeated over and over again, "It's not your fault, it's not your fault, it's not your fault." He said he felt that the overarching message was that it was okay to be imperfect. He felt a profound change after the film and said that he had come to recognize that his father's abuse of him as a child was *not* his [own] fault. He also said he no longer felt the need to prove himself or justify his actions to others because to do so would take on others' expectations as his own undue burden. He told his therapist that he was now willing to talk about daily struggles but no longer felt any need to explore past events. He announced himself "cured" by the movie of any deeply rooted issues.

Certain depictions of psychotherapy in the cinema may be a perfect fit for a patient's idiosyncratic fantasy of how therapy works. In this case, the young man had a model of therapy in mind that involved absolution. In other words, if the therapist would only reassure him that what happened in the past was not his fault and that he had no need to bear that responsibility, a magical cure would take place. The film *Good Will Hunting* depicted just such a method of cure, and the patient was convinced that his problems were over. As one would expect, the "cure" lasted only about a month and served as a resistance to more painful explorations of the past with all their ramifications in the patient's current life. He gradually realized that it was impossible to simply shut down the traumatic memories from his childhood.

These clinical vignettes illustrate how psychiatric patients leave movies with conscious and unconscious expectations of certain behavior from their therapists. But is it only the patient who is affected by these depictions? To some extent, characters in movies teach us all how to function in our respective roles in society. John Wayne showed generations of men how to be manly. Marilyn Monroe taught women how to be sexy. Even though we may abhor these stereotypes, we cannot question their influence on how people function with one another and how they view themselves. Psychiatrists have no professional immunity from this influence. A resident psychiatrist told his psychotherapy supervisor somewhat sheepishly that he had been so taken by Judd Hirsch's engaging portrayal that he had tried to affect some of those qualities in his own behavior toward patients. He even confessed that he had borrowed some lines from the character of Dr. Berger verbatim! An elderly analyst admitted that he had originally chosen psychiatry because of Claude Rains's portrayal of Dr. Jaquith in *Now, Voyager*. Most likely he was responding to the character's aura, since Dr. Jaquith engages in virtually no psychotherapeutic work in the film. Another middle-aged psychiatrist acknowledged that his viewing of *The Three Faces of Eve* as a teenager had convinced him to become a psychiatrist. The same psychiatrist recalled his early disenchantment with the painstakingly slow pace of psychotherapy compared with his expectation that its effects would be as dramatic as those depicted in the movies of his adolescence. One can only speculate on how many therapists secretly have nagging doubts that they are not living up to the standards of their favorite movie psychiatrist. The influence of cinematic portrayals of psychiatry cannot, then, be dismissed as trivial. The impact on patient, therapist, and the treatment itself may be protean and elusive at times, but it is significant and far-reaching.

The Image of Psychiatry

Psychiatry's image problem in the thirty-five years since the Golden Age has certainly not been confined to the movies. Statistics reflecting the trends in recruitment of medical students into the specialty of psychiatry are particularly revealing in terms of the decline in respect for the discipline. A consistent figure of 7% of medical school graduates entered psychiatry from the post–World War II period through the 1950s and into the early 1960s (Nielsen 1980). Beginning in 1965 a noticeable drop occurred in the number of medical school graduates specializing in psychiatry. This decline continued gradually right on through into the 1970s, and a 50 percent decrease in the percentage of graduates entering psychiatry was recorded by 1980. Although psychiatry, particularly psychoanalysis, is one of the least remunerative medical specialties in terms of rewards for time spent in training, there are other reasons for the decline of interest among medical students. Yager and Scheiber (1981) found that a primary reason that students were shunning psychiatry as a specialty was psychiatry's negative public image. The authors specifically cited media images of evil or foolish psychiatrists as contributing to these negative feelings.

A corresponding decrease in federal funding of psychiatric research and education can be documented in the same historical pattern. Adjusting for inflation, grant support from the National Institute of Mental Health leveled off around the mid-1960s, following almost two decades of dramatic increases (Pardes and Pincus 1983). From this plateau, support steadily declined from the mid-1960s to 1980. A parallel but even more dramatic pattern can be traced for the amount of money NIMH set aside for its clinical training budget designated for psychiatric education (Pardes and Pincus 1983). Throughout the 1980s and 1990s, recruitment of medical students into psychiatry has remained extremely low.

These declines in the public image of psychiatry, in the career interest of medical students, and in the funding of psychiatric research and education parallel the historical trend we have outlined in the cinematic attitude toward psychiatrists with uncanny synchrony. Whether the fall from grace in the movies is the partial cause or the partial result of the parallel pattern in society at large is a chicken-egg question that is probably unanswerable. Presumably, both processes influence each other. Students clearly come to medical school with the same biases against psychiatry that characterize most graduating medical students. In another study, Yager and colleagues (1982) found no significant differences between the attitudes of first- and fourth-year medical students toward the specialty; the students surveyed viewed psychiatry as unscientific and imprecise as well as less prestigious than other medical specialties. These preconceived biases apparently are further reinforced through the negative opinions expressed by other specialists during their training years. If these negative views are preexisting, one can assume that they must, at least in part, stem from negative portrayals in the media, including movies. As Linter (1979) has pointed out, while the electronic media cannot be entirely responsible for the prejudicial attitudes toward psychiatrists, they play a prominent role in perpetuating and broadening the stigma.

Since this book's first edition in 1987, some empirical data have shed further light on the extent to which movie portrayals may influence the perceptions of the public and of potential patients. Bram (1997) surveyed 265 undergraduate students regarding their attitude toward psychotherapy and psychotherapists. He constructed fifty-two statements related to views of psychotherapy and psychotherapists, based in part on hypotheses emerging from our book's first edition. What emerged from this survey was a striking and disconcerting tendency to view therapists as prone to act on countertransference erotic and aggressive feelings. Of the total sample, 26.8 percent believed that an insulted therapist would attempt to retaliate against his patient in some way. In addition, 31.8 percent believed that a therapist would violate professional boundaries and respond to sexual overtures from a patient. Of particular interest was the finding that not a single subject in the study responded with the idea that a therapist who experienced intense erotic feelings toward a patient would seek out a consultation or attempt to understand the countertransference in a way that would ultimately be helpful to the therapy. The survey found that in spite of generally favorable views about mental health professionals, exposure to movies, books, and talk shows significantly predicted particular perceptions of psychotherapists.

Another study is relevant to movie portrayals of female therapists, as we have described in chapter 5. Mayer and De Marneffe (1992) studied referral patterns for 170 analysts from four institutes in the American Psychoanalytic Association. They found that analysts and nonanalysts alike demonstrated a reluctance to refer male patients to female analysts. Moreover, analysts' behavior with regard to making referrals did not correspond to explicit clinical theory regarding how analysts make referrals. The investigators speculated that the cinematic myth that we describe in chapter 5 may be a manifestation of a wider myth pervasive in the culture—namely, that women cannot or should not treat men.

Despite the historical trends that we have outlined in the cinematic portrayal of psychiatrists, the public at large has always maintained a split view of psychotherapists and psychoanalysts. On the one hand, people express awe at therapists' and analysts' perceived knowledge of the mysterious workings of the unconscious mind. Existing side by side with this idealization and reverence is contempt for mental health professionals' limitations, disappointment related to their failure to solve all the social ills of the world, and devaluation associated with their inability even to solve the personal ills of individuals. Depending on the social and psychological forces ascendant at the time, the idealized or the devalued aspect of the specialty may predominate, but underlying all historical epochs is this pervasive contradiction in our attitudes toward psychiatrists. Their perceived omniscience is envied and feared, so mental health professionals must be continually ridiculed and put in their place to neutralize these negative feelings. Movies reflect this process by continually seeking to demonstrate that psychiatrists, and analysts in particular, are vulnerable to the same human frailties as everyone else. Those of us in the mental health professions may simply respond with, "So what? We already knew that." However, the fantasy that psychoanalysts and psychotherapists are somehow perfect or superior to everyone else dies hard, and there seems to be a need to confirm repeatedly that they are not perfect. One is reminded of the humorous definition, "A psychoanalyst is someone who pretends he doesn't know everything."

When psychiatrists react with hurt and defensiveness to celluloid images on the screen, they probably do little to help their cause. The choice of psychotherapy as a profession entails the acceptance that one must serve as a target for a variety of primitive feelings in one's patients. If therapists can accept that their role as transference object transcends the consulting room and spreads onto the movie screen, they can view the distortions with detached curiosity, with empathy, and with understanding, just as one approaches transference reactions in patients. Surveys of public attitudes convey a predominant message that a basically positive image of the profession prevails, despite all the negative publicity. In the meantime, psychiatrists and other psychotherapists can be content with the fact that the rash of films made about them reflects an intense interest in psychiatry on the parts of filmmakers and film audiences. To paraphrase Oscar Wilde, the only thing worse than being negatively portrayed in movies is not being portrayed in movies at all.

PART TWO

THE PSYCHIATRIST
AT
THE MOVIES

CHAPTER 7

Methodology and Psychoanalytic Film Criticism

As Robert B. Ray (1985) has noted, American movies are "massively overdetermined." Numerous overlapping forces such as technology, politics, the star system, the studio system, censorship, and advertising strategies have helped determine what Americans see at the movies. In Part One we attempted to explain the changing images of psychiatrists in American movies in terms of many of these forces. In doing so, we occasionally made use of psychoanalytic interpretations, suggesting, for example, that Freud's understanding of displacement in the dream work can explain how movies often shift forbidden subjects such as sex and politics into the less controversial realm of melodrama. But as we hope the first six chapters have demonstrated, many other forces have informed the repertory of conventions with which the American cinema has portrayed the psychiatrist.

In the six chapters that follow, we rely almost exclusively on psychoanalytic thinking to interpret a number of recent films. These films address unconscious forces so compellingly that we have found psychoanalytically informed methodologies to be the most effective means for understanding them. The best complement to a study of the cinema's mythology of psychiatry is a psychoanalytic inquiry into how movies actually play on the mind.

The application of Freudian and post-Freudian thought to movies, however, has been a controversial subject at least since the 1970s, when film scholars began relying on semiotics and poststructuralism, especially in France and England. When film study first became a recognized discipline in American universities in the early 1970s, few American writings about cinema could be considered theoretical in the contemporary sense. The principal film theorists were Europeans such as Eisenstein, Pudovkin, Bazin, and Kracauer, but in the United States serious viewers had little to turn to except the films themselves. For example, the theoretical writings of D. W. Griffith seem absurd today: the most important principle of filmmaking, according to Griffith, was matching the action to the "human pulse beat" (Monaco 1998).

Most of what Americans wrote about films before the mid-1970s was not anchored in larger theoretical systems. (The most influential statements by American film critics and theorists, among others, are now available in Nichols [1985], Rosen [1986], and Mast, Cohen, and Braudy [1992].) More ambitious examinations of American movies first began to appear in French periodicals in the 1950s, most notably in *Cahiers du cinéma* (Hillier 1985). The early contributors to that journal were a variegated lot. The more famous included François Truffaut, Jean-Luc Godard, Jacques Rivette, Claude Chabrol, and Eric Rohmer, all of whom would go on to make movies, many of which engaged in some kind of dialogue with the classical Hollywood cinema. These filmmakers took American movies much more seriously than did Americans themselves, largely because they saw film in terms of "la politique des auteurs" rather than as entertainment or sociological document. The auteur theory of cinema—which basically sees the director as the true author of a film—can be understood as another way of "centering" the reading of a film on a single artistic vision, giving movies the same aesthetic legitimacy as, for example, a Beethoven symphony or a painting by Van Gogh. Later, when film study became an academic discipline in American universities, the auteur theory was crucial in legitimating the entry of films into an aesthetic canon.

In addition to auteurism, the *Cahiers* theorists incorporated ideas from thinkers who worked at "decentering" critical study away from a unifying subject. They appropriated Italian semiotics as well as the work of French-speaking theorists such as Ferdinand de Saussure, the founder of modern linguistics, and the structural anthropologist Claude Lévi-Strauss. After France was struck by the cultural upheavals of 1968, some of the *Cahiers* critics incorporated the more politically charged ideas of Louis Althusser, Roland Barthes, Julia Kristeva, and that most eminent philosophical critic of centers, Jacques Derrida. They also began reading the post-Freudian psychology of Jacques Lacan, whose ideas were a major influence on the thinking of Christian Metz (1982), an important French film theorist.

In one way or another, all of these thinkers practiced a "hermeneutics of suspicion"; they were less interested in seeing a work of art as an aesthetic whole than as an element in a larger cultural matrix. The *Cahiers* critics have been extremely successful, if only in terms of their influence. By the mid-1970s a new generation of film scholars with roots in French theory and semiotics was writing prolifically about film in England and the United States as well as in France. Other journals, such as *Screen* in England, *Communications* in France, and *Camera Obscura* in the United States, began printing articles that drew almost exclusively upon methodologies established by the *Cahiers* critics.

One of the most fascinating effects of the semiotic revolution in film criticism has been the rediscovery of Freud in the academy. Many professors of psychology were telling their students in the 1960s and 1970s that Freud's writings were obsolete at the same time that, as we have demonstrated in chapters 1–6, the prestige of psychoanalysis was declining in Hollywood cinema. Curiously, attacks on analysts in the movies were most pronounced during the same years that Freud was becoming increasingly important to film theorists. The writings of Lacan still intrigue professors in a variety of disciplines, and Metz and his followers have made Freudian thought a crucial ingredient in semiotically based film theory. Certain aspects of Freudian and post-Freudian film theory are still part of the orthodoxy in many university cinema study programs.

The psychoanalytic film criticism of the 1970s was controversial in its day because of its incompatibility with the more familiar modes of film criticism. Compared with the rigorous theoretical models developed for a psychoanalytic semiotics, most American film criticism appeared impressionistic and unsystematic, borrowing haphazardly from disciplines such as theater, sociology, and literary study. Writing with a degree of ambivalence in 1974, the American film theorist Charles Eckert described the new methods entering his discipline: "there is a stiff, cold wind blowing against partial, outmoded, or theoretically unsound forms of film criticism—and it just might blow many of them away" (1974b, 65).

Perhaps the most important contribution of the French theorists and their disciples has been the creation of an intellectual climate that compels critics to lay their methodological cards on the table, robbing them of the assumption that their readers share the innumerable unspoken judgments that are made long before the actual writing takes place. In this spirit, we will lay out our own methods later in this chapter, but it is necessary first to survey the important psychoanalytic elements of contemporary cinema semiotics in order to establish how our approach is different. It is difficult, however, to locate the precise boundaries of current trends in psychoanalytic film theory because so many writers have thoroughly incorporated Freud's legacy into the larger semiotic project. And although many writers engage in psychoanalytic criticism, they do not always openly proclaim themselves to be "psychoanalytic critics." On the one hand, this tendency can be attributed to the reluctance of critics to take sides within the current politics of the discipline. On the other, it is just as likely that psychoanalysis has become so conventionalized and familiar that a critic need not engage in polemics when psychoanalysis plays some role in his or her pluralistic methodology. For example, in the opening section of *Flashbacks in Film: Memory and History* (1989), Maureen Turim sketches in the various approaches to understanding flashback narration—formalism, structuralism, semiotics, theories of ideology, philosophies of memory and consciousness, as well as psychoanalysis. She then proposes to leave behind the exposition of her theoretical apparatus in order to apply it to flashbacks, even if the various methods might seem to be in conflict.

> [O]ne theory will come to the foreground temporarily, while another recedes. This ebb and flow of points is in part a response to the historical shifts that the flashback undergoes, but it is also a product of my desire not to fix on a single theoretical vantage point that ignores others. Rather than seek to hold on to all perspectives simultaneously throughout this analysis, an impossible and immobilizing task, it is better, I believe, to allow the vantages to shift and comment on one another self-consciously. (20)

It would be unfair and incomplete to regard Turim's work on flashbacks as simply an example of "psychoanalytic film study" just as it would be inaccurate to say that she has moved beyond or in some way abandoned psychoanalysis.

Any survey of the psychoanalytic currents in contemporary film theory must begin with the impact of Jacques Lacan. Unfortunately, his work presents problems for even the most advanced student of contemporary film criticism. As devout a reader as Kaja Silverman has written: "Lacan's prose is notoriously remote, and his presentation deliberately a-systematic. Many of the terms to which he most frequently returns constantly shift meaning. These qualities make it almost impossible to offer definitive statements about the Lacanian argument; indeed, Lacan himself almost never agreed with his commentators" (1983, 150). It is therefore difficult to define clearly the terms from Lacanian theory that have proved the most useful for semiotic film criticism. Without attempting even a superficial survey of his work, we nevertheless will touch on his concepts of the "mirror-stage," the "Imaginary," and the "Symbolic," and the subsequent use of his ideas in the concept of "suture" in the cinema.

In his revision of Freudian theory, Lacan locates the Imaginary in the new-born child's pleasure in the sense of complete union with its mother. The child makes no differentiation between itself and its surroundings—blankets, pillows, milk, or nurse as well as mother. "At this point the infant has the status of what Freud describes as an 'oceanic self,' or what Lacan punningly refers to as 'l'hommelette' (a human omelette which spreads in all directions)" (Silverman 1983, 155). Somewhere between the ages of six and eighteen months, the child sees its image in a mirror and experiences this reflection as the first illustration of a unified self-concept (Laplanche and Pontalis 1973, 250–52). The child, however, *misrecognizes* its image in the mirror as more coordinated and focused than it actually is, projecting this reflected body outside itself as an ego-ideal. Later, when this ego-ideal has been introjected, the child acquires the desire to identify with others, a crucial aspect in the experience yet to come of finding pleasure in identifying with characters in movies.

For our purposes, the most important element in this formulation is the child's exclusive understanding of itself through projection and hence its inability to see itself except in terms of the Other. Lacan also suggests that the infant develops a dramatically ambivalent relationship with this reflected self, both loving it (for possessing the child's ideal image) and hating it (for being outside the child's body). Consequently, the child gains a facility that it will later use at the movies, the ability to identify alternately with the exhibitionist and the voyeur, the master and the slave, the victim and the victimizer. Lacan has called this ambivalent order, with its extremes of love and hate, "the Imaginary." Metz takes one of his most important titles from this concept. *The Imaginary Signifier* (1982) suggests that identifying ourselves with the visual images we encounter in the cinema replicates our childhood experiences. The irresistible appeal of movies resides in their close relationship with the mirror stage, a moment in our development when we begin confusing self with Other.

Only when we acquire language and the structures that go with it do we enter into what Lacan calls "the Symbolic," even though the images produced during the Imaginary stage are still present. The Symbolic serves merely to control these images and to derive meaning from them. Lacan posits a close association between the Symbolic order and the oedipal crisis; in fact, he even goes so far as to suggest that the primordial law of the Oedipus complex is identical with the order of language (Lacan 1976, 66). Since language is the means by which we structure the world, and since the oedipal crisis is only resolved by assimilating the patriarchal values by which this structuring takes place, the child acquires a controlling awareness of sexual difference along with the Symbolic order. In particular, Lacanian discourse involves the concept of "lack," both as the phallocentric key to sexual difference and in the more symbolic sense of seeing the world in terms of absence and presence.

Over the last few decades, semiotics has influenced numerous disciplines by deflecting study away from the "meaning" of a text and toward the processes through which any assumed meaning is generated. Similarly, the appropriation of Lacanian psychoanalysis by cinema semioticians centers on how audiences experience movies, particularly the narrative films of classic Hollywood. Rather than psychoanalyzing the characters or the filmmakers, students of Lacan address the complex means by which the cinematic apparatus invokes the Imaginary and Symbolic orders of the typical viewer. The key word in this process is *suture*, a term that was first applied to cinema in a pair of articles published in 1969 in *Cahiers du cinéma* by Jean-Pierre Oudart (1978). Suture is usually understood in terms of a medical metaphor implying that cinematic gaps created by cutting or editing are "sewed" shut to include the viewers, who identify themselves with some aspect of the "gaze" created by the camera (Dayan 1976, 451–59). Instead of asking, "Who is watching this?" and "Who is ordering these images?" viewers accept what they see as natural, even when the camera's gaze shifts most abruptly from one character or scene to another. Suture works because of the cinematic code that makes each shot appear as the object of the gaze of whoever appears in the shot that follows, the most commonly cited example being the "shot/reverse shot" formulation in which each of two characters is viewed alternately over the other's shoulder. We do not ask, "Who is watching?" because each shot answers the question for the previous shot. The Israeli theoretician Daniel Dayan calls this "the tutor-code of classical cinema": "Unable to see the workings of the code, the spectator is at its mercy. His Imaginary is sealed into the film" (1976, 449).

The operation of suture within a particular film determines the unique way that we experience that film, especially how we are affected by its subtext. Two films from the Golden Age of the psychiatrist in cinema, *Suddenly, Last Summer* (1959) and *Psycho* (1960), contain scenes in which viewers are sutured into the narrative. At a crucial moment in *Suddenly, Last Summer*, Dr. Cukrowicz (Montgomery Clift) first meets Catherine (Elizabeth Taylor) while she is under the supervision of a nun in a mental hospital. Clift is in the foreground of the shot when Taylor enters without seeing him.

He drifts out of the frame to the left, stationing himself behind a bookcase while he observes an exchange between the victimized Taylor and the victimizing nun. Although the audience cannot see Clift, and although the camera shifts back and forth between Taylor and the nun, the entire scene is played out under his gaze. When the tormented Taylor unintentionally burns the nun's hand with a cigarette, Clift emerges from the left side of the frame and saves Taylor from imminent punishment. Later on, when the corrupt hospital director, Hockstader (Albert Dekker), demands that Taylor be lobotomized, he cites the hand-burning incident as evidence of her violent behavior. Clift insists that "she was provoked," a judgment that the audience can verify, having seen the entire episode from his point of view. We identify with Clift because we have become him, watching the same scene with his compassionate perspective and projecting him as our surrogate into the action to rescue the helpless and pulchritudinous heroine.

The work of Mulvey (1975), Doane (1982), and de Lauretis (1984) establishes the basis for a feminist/Lacanian reading of the scene we have just described. The cinematic apparatus of the commercial cinema has historically served the interests of patriarchy, privileging the gaze of the male hero and subordinating the heroine as the object of the gaze. When Montgomery Clift emerges from behind the camera to save Elizabeth Taylor, he is part of a system that dominates and determines the behavior of the female while simultaneously using her for voyeuristic pleasure. One of the most essential—and one of the most controversial—elements in the feminist appropriation of Lacanian psychoanalysis is the suggestion that the female body creates anxiety for men because it represents the possibility of castration. As we noted in chapter 5, Laura Mulvey (1975) has suggested in her extremely influential essay "Visual Pleasure and Narrative Cinema" that the patriarchal camera style of classical Hollywood can assuage this anxiety only by submitting women to the male order or by fetishizing their bodies. Although Mulvey devotes her attention primarily to films by Josef von Sternberg and Alfred Hitchcock, her thesis has been used to explain the fetishistic display of women's bodies that takes place throughout the history of the American cinema.

Psycho provides a more complex example of suture. As in Busby Berkeley's fanciful dance sequences, Hitchcock's camera seems to take on a life of its own, even though we are expected to understand Hitchcock's films as a much closer replication of the "real" than is the case with Berkeley's production numbers. Specifically, Hitchcock's camera seems to perform feats that destroy any possibility that it might possess the gaze of a character in the film. In fact, *Psycho* begins with several establishing shots of Phoenix, Arizona, in which the camera seems to float across the city, searching for one specific window. It ultimately closes in on this window, finding a small opening beneath the venetian blinds, which have been pulled down almost all the way. The camera then appears to glide through this tiny space and into a hotel room occupied by two partially clad lovers (Janet Leigh and John Gavin). Not only has the camera (and the spectator) violated the laws of gravity; the impossible entrance into the room also constitutes a violation of the lovers' privacy, one that recalls the primal scene and its subsequent anxieties. We identify at our own peril with the camera's gaze.

Another example of a purposeful camera operating in *Psycho* without the gaze of a predetermined character takes place just after the famous shower murder. A close-up of the dead Marion (Leigh) alone in her motel room is the point of departure for a tracking shot that leaves the bathroom, traverses the bed, pauses to glance at the newspaper containing the stolen money, and then looks out the window to the house where Norman Bates (Anthony Perkins) can be heard shouting, "Mother! Oh, God, Mother! Blood, blood!" Silverman has described this shot as essential to the complex system of suture, keeping the narrative going after we have lost our heroine. We identified with her in the shower, even though the camera frequently threw us back into the Imaginary by letting us experience the murder from several points of view, from that of the victim, the victimizer, and even the showerhead. The extent of our complicity in the murder becomes clear when the camera becomes the only "living" thing in the bathroom. Silverman describes the tracking shot that closes momentarily on the stolen money as the promise that the narrative will continue. "What sutures us at this juncture is the fear of being cut off from the narrative" (Silverman 1983, 212). To satisfy us, the shot continues out the window to the house from which Norman appears, the next object with whom we can identify. Spectators at a screening of *Psycho* are so hungry for suture that they do not rebel against a film that not only implicates them in murder and voyeurism but even exposes its own workings. What they eventually get for their trouble is narrative closure, the comforting statements of a psychiatrist who exorcizes their terror with the authority of science. Critics who scoff at Dr. Richmond's pronouncements call attention to the transgressions into which we have voluntarily let ourselves be sutured as well as to the final shot of Anthony Perkins, which once again makes us identify with a missing Other. This Absent One (Oudart 1978) is the same unattached camera that has brought us into the terror of the Imaginary and that is completely outside the psychiatrist's discourse.

The most interesting theoreticians of suture, such as Dayan and the *Screen* critics Stephen Heath (1981) and Colin MacCabe (1976/1985), have expanded the concept to include a Marxist perspective, particularly Althusser's reading of Lacan. In "Ideology and Ideological State Apparatuses (Notes To-wards an Investigation)" (1971), Althusser argues that ideology represents the Imaginary relationship of individuals to their material conditions. The system of suture, relying on a complex technology manipulated by a major commercial industry, is responsible for "naturalizing" the ideology articu-lated artificially but persuasively by this industry. These critics frequently succeed in demystifying Hollywood movies, revealing the psychological means by which they bind audiences to their cultures. The *Screen* critics may have made the most important contributions to film theory in the 1970s and 1980s. Despite the fact that their prose often rendered their writings inac-cessible to many film students, their theoretical positions have been ex-tremely influential, providing critics with the basis for many of the most thorough readings of American films.

We should point out that many critics who rely on psychoanalysis do not depend exclusively on the semiotic methodologies of Lacan, Metz, and Althusser. Stanley Cavell (1981b) and Robin Wood (1986) use Freud for quite different purposes, but both have worked psychoanalytic thought into original and convincing readings of specific films. Some of the most interest-ing work in the 1980s examined the relationship between film and the "dream screen," an area researched by Bruce Kawin (1978), Marsha Kinder (1980), and Robert Eberwein (1984). Jane Feuer (1982) has even appropri-ated dream analysis into a study of the Hollywood musical. Critics such as Robert B. Ray (1985), Dana Polan (1986), and Patrice Petro (1989) have transcended the rigidly theoretical orientations of the *Screen* and *Cahiers* critics, taking from them what they need while writing scrupulously re-searched film histories. These critics have adopted a pluralistic approach based primarily in the deep structures identified by Freud, Althusser, and Lévi-Strauss.

Shortly after the publication of the first edition of this volume, psychoana-lytic film study in the university came under sustained attack in two books, Noël Carroll's *Mystifying Movies: Fads and Fallacies in Contemporary Film Theory* (1988) and David Bordwell's *Making Meaning: Inference and Rheto-ric in the Interpretation of Cinema* (1989). The writers took different paths to their complementary conclusions. Carroll, who holds doctorates in both philosophy and cinema, was once a strong advocate of the value of psycho-analysis for film studies but has since rewritten earlier essays to eliminate all psychoanalytic methodologies; Bordwell, for many years the *capo di tutti capi* among cinema scholars, seems to have read every book and article in film studies since the 1960s while developing an approach that he calls a "histori-cal poetics." Ultimately, both Carroll and Bordwell urge film scholars to abandon or at least to rethink radically the dominant strains of psychoanalytically inflected film study, dubbed "SLAB theory" (as in *S*aussure, *L*acan, *A*lthusser, *B*arthes) by Bordwell.

For Carroll, the central metaphors of film theory can be refuted by appeals to simple empirical logic; the idea that "films are dreams" fails to account for the chatting, changing of seats, and visits to the concession stand that are an inevitable part of audience activity in movie theaters. For Bordwell, psychoanalysis is one of several inefficient machines for manufacturing dubious meanings in films primarily for the sake of professional advancement for university professors. Bordwell advocates a return to the archives for more film history along with a more traditional mode of formalist analysis based on small-scale theorizing rather than on the "grand theory" of the "SLAB" discourses.

Carroll's and Bordwell's books by no means marked the end or the beginning of debates about psychoanalytic film theory, but they did draw attention to a number of issues that had dwelled at the margins of film study. The *Chronicle of Higher Education* subsequently contributed to the popularization and polarization of these debates by interviewing feminist theorist Tania Modleski for a response to Bordwell's arguments (Heller 1990). The *Chronicle's* article suggests that the debate about psychoanalytic theory in film study was part of a political struggle, placing feminists against male formalists, and advocates of "SLAB theory" against the small group of historians that Bordwell praised in the conclusion to his book. The debate became even more intense when Lloyd Michaels, the editor of *Film Criticism*, devoted an entire issue of his journal to Bordwell's *Making Meaning* (Michaels 1993), inviting several film scholars to take issue with Bordwell's critique.

Perhaps coincidentally, perhaps not, debates over the application of psychoanalysis to film study during the early 1990s took place at the same time that a number of scholars moved away from film theory and toward more historical and/or text-oriented work. In the most dramatic defection from the community of psychoanalytic film study, Ben Brewster, a translator of Christian Metz and Louis Althusser and an early member of the *Screen* collective, embraced early cinema research over theory (Brewster 1998). Constance Penley, one of the founders of the feminist/psychoanalytic film journal *Camera Obscura* and an assiduous student of psychoanalysis's heuristic potential for both avant-garde and mainstream film, has written extensively on the phenomenon of underground writing by devotees of television's *Star Trek* (Penley 1995). And with the publication of *Babel and Babylon* (1991), Miriam Hansen effectively changed her job description from film theorist to film historian. It may also be no coincidence that these transformations within academia took place at roughly the same time that the *New York Review of Books*, a journal on the cusp of academia, was publishing Frederick Crews's hyperbolic attacks on Freud and the entire Freudian project.

But psychoanalytic film study in the university has not died. And the publication of scholarly books by Lear (1998), Buhle (1998), Forrester (1997), and Rand and Torok (1997), not to mention Daniel Menaker's novel *The Treatment* (1998), may indicate that Freud's reputation is on the rise once again as we enter a new millennium. Many film scholars in the 1990s have used Freudian and post-Freudian methods to close-read individual films, to explore changes in a culture's zeitgeist, to map the inner world of a director, and even to psychoanalyze film scholars. As we have suggested, however, critics no longer feel the need to declare their allegiances to psychoanalytically informed methods because so many of these methods have become standard components in the analyses of films. The work of Adam Knee provides an especially striking example of the almost invisible presence of psychoanalytic concepts within the mainstreams of film criticism. In his work on science fiction films, Knee (1996) uses the Freudian notion of displacement to explain how cold war anxieties were transformed in the plots of science fiction films at the same time that he specifically disavows his reliance on psychoanalytic readings.

Whether psychoanalysis is acknowledged, unacknowledged, or partially acknowledged in film study today, one thing is certain: psychoanalytic film criticism has long ceased to be monolithic. Freud's theories were being radically revised and rethought long before his ideas entered the armamentarium of the film critic. Although some strains of psychoanalysis may have led film theorists to dead ends, they have also been responsible for inspiring theorists to develop alternative paradigms. This is surely the case with Mulvey's "Visual Pleasure and Narrative Cinema" (1975). Mulvey relied on Lacanian models to characterize the gaze of the camera as patriarchal, scopophilic, and sadistic, while her understanding of the fetish was High Church Freudian. Although Mulvey's argument held sway for several years during the 1980s, it eventually provoked a number of responses, including some of the most important books in the field of psychoanalytic film study. Gaylyn Studlar's *In the Realm of Pleasure: von Sternberg, Dietrich, and the Masochistic Aesthetic* (1988) argued that the films of Josef von Sternberg invite a masochistic rather than a sadistic order of spectatorship. Mulvey's reading of Hitchcock's *Vertigo* in terms of Scottie's (James Stewart) sadism and voyeurism was extensively addressed in a book on Hitchcock by Modleski (1988), who found striking parallels between the mad Carlotta, wandering the streets looking for her dead child, and the deranged Scottie, wandering the streets looking for his dead Madeleine. For Modleski, the spectator of films such as *Vertigo* may be constructed, as Mulvey suggests, from a male point of view, but this same spectator "is as much 'deconstructed' as constructed by the films, which reveal a fascination with femininity that throws the masculine identity into question and crisis" (Modleski 1988, 87).

Mulvey's implication that spectators are strictly gendered as they watch mainstream films has been called into question by Carol Clover (1992), who found that slasher films from *The Texas Chainsaw Massacre* to *Halloween IV* invariably invite an audience made up largely of adolescent boys to identify with "the final girl" as she does battle with a male killer. Steven Cohan (1993) and Peter Lehman (1994) have problematized Mulvey's notion that the object of the cinematic gaze is exclusively female by analyzing films in which the bodies of male stars such as William Holden, Fred Astaire, and Richard Gere are held up for display and fetishization. We also should mention Linda Williams's *Hard Core: Power, Pleasure, and the "Frenzy of the Visible"* (1989) and D. N. Rodowick's *The Difficulty of Difference* (1991) as sophisticated responses to what were once the mainstreams of psychoanalytic film theory represented by Mulvey's contributions.

Perhaps the most striking developments in film theory of the 1990s occurred in the area of "gender studies," a term first developed to expand the field of women's studies and that has since grown to encompass gay and lesbian, or "queer," theory as well as much of what is now called "men's studies." One of the more fortuitous projects of gender studies has been the rejection of the notion that masculinity is monolithic and clearly defined in popular media. As Frank Krutnik (1991) has argued, in the hard-boiled genres associated with film noir, the masculinity of actors is regularly undermined, even that of actors such as Robert Mitchum, Humphrey Bogart, and Kirk Douglas, whose maleness in other kinds of films is seldom if ever questioned. Dennis Bingham (1994) has found elements of bisexuality lurking beneath the carefully sanitized public image of James Stewart. Thomas DiPiero (1991) has even gone so far as to suggest that *any* display of masculinity is essentially hysterical. Many of these theorists have relied on classically psychoanalytic works such as Joan Riviere's "Womanliness as Masquerade" (1929/1966) as well as texts such as Judith Butler's *Gender Trouble* (1990) to argue that masculinity, like femininity, is essentially a masquerade and that no one is *essentially* male or female. As she suggests in the title of her book *Male Subjectivity at the Margins* (1992), Kaja Silverman has looked to the boundaries of what is normally considered male—for example, the work of the gay German director Rainer Werner Fassbinder—to rethink concepts of spectatorship and the masquerade.

One strength of Silverman's work from the early 1990s was her attention to issues of race and class, both of which have been neglected in much psychoanalytic theory, including recent gender-based revisions of Freudian and Lacanian paradigms. E. Ann Kaplan (1994) also has undertaken the project of applying psychoanalysis to films such as *Imitation of Life* and *Home of the Brave* in which issues of race are central. Nevertheless, film scholars interested in the emerging discipline of cultural studies regularly charge that psychoanalysis is inevitably ahistorical and blind to race and class. We might see the cultural studies critique as coming from the political left and Bordwell's call for a return to formalist analysis as coming from the political right. Certainly, these developments can be credited with reducing the influence of Lacan for film study in the 1990s. Still, one of the most widely quoted theorists among cinema scholars in the 1990s is Slavoj Zizek, who has rediscovered and perhaps even resuscitated Lacan for the discipline.

Paradoxically, Zizek is less interested in the interpretation of films than in the critique of self-consciousness since the Enlightenment as practiced in the works of Kant, Hegel, Derrida, and other Western philosophers. He sees Lacan's writings as an appealing response to, and continuation of, this tradition. Unlike many scholars who have wrestled with Lacan's shifting vocabularies, Zizek has embraced the French analyst's system because of its supple playfulness. Although Zizek, originally from Yugoslavia, claims that he arrived at Lacan through the works of Louis Althusser, many of his writings seem apolitical. Furthermore, his references to cinema tend to illustrate theories about the intricacies of subjectivity and consciousness that ultimately take the reader back to discourses on Hegel. Zizek (1994) has explicitly acknowledged that he uses references to films and popular culture only to make his ideas accessible to his readers as well as to himself. But for many who practice film theory, Zizek's readings of films as diverse as *Blade Runner* (Zizek 1993), *Psycho* (Zizek 1992), and *Short Cuts* (Zizek 1994) have been especially rewarding. If nothing else, the importance of Lacan for Zizek shows that the discipline of film studies has become sufficiently established to have experienced the rise and fall as well as the reappearance of psychoanalytic paradigms.

In the remaining chapters, we hope to illustrate the potential for pluralism in psychoanalytic film criticism. We have based our work in this section on concepts derived from a wide array of clinical psychoanalytic writings. Like the clinician who adopts different theoretical positions according to the needs of different patients, we have used a variety of perspectives to illuminate a number of markedly different films. While the Lacanian approach has produced intriguing accounts of film as process, we are more interested in the films themselves—in their texts, subtexts, themes, and characters. Each film invites different degrees of explanatory power from a variety of theoretical formulations. In addition, we have fleshed out our interpretations by drawing on relevant information that may not always be grounded in psychoanalysis. For example, we frequently quote statements that the filmmakers have made to interviewers, realizing that the artists themselves may have much to tell us, even if we do not subject their statements to psychoanalytic interpretation.

The methodological problems encountered in the psychoanalytic understanding of film are essentially no different from those problems intrinsic to applied psychoanalysis as a whole field. This love child of clinical psychoanalysis and practical criticism has always been viewed ambivalently by critics within psychoanalysis itself, especially those most skeptical of Freud's work. Clinical psychoanalysis is anchored to the here-and-now phenomena of transference and resistance and to the associations of a patient who attempts to put aside his or her psychological censor and say whatever comes to mind. Applied psychoanalysis runs the risk of losing its way once the consulting room has been left behind. From Freud's earliest forays into applying psychoanalytic ideas to art, literature, and biography, these difficulties have regularly been acknowledged. Artistic creations, books, letters, and diaries have been used as substitutes for free associations and transference material. As Freud himself realized, these substitutes could in no way compare with bona fide clinical data from the consulting room. He noted in *Moses and Monotheism:*

> I am very well aware that in dealing so autocratically and arbitrarily with Biblical tradition—bringing it up to confirm my views when it suits me and unhesitatingly rejecting it when it contradicts me—I am exposing myself to serious methodological criticism and weakening the convincing force of my arguments. But this is the only way in which one can treat material of which one knows definitely that its trustworthiness has been severely impaired by the distorting influence of tendentious purposes. It is to be hoped that I shall find some degree of justification later on, when I come upon the track of these secret motives. Certainty is in any case unattainable, and moreover it may be said that every other writer on the subject has adopted the same procedure. (1939, 27)

Joseph Coltrera (1981), in an elegantly argued essay on the methodological problems inherent in the application of psychoanalytic principles to biography, emphasizes that Freud never claimed that his proposed reconstructions regarding historical figures such as Leonardo (Freud 1910) were meant to be taken as historical facts. Critics tend to overlook, Coltrera argues, that Freud's only claim was psychoanalytic validity rather than historical truth, a critical methodological distinction. From Freud's point of view, the Leonardo construction was best viewed as a *Romandichtung*, a fiction intended to be understood as analogical rather than as a reconstruction of the artist's actual childhood. "The point is really that Freud's construction is a psychological explanation meant to facilitate understanding and is not an empirical statement about causality. As such, it is valid in that it is consistent within the conditions of its premises; but one may fairly ask whether it is useful as a biographical construction" (Coltrera 1981, 19). Like the semioticians, we make no claims that we have arrived at the definitive reading for each of the films we will discuss. We are more interested in providing a variety of means for making sense of particular characters or particular movies. More specifically, our emphasis is on how clinical psychoanalytic theory can illuminate the text, the characters, and the subtext of a film as well as the way in which an audience experiences it. Following Coltrera, our aims are to be psychoanalytically valid and internally consistent.

CHAPTER 8

Play It Again, Sigmund: Psychoanalytic Approaches to the Classical Hollywood Text

Film writers often express bewilderment when faced with *Casablanca*'s enduring appeal or, more specifically, with their own slightly embarrassed affection for the Warner Bros. relic. "Some undefinable quality in *Casablanca* seems to make it better with each viewing," write Don Whitemore and Philip Alan Cecchettini (1976, 197) in their essay on Michael Curtiz, the film's prolific director, while Harvey Greenberg (1975) calls his essay on the film, "If It's So Schmaltzy, Why Am I Weeping?" (79–105). In his famous gloss on the film, Andrew Sarris (1968) throws up his hands and calls it an "accident," singling out the work of "lightly likable" Curtiz as "the most decisive exception" to his own application of the auteur theory (176). Richard Schickel (1973) is probably not alone in declaring *Casablanca* to be his favorite film, even while acknowledging its limitations as "a somewhat better-than-average example of what the American studio system could do when it was at its most stable and powerful" (114).

Even the film's cult status is problematic. *Casablanca* reached the full flowering of its culthood only in the 1960s when Harvard students regularly attended Humphrey Bogart film festivals during finals week (Hoberman and Rosenbaum 1983, 30). More than a decade before *The Rocky Horror Picture Show*, *Casablanca* initiates would shout, "The Germans wore gray; you wore blue" and "Is that cannon fire, or is it my heart pounding?" along with the projected images of Rick (Bogart) and Ilsa (Ingrid Bergman). *Casablanca* needed twenty years to become a cult item, perhaps because it did not take the usual route to that status. The film's success within the industry—it won the 1943 Academy Award for best picture—was helped in no small part by the Allied invasion of North Africa, which preceded the film's initial Thanksgiving Day release by only three weeks, and the meeting two months later of Roosevelt and Churchill in Casablanca, which took place during the film's national release. Later, more "conventional" cult films like *The Rocky Horror Picture Show*, *Pink Flamingos*, and *Eraserhead* had much less auspicious beginnings. How can a popular wartime melodrama, promoted initially as home front propaganda, continue to find such devoted audiences?

For Umberto Eco (1985), the key to *Casablanca* is its "glorious incoherence," producing enough contradictory material to support new meanings for each new audience. Not only does *Casablanca* contain several archetypal situations, writes Eco: "When all the archetypes burst in shamelessly, we reach Homeric depths. Two clichés make us laugh, but a hundred clichés move us because we sense dimly that the clichés are talking among themselves and celebrating a reunion" (11). If Eco had watched more products of the American studio system, he might have observed that, from the beginning, Hollywood films have constituted a never-ending reunion of archetypes. We suspect that the film's appeal has more to do with its ability to tap into the unconscious concerns that regularly drive audiences to the movies. Psychoanalytic theory provides the royal road to understanding the American cinema, especially the films of the "classical" period that began with the acceptance of sound films around 1930 and culminated about the time that *Casablanca* was made in 1942. But since psychoanalysis in the last two decades has ceased to be a monolithic method for film scholars, we have adopted a pluralist approach, deploying a range of psychoanalytically based methodologies around *Casablanca*. We share Donald Kaplan's view (1988) that "a psychoanalytic reflection on any phenomenon is incisive to the extent that it employs more than one dimension" (283). The "star" performances of Bogart and Bergman, the music of Max Steiner, the romantic tensions of the narrative, even the film's handling of American politics can be approached through psychoanalytic thought. We are as interested in illustrating the heterogeneity of psychoanalytic film theory as we are in offering a thorough reading of *Casablanca*.

Oedipus in North Africa

A wealth of oedipal material awaits anyone wishing to interpret the film along classical Freudian lines. Like Sophocles' Oedipus, Rick Blaine is an outcast from his home country. At least in the fantasies of Captain Renault, Rick may have fled because he killed a man. In fact, as Greenberg has observed, Renault's speculations have a great deal of oedipal resonance. Because Rick will not divulge the real reasons that brought him to Casablanca, Renault wonders if Rick absconded with the sacred money of the church, or if he ran off with a senator's wife. Renault says that the romantic in him would like to believe that Rick took a man's life. Rick's response that he left the United States because of a combination of all three can be read as more than a glib piece of verbal sparring. Greenberg (1975) suggests that "the sacrosanct stolen treasure [is] the wife of a preeminent older man; her husband is the one murdered—and by the love thief. Thus, the essence of the 'combination' of offenses is the child's original desire to kill his father and possess his mother" (88). (Contrast Greenberg's interpretation with Richard Corliss's (1974) ingenious but nonpsychoanalytic reading of Rick's response to Renault's interrogations about his past: "But if Rick's sardonic evasion doesn't tell us about his past, it does portend future events which only he can control. The film's climax will have Rick 'abscond with the church funds' by selling his saloon to Ferrari, 'run off with a Senator's wife' by leaving Casablanca in the company of the coquettish representative from Vichy, and 'kill a man'—Major Strasser" [110].)

In *Casablanca*'s one flashback, Rick's Parisian interlude with Ilsa can be understood as the realization of this desire to possess: the blissful union with an all-good, nurturing woman completely unattached (at least in Rick's mind) to a threatening paternal figure. We doubt that any other actress could have fulfilled this role as completely as Bergman, whose screen image projects the most desirable qualities of mother and lover. Whenever Curtiz's camera closes tightly on her face, she appears to be as innocent and nurturing as she is sensual and compliant. Rick was not the only one who responded to Bergman's face in this way. Seven years later, the American media worked itself into a frenzy when Bergman bore a child out of wedlock to the Italian film director Roberto Rossellini. After years of being portrayed in the press as the ideal wife and mother, Bergman so thoroughly flouted American mythology that she was denounced on the floor of the U.S. Senate, and a legislator in the Maryland state senate introduced a bill to condemn *Stromboli* (1950), Bergman's first film with Rossellini (Leamer 1986, 206–7).

Rick's flashback at first depicts a dreamlike paradise of prewar, pre-oedipal Paris, where he toasts Ilsa amid romantic settings. The lovers exist in a passionate romance that comes to its inevitable end with the arrival of Nazi armies, a nightmare image of the jealous, castrating father. Ilsa, as nurturing mother, has even warned Rick that the Nazis will take special pains to look for him. Later on, in Casablanca, Rick enters a more advanced stage of development when he comes face to face with Ilsa's husband, Victor Laszlo (Paul Henreid). Although some viewers may consider Henreid's Laszlo something of a cold fish, there is no question that the intellectual freedom-fighter manages to be more heroic, virtuous, understanding, and forgiving than the most idealized hero of romance fiction. Laszlo's entrance presents Rick with a typical conflict of the oedipal phase male child: Does he challenge and attempt to *replace* his rival, or does he renounce the forbidden object of his love and *identify with* his father?

Unlike Oedipus, whose entire, undisplaced story has never really been taken up by Hollywood, Rick negotiates the oedipal phase with success. He renounces his incestuous object of desire and identifies with father/Laszlo, Ilsa's original mate, whose place Rick could only temporarily usurp. When he guns down the evil Nazi Major Strasser (Conrad Veidt), Rick kills the principal enemy of his father surrogate, thereby becoming a man himself. Alternatively, we might also regard the killing of Strasser as the displacement of Rick's oedipal rage onto a less stigmatizing individual, but one who is nevertheless associated with the pre-oedipal disruption brought about when the Nazis entered Paris. Like Ernest Jones's Hamlet (Jones 1964), Rick is an indecisive, passive individual until he renounces mother, identifies with father, and kills the villain. In terms of the film's political/oedipal nexus, Rick's decision to fight the Nazis corresponds with his realization that the paradise he has lost was an illusion sustained only by a refusal to acknowledge the existence of father. *Casablanca* resembles most Hollywood films of the classical period in its highly involving combination of myth and politics with melodrama.

Another aspect of Rick's dilemma is that the man he wishes to replace is a figure of unimpeachable integrity and virtue, thus complicating his efforts to integrate his positive regard for Laszlo with his murderous wishes toward him. Similarly, it is difficult for Rick to view this forgiving and saintly leader of the Resistance as a castrating, punitive father who will retaliate against Rick for his lustful yearning toward Ilsa. Because of Rick's difficulty in integrating these representations of himself and Laszlo, he appears to regress from the task of integration that accompanies the oedipal phase. The result is a splitting of the father figure into the benevolent Laszlo on the one hand and the sadistic Major Strasser on the other. Even the ultimate identification with Laszlo at the end of the film comes at the expense of his murdering the disavowed and split-off "bad" aspects of the internalized father. One could argue, then, that resolution of the oedipal conflict is only partial since a true integration of "good" and "bad" aspects of the father has not been achieved.

"Here's *Looking* . . ."

These classically psychoanalytic readings of *Casablanca* are not typical of the theoretically oriented writing that currently fills most academic film journals. By isolating the characters as case histories, this application of Freudian theory casts the viewer in the role of ideal analyst, completely free from any countertransferential reaction to the images on the screen. As Shoshana Felman has observed, the actual experience of texts puts the reader/viewer in the dual position of analyst *and* analysand, attempting to take charge of the story at the same time that the story takes charge of its consumer (1982, 7). Lacanian alternatives to more conventionally Freudian readings, however, have shortcomings of their own. In particular, they tend to ignore the specificity of actors: Bogart and Bergman, for example, are virtual texts unto themselves, and any thorough reading of *Casablanca* must account for how their star qualities, their histories, and the meanings encoded in their cinematic images transform the films in which they appear. We undertake a Lacanian reading of *Casablanca* to illustrate one of several possibilities in the application of psychoanalysis to the Hollywood cinema.

A major similarity between Lacanian analysis and classical psychoanalysis is an attention to oedipal triangles. Raymond Bellour, especially eminent among Lacanian theorists, has suggested that the Oedipus story is the masterplot of all Hollywood narrative (Bergstrom 1979, 93). A Lacanian reading of *Casablanca* would focus not so much on the dynamics among the characters, but on how the viewer is contructed within a larger discursive field that positions the viewer in a circuit of looks.

Richard Corliss (1974) has suggested that "Rick's famous toast—'Here's looking at you, kid'—can be read as meaning, 'Here's trying to look into your soul, kid, to figure out who you really are'" (111) A Lacanian would have no difficulty conceptualizing the remark somewhat differently—in terms of how the viewer is positioned through Rick, its surrogate. So long as the audience is in control of the gaze, looking at Ilsa but also at everyone else, it need not acknowledge the range of differences that the classical realist text works so hard to conceal. The possibility that someone or something may be looking at Rick raises the possibility of difference and the possibilities of castration that mark the entry of the subject into the symbolic register. As long as the viewer controls the look, the viewer can safely remain in the imaginary register where there is no difference between itself and mother.

Significantly, when Rick's looking toast is interrupted in the flashback by Gestapo loudspeakers, Sam (Dooley Wilson) warns him that the Germans will soon be in Paris, "and they'll come lookin' for ya." The invading Nazis represent not only the castrating father but the castrating gaze of the Other as well. The coincidence of the Nazi's arrival with the baffling disappearance of Ilsa leaves Rick as an object in someone else's plot, his previously ominiscient gaze reduced to a limited point of view. Similarly, the oedipal trajectory that leads Rick to the reconciliation with Laszlo and the elimination of Strasser restores him to a sense of origin and identity offered by the father. Rick surrenders Ilsa to Laszlo only after he has completely regained control over the narrative, writing a script to which he holds the only copy. As a result, he has regained the right to utter the looking toast once again. His newly found father, unjealous and supportive to a fault then tells him, "This time I know our side will win." (For this reading, we have relied most heavily on Colin MacCabe's 1976 account of *American Graffiti*.)

"... At You, *Kid*"

As we noted in chapter 7, Lacan's theses on the look and castration have been central to feminist film theory. According to Mulvey and the many writers who have followed in her wake, the patriarchal order of the Hollywood cinema provides two basic solutions to the fear activated in men by women's implied threat of castration: either the woman's lack is part of her punishment for some wrongdoing, usually sexual transgression, or she is fetishized so that a portion of her body (breasts, hair, face, legs, bottom, even the entire body) becomes important enough to compensate for the lack of a penis. Male viewers can then derive voyeuristic pleasure from a cinema that provides fetishized images of women to exorcise male castration anxiety.

The plot of *Casablanca* consistently emphasizes Ilsa's sufferings, carefully placing the burden of transgression on her more than on the two male leads. Both Rick and Laszlo have loved her unselfishly, but she has been unfaithful to both. Although the film finds narrative means for repressing her guilt, justifying her conduct in terms of a legitimate romantic dilemma, there is no question that she has deceived Laszlo through her silences as much as she has deceived Rick by concealing her marriage. As Greenberg has observed, the

Laszlos' decision to keep their marriage a secret to protect Ilsa from the Gestapo makes little sense (1975, 97). It would be just as logical for the Germans to interrogate a lover as a wife, perhaps even more logical. Ilsa has no real justification for not telling Rick of her marriage, just as she has no sound reason for concealing her affair with Rick from the infinitely forgiving Laszlo.

Significantly, Ilsa's sins are those of omission rather than commission, resulting from the absence of, rather than from too much, voice. Kaja Silverman (1988) has extended Mulvey's work on the role of women in the visual register to a study of woman's cinematic voice. Classical cinema does not stop at confining women to an interior function in which a male-driven diegesis stops so that the woman may be exhibited. In addition, the voice of a woman is seldom given the powerful position of voice-over narration. With rare and problematic exceptions such as Hitchcock's *Rebecca* (Modleski 1988), extradiegetic voice-over is inevitably male in Hollywood films, including *Casablanca*, which begins with voice-of-god newsreel intonations. The subordination of women in patriarchal cinema has even been extended to situations in which heroines are literally deprived of voice, the most often cited examples being *The Spiral Staircase* and *Johnny Belinda*. Appropriately, at the end of *Casablanca*, Ilsa has little to say to either Rick or Laszlo, her lying silences giving way to a continuing renunciation of voice after the crucial love scene "up a flight" in which she asks Rick to do the thinking—and speaking—for both of them.

The film's sadistic treatment of Ilsa takes a substantial toll in tears, often revealed in tight close-ups of her fetishized face. The almost kittenish sexuality of Ingrid Bergman's face, combined with her country girl wholesomeness, provides the male viewer with an object of aesthetic perfection sufficient to ward off the thought of castration. Significantly, the first Mount Rushmore close-up of Bergman in *Casablanca* takes place as she listens, lost in thought, to Sam playing "As Time Goes By." Mulvey points out that musicals are typical of the patriarchal order of classical cinema in their careful separation of performance numbers—often featuring scantily clad females—from the diegesis so that the viewer can divert all his attention to contemplating the female body. A risk always inheres in interrupting the diegesis, however, because the involving flow of the story effectively stops. Mulvey mentions the "buddy movie," in which the eroticized display of women is entirely eliminated, as one solution to this problem. The long close-up of Bergman's face as she listens to the music is perhaps an even better solution, integrating a moment of fetishized display into a diegetic sequence that prepares us for her climactic reunion with Rick.

"Moonlight and Love Songs
Never Out of Date"

Until recently, little work had been done on the importance of background
music in classical cinema. Claudia Gorbman (1987) is one of a handful of critics who have productively brought psychoanalytic theories of music into film
study. She cites a number of Lacanian writers such as Guy Rosolato (1974)
and Didier Anzieu (1976) who have associated music with a pre-oedipal stage
in which the child lives in a "sonorous envelope" dominated by the pleasingly
rhythmic sound of the mother's heart and, later, by the soothing, musical
sound of her voice. By promoting "benign regression" to the blissful time before the child senses that it is separate from the mother, movie music "invokes the (auditory) imaginary" (62). Furthermore, music is free from
linguistic signification and other kinds of representation, and thus it can more
easily bypass defense systems and penetrate to the unconscious. Gorbman accepts the arguments of Metz and others that dominant cinema attempts to
erase the signs of its workings by casting the viewer as the subject rather than
the object of the film's enunciation. "Music greases the wheels of cinematic
pleasure by easing the spectator's passage into subjectivity" (69).

Although she does not dwell on *Casablanca*, Gorbman devotes an entire
chapter to the work of Max Steiner, the prolific composer who scored *Casablanca*, in order to illustrate "classical Hollywood practice" (70–98). After
establishing a set of principles for the use of music in Hollywood films (invisi-
bility, "inaudibility," signifier of emotion, narrative cueing, continuity, unity,
and the legitimate violation of any principle at the service of another),
Gorbman undertakes a discussion of "the epic feeling" of music that is especially relevant to *Casablanca*'s appeal. Remarking on the anthropological
analysis of musical elements in rituals that bind together human communities, she notes how music in classical cinema can be put to use for the
pleasureful creation of the sense of commonality. The most obvious example
of this phenomenon occurs diegetically in *Casablanca* when Laszlo leads the
non-German patrons of Rick's Café Américain in a performance of "La Mar-
seillaise," eliciting patriotic tears even from the sexually collaborationist
Yvonne (Madeleine LeBeau). The extradiegetic music in *Casablanca* is carefully constructed to elicit appropriate emotions from the audience, usually
the same emotions that the film attributes to Rick. The most striking example is the string orchestra voicing of "As Time Goes By" that is superimposed
on Sam's diegetic piano after Rick insists on hearing the song. Steiner's music
intrudes "inaudibly" at this crucial moment in order to seal us into
Rick's—and the film's—Imaginary, the pre-oedipal scenes in Paris before the

arrival of the Germans and the departure of Ilsa.

Citing an example from Steiner's score for Curtiz's *Mildred Pierce* (1945), Gorbman has written, "[T]he appropriate music will elevate the story of a man to the story of Man" (81). Much the same can be said for the long close-up of Bergman as she listens to "As Time Goes By." With Ilsa's face providing additional validation, Sam's interpretation of the lyrics elevates a love song to a song about Love. Surprisingly, the song was almost excised from the film. "As Time Goes By" was written by Herman Hupfeld and first performed in 1931 in the Broadway show *Everybody's Welcome*. The song is central in the unproduced play on which the script for *Casablanca* is based. When shooting was completed and an edited print of the film was presented to Steiner, he objected to the use of "As Time Goes By" and asked to substitute a song of his own composition. Steiner said that he disliked the song, but he also knew that he would surely benefit from the royalty checks if his own song became popular. At first, producer Hal Wallis consented to cut the scene in which Bergman requests "As Time Goes By" by name and to shoot additional scenes in which Steiner's song would be used. But since Ingrid Bergman had by this time received a severe haircut for her role in *For Whom the Bell Tolls*, Wallis realized that a new scene with Bergman and Wilson was out of the question. Steiner subsequently learned that he would have to work with the original scene and hence with "As Time Goes By" (Behlmer 1982, 172–74).

It is as difficult to imagine *Casablanca* without "As Time Goes By" as it is to imagine the film with Ronald Reagan, Ann Sheridan, and Dennis Morgan, the leads who were, according to legend, originally projected for the film (Corliss 1974, 104). In its day, the film gained an element of nostalgic power by using a well-known song. Many in the audience may have associated a romantic experience of their own with the music, thus adding an additional level of audience subjectivity to Ilsa's, and later Rick's, reaction to the song. For a moment, Ilsa *and* the viewer return to an earlier time, but the audience has the larger-than-life face of an idealized maternal figure to facilitate regression to a moment even more pleasant than the one recalled by the heroine. Although more contemporary audiences are likely to associate the song with the same era as the film, the music is still crucial in associating the experience of the film with a simpler, more romantic era to which the viewer can blissfully return.

The Death of the Author/Father

One of the consequences of feminist film theory's ascendancy is an undermining of "la politique d'auteur," which observed its thirty-fifth anniversary in American film criticism in 1998 (Sarris 1988, 66). As we pointed out in chapter 7, the auteur theory of cinema associates each film with the singular artistic vision of the director. But by characterizing classical cinema as funda- mentally a transmitter of the dominant (patriarchal) ideology, feminist theory has "decentered" film study, granting less importance to the director's vision. One of the more intriguing developments in feminist criticism involves postauteurist approaches to male directors, such as Modleski's study of Hitchcock (1988), as well as to female directors, such as Kaja Silverman's work on Liliana Cavani (1988).

We doubt, however, that there will ever be much interest—among male or female critics—in reading *Casablanca* across the life and career of its direc- tor, Michael Curtiz. In fact, the life of Curtiz is a dark continent on the globe of film history, especially considering his voluminous filmography. According to Kingsley Canham (1973), Curtiz began his career by working on more than thirty silent films in Hungary. In Sweden, Germany, Italy, France, and Austria, he directed more than twenty films before leaving for the United States in 1926. Between 1930 and 1939, when he was most productive, Curtiz directed forty-four films for Warner Bros. Before his death in 1962, he had signed nearly a hundred American films, many of them considered genre masterpieces: *Captain Blood, The Sea Hawk, Yankee Doodle Dandy, Mildred Pierce, Mystery of the Wax Museum, The Kennel Murder Case, Ad- ventures of Robin Hood, Angels with Dirty Faces*, and *Casablanca*. Perhaps the sheer bulk of his output has intimidated scholars who might search out the signature and obsessions of a less prolific director.

Nor is enough known of Curtiz's life to anchor the kind of psycho- biographical studies that directors such as Chaplin (Weissman 1987), Hitch- cock (Spoto 1983), and Welles (Leaming 1986) have inspired. Even the substantial bibliography on *Casablanca* makes no connection between the expatriate American Rick Blaine living in exotic Morocco and the expatriate Hungarian director living in exotic Hollywood. It should be remembered that directors like Chaplin, Hitchcock, and Welles have provoked psychobio- graphical speculation not so much because of the stories they told but be- cause of stylistic eccentricities that separate them from the Hollywood mainstream. From the beginning of his Hollywood career, Curtiz learned to submerge himself in the conventions of his craft, *intentionally* becoming the transmitter of ideology that antiauteurists have sought to find in all Holly- wood directors. But the willing denial of his own subjectivity, especially in terms of his identity as a Central European Jew, suggests interpretive possi- bilities. So does Curtiz's long working relationship with Errol Flynn: after di- recting Flynn in twelve films, Curtiz and the actor ended their relationship in

1941 during the filming of *Dive Bomber*, possibly because of statements that Curtiz made about Flynn's estrangement from his wife, the French actress Lily Damita (Whitemore and Cecchettini 1976, 195). Curtiz made an international star of Damita while directing her in three films just before his departure for the United States in 1926. Curtiz's self-effacing style may explain the absence of critical speculation on Curtiz's handling of the Rick-Ilsa-Laszlo triangle just one year after he severed his own triangular relationship with Flynn and Damita.

America Dreaming

Psychoanalytic thought is relevant to the political gambit of *Casablanca* as well as to the film's expression of American ideology. We are most concerned here with the extent to which the "dream work" of the film censors or displaces political material that may be intrinsic to American mythology but incompatible with the war effort. Michael Wood (1975) was one of the first critics to observe that Rick is portrayed as a patriot ultimately dedicated to fighting the Nazis even though he represents a well-established breed of American heroes who are more suspicious of compromising entanglements with friends than with the predictable hostility of enemies. According to Wood, the well-known poster of Bogart as Rick, "staring into the middle distance, a glint of heroic self-pity in his eyes . . . is a picture of what isolation looks like at its best: proud, bitter, mournful, and tremendously attractive" (24–25). When Rick gives over Ilsa to Laszlo, he tells her "where I'm going, you can't follow," and yet if Rick and Laszlo now share the same cause, why is it suddenly so essential that she follow Laszlo and not Rick?

In categorizing it as "*the* most typical" American film (5), Ray (1985) uses *Casablanca* as a tutor text for what he calls the "formal paradigm" of classical Hollywood as well as the "thematic paradigm" that addresses the conflict between isolationism and communitarian participation. Thematically, the film is typical in its appropriation of an official hero (Laszlo), who stands for the civilizing values of home and community, and an outlaw hero (Rick), who stands for ad hoc individualism. Although these mythological types at first appear to be at odds, they share a common purpose by the end, just as they do in films as generically dissimilar as *Angels with Dirty Faces*, *Shane*, and *Star Wars*.

Formally, *Casablanca* abundantly illustrates the importance of a number of "centering" techniques that create the illusion of realism while at the same time disguising the complex apparatus that lies behind each shot. Although Ray does little to develop a Lacanian reading of *Casablanca*, he relies on the

Lacanian-inflected writings of the *Screen* critics such as Stephen Heath (1981) and Colin MacCabe (1976/1985) to develop his thesis of the formal paradigm. Ray, however, is less interested in castration and the gaze than he is in adapting psychoanalytic thought to a theory of how "the concealment of the necessity for choice" (32) determines the sequence of shots in classical cinema. By pinning the viewer's consciousness to Rick's, most of what happens takes its logic from his point of view. The fusion of Rick and audience begins when we first catch a glimpse of nothing more than Rick's hand as it signs a check. Ray observes that the shot is striking, however, because the hand comes directly out of our space, as if a (right-handed) viewer were to reach up to the screen and sign the check himself (54). Shortly after this shot, Rick's entire body emerges from the viewer's space as he walks into the frame to confront the arrogant German who tries to force his way into Rick's inner sanctum.

Earlier, Rick's personal magnetism seems to exert an inexorable pull on the camera. After being told that "everyone comes to Rick's," and having seen the sign with his name above the café door, the viewer enters the café and is drawn steadily toward Rick as the camera drifts always to the left in tracking shots. The camera pauses first to close in slightly on Sam, allowing him to be centered against a background that loses a bit of the definition that deep-focus cinematography usually grants to establishing shots in this and most other classical Hollywood films. The tracking shots eventually arrive at Rick's table, where he is engaged in a solitary game of chess. The audience is then granted its first good look at Bogart's face, a visage that *Casablanca* cultists have called "existential."

Immediately after Rick/Bogart has received the film's first star close-up, *Casablanca* yields its first shot from the point of view of a single individual at nine minutes into the film when Rick observes the German's attempt to enter. For most of the remainder of the film, Rick's point of view is privileged, and his face and body are centered. This is especially true when he is in the company of Victor Laszlo, who is regularly consigned to the margins of the frame throughout the sequence when Rick first encounters Ilsa and her husband at the café. All of this seems natural because the film has so carefully constructed the viewer as a secret sharer in Rick's vision. The innumerable choices that are made in the production of each shot in *Casablanca* are concealed by our acceptance of Rick as our surrogate. Although few would find reason to object, the film chooses to deprive Laszlo of a flashback, not to mention an "As Time Goes By" to unite him with Ilsa.

Ray points out that this concealing of the necessity for choice also governs the thematic paradigm in *Casablanca*. The film invites the audience to identify with Rick rather than Laszlo, even though official American wartime sentiments are consistently voiced by Laszlo. Rick regularly insists upon unmediated self-interest ("I stick my neck out for nobody," "I'm the only cause I'm interested in"), a position that Ferrari (Sidney Greenstreet) explicity identifies with a discredited American tradition: "My dear Rick, when will you realize that in this world today isolationism is no longer a practical policy?" *Casablanca* is typical of classical Hollywood in its willingness to confront, at least initially, its audience's most important concerns, in this case, "the deep-seated, instinctive anxiety that America's unencumbered autonomy could not survive the global commitments required by another world war" (Ray 1985, 91). Although the film never puts Rick in a position to retract his innately American reluctance to give up his independence, he ultimately does exactly what Laszlo—and the U.S. government—would have him do. Of course, Rick's decision to fight the Nazis is related to his feelings for Ilsa rather than a change of heart about being an isolationist. By means of this well-established Hollywood pattern of reconciliation, *Casablanca* could support the war effort without disturbing the foundations of American myth. (Although the film suggests that Rick *has* been actively involved in political causes, the ideological work of the script tries hard to cast him as an apolitical loner. We might attribute Rick's rejection of commitment to screenwriters Julius and Philip Epstein and his activism to the film's other credited screenwriter, Howard Koch. While the Epsteins dutifully created Hollywood myth, Koch was a committed leftist.)

Ray acknowledges a debt to an essay by Charles Eckert (1974a) on the gangster melodrama *Marked Woman* (1937). Eckert argues that the corrupt, conspicuously affluent movie gangsters of 1930s' Hollywood provided depression-era audiences with ideologically sanctioned objects for the hatred that they felt toward the rich. Although Eckert uses Marxist and Lévi-Straussian methodologies to uncover the class conflict and mythmaking that is submerged in *Marked Woman*, he also is interested in how Freudian concepts of the dream work can explain the process by which politically proscribed class hatred is *displaced* into familiar conventions of melodrama. We should also mention Brian Henderson's (1980–81) work on John Ford's *The Searchers* (1956) that reveals how the film's dialectic on the assimilation of Indians is also a displacement for American concerns about black integration in the months just after the "separate but equal doctrine" was struck down by the U.S. Supreme Court in 1954. Although Eckert and Henderson have both cautioned against reductive readings that ignore the overdetermined polysemy of Hollywood films, they have both acknowledged the importance of psychoanalysis in their larger semiotic project.

Casablanca's audience must never be asked to choose between Rick and Laszlo because everything in the film has prepared them to choose Rick, who represents the rejection of America's involvement in world politics. Instead, the film relieves the audience of the necessity of choice by displacing the film's political conflict into melodrama, where familiar emotions overwhelm ideas. To the extent that films resemble dreams, the film's latent political content—should America risk entering the war?—appears in the manifest content as whether or not Rick should help Laszlo. Although Victor Laszlo is always in Rick's shadow, he stands for the values of the father *and* the prevailing American belief in 1942 that freedom is worth fighting and dying for. By censoring the theme of American reluctance to give up its autonomy, the film spares the audience the agony of siding against the values of the father, condensing the oedipal resolution to another shared experience between Rick and the viewer.

What Makes a Cult Film?

Once a cult is established, it can often sustain itself by means of its own inertia. After becoming a camp item in the 1960s, *Casablanca* attained the status of a classic by an alternative system of canon-building. Usually, a work of art finds its validation in the academy. Even though popular film is currently an accepted subject of university study, films like *Casablanca* need not establish their importance by impressing faculty committees as masterpieces. Although it existed briefly as a television series during the 1955–1956 season (McNeil 1980), *Casablanca* did not become a fetish object until the Rick/Bogie poster became popular and Woody Allen subsequently wrote the play (and movie) *Play It Again, Sam* (Hoberman and Rosenbaum 1983, 30). Allusions regularly appear in films and TV shows; in the same week in 1988, for example, audiences could see a full-dress, five-minute parody of *Casablanca* as the dream of Bert Viola (Curtis Armstrong) in an episode of *Moonlighting* and, on *Miami Vice*, a lovable crook attempting to corrupt Detective Sonny Crockett (Don Johnson) by telling him that a suitcase full of contraband was their "letters of transit," prompting Crockett to reply, "This is *not* the beginning of a beautiful friendship." Canonized in 1998 by the American Film Institute as second only to *Citizen Kane* as the greatest American film, *Casablanca* is certain to continue as a universal signifier of romantic love, doing the right thing, and painful sacrifice.

As for the qualities that made *Casablanca* a cult film and have made its appeal "never out of date," we can point to all the psychologically resonant

aspects of the film discussed in this chapter. Probably the most crucial ingredients in the film's success are 1) the star presence of Bogart and Bergman; 2) the subliminal but nostalgically potent music, both diegetic and extra-diegetic; 3) the satisfyingly resolved oedipal material; and 4) the reassuring message that the American outlaw hero can survive even World War II. This last message may seem specific to the film's 1943 audience, but movies have been unusually successful in keeping myths alive, and when reconfigured for the era of Reagan, Bush, and Clinton, these myths can be more vital than ever. *Star Wars* was the first in a cycle of "disguised westerns" that have achieved extraordinary popularity by reviving the outlaw hero/official hero plot. Since then, *Beverly Hills Cop I* and *II, Top Gun, Rambo III,* and the *Lethal Weapon* films have recycled the same basic myth with enormous success.

As for the audience today, *Casablanca* has an extra level of appeal, offering a sense of control to repeat viewers. Just as "As Time Goes By" eased the 1943 viewer into a nostalgic Imaginary, the film itself now grants the viewer "benign regression" to a lost moment when right and wrong were clear-cut and going off to war could be a deeply romantic gesture.

CHAPTER 9

3 Women: Robert Altman's Dreamworld

In the fairy tale "Beauty and the Beast," a young girl must leave her father and journey to a remote kingdom where she is to live as the captive of a beast with a hideous aspect. Although she finds the monster terrifying, she also discovers him to be a most gracious host. He treats Beauty with kindness and consideration, catering to her every whim. The peace is disrupted only when the Beast makes his daily visit to Beauty to ask in vain if she has grown to love him. Finally, as the creature lies dying, Beauty acknowledges her love for him, and he is transformed into a handsome prince. If this enchanting fairy tale were a dream recounted by a young girl blossoming into womanhood, one might well speculate that the dream revealed the young girl's unconscious attempts to reconcile her anxieties about male genitality. The dream could be interpreted as a wish fulfillment in which the violent fantasies connected with the male genitals prove to be totally unwarranted, and sexual fears are conquered through the healing power of love.

3 Women (1977), written and directed by Robert Altman, can best be understood as another variation of the same dream, in which a girl verging on womanhood attempts to come to terms with the phallic aspect of male sexuality and to forge a new identity as an adult woman. Altman has in fact said that the movie came to him in a dream. His statement is useful because the film defies understanding when approached on the secondary-process level of rational, left-hemispheric thinking. *3 Women* becomes comprehensible only when viewed at the primary-process level of condensation, displacement, symbolization, dramatization, and the mobile cathexes of the dream work described by Freud (1900), Sharpe (1937), and others.

In interviews conducted just after the release of *3 Women* (Ciment 1977; Jameson and Murphy 1976), Altman seemed genuinely uninterested in explaining the meaning of his film, a position consistent with his reputation as a thoroughly intuitive artist. In fact, Pauline Kael (1973) has said that Altman, more than any other film director, is able to make contact with his unconscious. In a conversation with Roger Ebert, Altman explains how *3 Women* took shape. "I dreamed of the desert, and I dreamed of these three women, and I remember that every once in a while I'd dream that I was waking up and sending out people to scout locations and cast the thing. And when I woke up in the morning, it was like I'd *done* the picture. What's more, I *liked* it. So I decided to do it" (Ebert 1978, 197). In an interview with the French critic Michel Ciment (1977), Altman also explains that the three women of the film's title were originally Millie, Pinky, and a synthesis of the two. However, the third woman, Willie (played by Janice Rule), originally an unnamed barmaid at the saloon visited by the other two women, developed into a central character as the production got under way. Nevertheless, the statements that Altman has made about the film suggest that a good deal of what appears on the screen in *3 Women* comes directly from his dream. The film is best understood as the dream of a young girl who is regressing from the pressures of fully sexual adulthood into a strange trio of roles that parody various stages of womanhood as well as familial relationship paradigms. Obviously, we are aware that what appears to be a young girl's dream originated in the mind of a middle-aged male. We could speculate here on how Altman and his coworkers may have reworked primary-process material—at least as it was reported by Altman—in order to create a viable cinematic work of art. On the other hand, it is just as important to emphasize that we do not hope to analyze Robert Altman or his dream. As we stated in chapter 7, our goal is to apply the methodology of dream analysis to a film, all the while realizing that this application is analogical rather than literal.

Regardless of how thoroughly Altman transformed images that originated in his sleep, few other filmmakers have been quite so successful in translating their dreams directly into cinema, a medium that always reflects the personalities of producers, writers, editors, cinematographers, set designers, costumers, composers, and actors as well as directors. It is all the more remarkable that Robert Altman has made this extremely personal film since Altman is more likely than most directors to let his coworkers inscribe their own visions onto his films. Consequently, critics have difficulty generalizing about Altman's "style" or "vision." As Robert Self (1985) has written,

Altman's films actually challenge notions of the self by which critics have conventionally established the identity of an auteur. Self singles out Altman's *Buffalo Bill and the Indians, or Sitting Bull's History Lesson* as "the most postmodern of Altman's films" because it "asserts the difficulty of any unified, coherent identity of the self" (1985, 10). A similar claim can be made for *3 Women*, the film Altman made immediately after *Buffalo Bill*. Psychoanalytically informed dream interpretation provides a privileged view of the shifting selves in *3 Women*, and it may help us understand the ambivalences in Altman's work that make the conventional auteurist signature difficult to find.

According to Sharpe (1937), the dream work can transform the dreamer's self into different characters in the dream. For example, murderous wishes may be attributed to another character as the dreamer herself innocently observes the murderer in action. In *3 Women*, three aspects of the dreamer's psyche are represented by three different female characters; and with the freely shifting cathexes of the primary process, the dreamer seems to be identified with different portions of her psyche at different times during the dream. As befits an action so closely tied to the secret wishes of the unconscious, the film frequently appropriates the dream work to tell its story.

3 Women was shot in and around Palm Springs, California, and the action begins at the "Desert Springs Rehabilitation and Geriatrics Center," where Pinky Rose (Sissy Spacek) has just taken a job. The childlike Pinky is immediately fascinated by Millie Lammoreaux (Shelley Duvall), an employee at the spa who is assigned to show Pinky the ropes. Although the two never become friends in the usual sense, Millie quickly wins the complete adulation of Pinky, who calls her "the most perfect person I've ever met." Millie does little to court Pinky's devotion, but since she is looking for a roommate, she invites Pinky to move into her apartment. Millie, whose ambition is to become the next Breck girl, has decorated her apartment primarily in yellow to match her car and her wardrobe. But none of the residents of the singles complex where Millie lives share Pinky's intense feelings about Millie. In fact, the building is called Purple Sage Apartments, and the other singles keep Millie as far away as yellow is from purple on the color wheel.

The third of the three women, Willie (Rule), paints bizarre murals (created for the film by Bodhi Wind) (plate 31) and wears dark eye makeup, gray clothes, and a floppy sun hat. She is the taciturn wife of Edgar Hart (Robert Fortier), owner of the Purple Sage Apartments and "Dodge City," a hangout with a bar, a shooting range, and a motorcycle track. The three women represent three aspects of the evolving self of the young female dreamer: Pinky is the prepubertal latency child, idealizing and emulating the women around

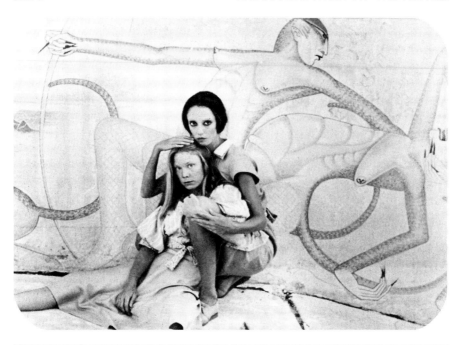

PLATE 31.   Sissy Spacek and Shelley Duvall posing on the set of Robert
Altman's *3 Women* (1977). Note Bodhi Wind's mural. Lion's Gate Films. The Museum of Modern Art/Film Stills Archive.

her, unconcerned about the perils of genital sexuality; Millie represents the
genital and sexually alive adolescent/young adult who is not afraid of her own
lust; and Willie, who is pregnant throughout most of the film, symbolizes the
maternal, "postgenital" woman who has successfully negotiated male sexuality and is now preparing to take the consequences of the genital consumma-
tion. The highly permeable boundaries of these three figures are evident in
the role reversals between Pinky and Millie halfway through the film and
among all three at the end. The interchangeability of the three characters is
reflected in the fact that both Millie and Pinky are Texans named Mildred
and in the obvious *Klang* association between the names Millie and Willie.

At the opening of the film the tension between the women and male
genitality is clearly drawn. Behind the titles and atonal theme music we see
Willie's gray-robed figure at the bottom of a dry swimming pool painting
strange, colored creatures with tails and angry faces. Three of the figures
have female breasts: two of them embrace, while the third, like Willie, is
pregnant. The fourth figure is male with a large, dangling penis. The same
four figures recur in at least two other murals that Willie has painted, includ-

ing the one in the swimming pool at Purple Sage Apartments, each time with a male figure represented as a satanic and victimizing creature.

Basically, the film has two parts. Although it often hints at the darker aspects of part two, particularly by means of Gerald Busby's ominous music, part one primarily invites us to laugh at the two naïve young women: Millie (Duvall) attempts to live out the two-dimensional life presented in slick magazines for women, while the infantile Pinky (Spacek) merely marvels at the other's sophistication. As Altman laughingly suggested to Jameson and Murphy (1976), the middle half of the film could be the antics of a comedy team, Pinky and Millie, who would later appear in a sequel "Pinky and Millie Move to the City." There is even a kind of Laurel and Hardy pathos in the quaint, slightly sad manner in which they mimic a mother/daughter relationship.

The film's second part takes on a completely different tone as it opens with Pinky's attempted suicide and the overtly symbolic rescue by Willie. The compelling image of the pregnant Willie shivering alone in the pool after Pinky has been removed establishes her as a new mother figure for Pinky. Altman himself has said that in this swimming pool scene, Pinky "floats in the water like a fetus in the maternal belly" (Ciment 1977, 14). Altman follows the image of Willie in the pool by cutting to Edgar walking down the stairs and then panning to the overbearing male creature that Willie has painted on the bottom of the swimming pool. This sequence is crucial because it unites Willie's painting with the characters of the drama at the same time that the film shifts away from satirical comedy and focuses on the conflict between Edgar and the three women. Henceforth, the women begin turning away from traditional roles as natural mothers, daughters, and wives toward an artificial family unit without a threatening male presence. Before reaching this goal, the women act out an elaborate drama in which sex, death, and birth are intimately related.

After introducing Willie and her paintings at the beginning of the film, Altman cuts to still another swimming pool, this one full of water, the symbol of birth, death, and renewal that recurs throughout the film. In the pool, aged bodies are guided about by much younger ones. It is a world dominated by pairs: the old people at the spa generally move in groups of two while the staff pairs off into sets of twins. Peggy and Polly, the blonde identical twin sisters, are only slightly better matched than the inseparable Doris and Alcira—one Chinese, the other Chicano. Both are dark and members of minority groups. Equally compatible are Dr. Maas and Vivian Bunweill, whose intimacy seems more than professional and who jointly supervise operations at the spa with equal degrees of officiousness. (To carry this device further, we later learn that Edgar was once Hugh O'Brian's "stunt double" on the set of television's *Wyatt Earp*.)

Into this world come two women who would seem to be another matched set. Millie even tells Pinky, "You're a little like me," as the newcomer is fitted for a bathing suit. But the girls are not headed for the closed self-sufficiency of the other dyadic units. Although Pinky idolizes Millie, she is always on the outside looking in, as when we first see her staring transfixed at Millie from behind a plate-glass window. Millie, too, is an alienated individual with no family and no prospect of a satisfying relationship either with the medical students, who barely tolerate her presence at lunch, or with the denizens of Purple Sage, who openly make fun of her.

Although Millie and Pinky may not be a perfectly matched pair, they consistently play at being big sister and little sister. Typically, when they first arrive at Dodge City, Millie expresses dismay when Pinky foreshadows her eventual symbolic death and rebirth by crawling in and out of a womblike te-pee and then miming her own hanging at a prop gallows. (Pinky had earlier forewarned her suicide attempt by dunking herself in the geriatrics center pool, again to the embarrassment of Millie.) Throughout the first half of the film, the sisterly relationship continues peacefully until the crisis of Edgar's late-night arrival with Millie. Pinky experiences something akin to the primal scene when she sees the two preparing to make love, but she receives the shock of a childhood nightmare when Millie rejects her for not being an adult: "You don't smoke, you don't drink, you don't do anything the way you're supposed to." In the context of the first half of the film, the remark is mildly amusing because it once again reveals the irony in Pinky's adulation of a woman who so completely misunderstands adulthood. Within the dream logic of the film, however, Millie's forbidden tryst and her outburst give substance to the worst fears of Pinky, who then attempts suicide.

Up to this point, despite the clear establishment of Pinky and Millie as doubles, their differences have been well-drawn. Pinky is the wide-eyed little sister in awe of her classy older sibling. Millie is engrossed in efforts to involve herself with young doctors but occasionally deigns to offer Pinky some worldly advice. No competitiveness exists between them, because they are in entirely different leagues. So far, so good. But with the arrival of Edgar in the bedroom, a major shift occurs. Edgar clearly symbolizes the father since he is married to the maternal (and pregnant) Willie. The oedipal crime of incestuous sexuality is shared by both Millie and Pinky, and as a result Pinky loses her innocence. Her introduction to male genitality and to sexuality is associated with the violation of an unspeakable taboo. While the manifest content of the film/dream indicates that Pinky attempts suicide because of her rejection by Millie, the latent content seems to be that she is punishing both herself and her double (Millie) for the oedipal crime of incest, just as Oedipus blinded himself. This portion of the film nicely illustrates the dream mechanism of dramatization, in that the dreamer, Pinky, can attribute incestuous sexual wishes to another character in the dream, Millie, rather than to herself.

After Willie rescues Pinky and becomes a new mother-surrogate, Millie undergoes a radical transformation as she seeks to do penance for her involvement in Pinky's trauma. We know the extent of Millie's transformation when she flatly rejects a sympathetic doctor who makes personal overtures outside Pinky's hospital room. Millie would have leapt at such an opportunity only the day before, but now her powerful desire to care for Pinky subsumes her previous longings. Her existence finally has a meaning greater than the one she created out of mail-order catalogs. She has found her true self in the role of Pinky's mother. Millie's selfless and guilt-ridden devotion to Pinky can be understood as an unconscious effort on her part to expiate her own guilt connected with the oedipal crime. Not only has she seduced father; she has almost killed off a female competitor in the process.

But when Pinky emerges from her coma, she first attempts to become Millie, even as Millie begins to mother her in earnest. The first thing that Pinky does upon awakening is disown her natural parents (Ruth Nelson and John Cromwell), whom Millie has summoned from Texas. At the top of her lungs she screams, "They're not my parents" and "I'm not Pinky," driving her parents from her hospital room. Here we see the family romance fantasy dramatically enacted. As Blum (1969) points out, when the child feels that his parents do not conform to the idealized and unconditionally loving roles he has attributed to them, he decides that his real parents, who have these features, have merely arranged for his adoption by those persons who claim to be his parents. This defense protects the child from the narcissistic injury of discovering that his parents do not love him in the way that he feels he should be loved. Moreover, Blum emphasizes how the genital/oedipal phase of development brings new significance to the family romance fantasy. By imagining himself to be a guest in the house of foster parents, the child eliminates the incest taboo in his relationship with his parents since biological relatedness is not an issue. The Oedipus myth, of course, would be the classical example of the family romance fantasy. Pinky's first words upon awakening from her coma, then, serve to announce the full flowering of this fantasy. Moreover, her words herald her passage from the pregenital quiescence of latency to the *reawakening* of the genital/oedipal phase of development associated with the onset of adolescence.

Back at the Purple Sage, Pinky takes over Millie's bed, her diary, her car, and her former lover, Edgar. In fact, Pinky is a great success at realizing the goals that eluded Millie: we see her at poolside attended by the same men who earlier scorned Millie. Meanwhile, Millie has changed from the impatient, disapproving big sister into the overindulgent, worried mother trying desperately to provide happiness and security for her child. Millie even loses her job to protect Pinky; she echoes Pinky's actions by rejecting *her* surrogate parents at the spa, Dr. Maas and Vivian. Since Millie has not seen her natural parents since she was eleven, Pinky is now the single focus of her familial life.

Pinky, on the other hand, wishes actually to replace Millie and in no way returns her devotion. Similarly, she seeks to replace both Willie and Millie by taking Edgar as her lover. Now Pinky acts like a daughter only in her wish to compete with Millie and Willie for the affection of Edgar, the father who by condensation is married to both Millie *and* Willie in Pinky's mind. Pinky's success in the competition for Edgar leaves Millie confused and humiliated, while Willie appears completely vanquished: after we see Pinky taking shooting lessons from an adoring Edgar (plate 32), who utters the prophetic line "I'd rather face a thousand crazy savages than one woman who's learned how to shoot," the camera pans to the empty swimming pool where Willie lies unconscious amid her paintings.

But Pinky cannot sustain her new role as the mother-vanquishing daughter, and after a bad dream she is again the insecure child asking to crawl into bed with Millie, whom she had earlier banished from the bedroom. At this moment, an intoxicated Edgar enters and announces that Willie is in labor. Neither of the women has any interest in Edgar now (Millie shouts, "Don't touch her" as he reaches for the cowering Pinky), and they both dash off to help Willie. They arrive just as Willie is giving birth, and Millie orders Pinky to go for help. Pinky, however, remains, watching while Millie attempts to deliver Willie's baby. After uttering what is perhaps the least encouraging series of lines ever delivered in the history of film to a woman in labor, Millie tells Willie that the baby is a boy and that it is dead. As Willie embraces the dead child, Millie sees that Pinky has not budged from her position outside the door. In a rage, Millie gives her the slap that should have gone to the newborn baby. After a brief period of trying to compete for men with the female rivals, Pinky has regressed to a phase of pregenital dyadic relationships in which she seeks to destroy baby brother in order to have sole possession of mother. Millie's displaced slap announces that Pinky has been reborn again, this time as the only child in the family.

The final scene of the film recalls the endings of Federico Fellini's *Juliet of the Spirits* (1965) and Ingmar Bergman's *Cries and Whispers* (1972), in

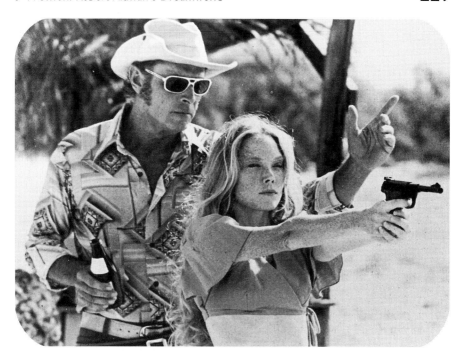

PLATE 32.   Edgar (Robert Fortier) teaching Pinky (Sissy Spacek) how to kill in *3 Women* (1977). Lion's Gate Films. The Museum of Modern Art/Film Stills Archive.

which the scene changes provocatively from darkness to broad daylight. The three women are now comfortably ensconced in roles that complete their previously unfulfilled characters. When men arrive at Dodge City to deliver Coca-Cola, a gum-chewing, girlish Pinky tells them, "I'll get my mom." We see her go after a gray-robed figure who is not Willie but a stern-faced Millie. She is wearing the same hat and makeup that once belonged to Willie, and her hair is now dark and straight in Willie's old style. On the porch of the house behind the bar sits a now grandmotherly Willie without her old makeup and with full, graying, wavy hair. Free at last from reticence, she says she has just awakened from "the most wonderful dream." In the last moments of *3 Women*, Millie appears to dominate the other two, and Willie gently urges her not to be so mean to Pinky (who is now called "Millie"). The three women show a sense of domestic contentment that none of them ever exhibited before. Edgar, by the way, has apparently died from a gunshot wound. Back in the bar, the Coca-Cola man remarks how odd it was that a man as expert with guns as Edgar should have died in what was presumably identified as a self-inflicted injury. The women, who are aloof to the personable young man, do not discuss the matter.

Although the script leaves the matter unresolved, it appears that all three women were involved in Edgar's death, just as all three were involved in the death of Willie's child. They all had something to gain by both deaths. Indeed, Edgar's and the child's deaths serve a similar purpose, and in the dream work of condensation, they could be the same event. Altman has said as much to a *New York Times* interviewer: "The death of the male child was as much a murder as the death of Edgar, and maybe they were the same thing. And I don't think it makes any real difference" (Demby 1976, 17).

Both Edgar and the child represent the threat of the male and his genitality, which stand between the three women and their desire to form a sexless, mother/daughter relationship. Phallic symbols abound in this context. Edgar is first introduced as a malevolent-looking fellow who draws his gun and pulls a snake from under a rock the moment he sees Millie and Pinky. Like the overbearing male figure in Willie's murals, the penis is Edgar's most characteristic possession, and he has sexual relations with all three women.

Nevertheless, the three women all act out their wish to be rid of Edgar and his phallus. Willie, who is closest to Edgar, makes sand paintings of snakes, which she ornaments with bullet holes. At Dodge City, when Pinky asks Millie to identify one of these works of art, Millie explains it in a most matter-of-fact way, although she suppresses the most important feature. "It's a sand painting with bullet holes," she says. Pinky too finds nothing unusual about the painting; in fact, she tells Willie that she likes it. Near the end of the film, after the Coca-Cola man leaves the bar, the camera comes to rest on the same sand painting hung on the wall as a kind of phallic trophy, indicating that Edgar and all other men in their lives have been effectively castrated. At one time or another, the film shows all three women on the shooting range putting bullet holes into the painted silhouette of a man, always in the phallic protrusion of the head. Edgar is further associated with phallic symbols when the sound of a rattlesnake accompanies the image of his face in Pinky's nightmare. Indeed, Pinky speaks for all three women when she expresses the irrational fear that she may have been raped while she lay unconscious in her hospital bed.

In a more general sense, Edgar represents the male-oriented values of the society in which the women are expected to live. Edgar and his companions (many of whom are policemen) ride dirt bikes, drink beer from bottles, fire pistols, and take or ignore women at their whim. Millie's ex-roommate,

Diedre, seems to be able to operate successfully in this world. Pinky, Millie, and Willie cannot. Pinky has a moment of success with men, which ends with her nightmare and her return to mother-Millie. Millie ineptly chases men through the first half of the film bur never with the determination with which she later indulges Pinky after the suicide attempt. Willie is so frustrated in her marriage that she never speaks, expressing herself only by drawing bizarre caricatures of herself and Edgar and by shooting bullets into phallic snake paintings. While the three women are multidimensional characters, none of the male characters are represented as anything more than part-objects. In other words, no persons are attached to the penises of the male characters, reflecting in part the anxiety and the inexperience in romantic matters of the pubescent girl dreaming the dream.

Only in the film's closing moments are the women free from male intrusions and able to lead the lives that, in one way or another, they were always seeking. Pinky has rejected her impossibly aged parents, who had brought her a plaque that urged her to become the traditional adult wife and mother. After also rejecting Millie's earlier conception of male-oriented adulthood, Pinky finds her true nature in perpetual childhood with not one but two mothers—one stern, the other beneficent. She will always have one mother to instruct her and another to indulge her. Altman's dream is unlike "Beauty and the Beast," however, because Beauty perseveres in the face of her genital anxiety to discover that men can be loving and three-dimensional human beings. Pinky retreats from the pressures intrinsic to fully genital, adult womanhood to a pregenital regressed state peopled with part-objects, symbolized by one good mother and one bad mother.

Millie has renounced her yellow-hued version of real life and accepted the role in which Pinky first cast her. In fact, Millie's brand of detached maternalism is something at which she had always excelled: at the spa, where the elderly occupants are treated like children, Vivian tells Pinky, "Millie's one of our best girls." Later, when she escorts Pinky's parents up the stairs to her apartment, she adopts a professional tone and tells them, "One hand on the rail." After Pinky's suicide attempt, Millie becomes more actively maternal, but she reverts after the death of the male child. As the stern mother figure in the film's final scenes, Millie first appears in the same place where we first saw Willie, but it appears that Millie is washing away Willie's paintings. Millie has not lost her eye for how a place should look, and in the women's new life there is no need for sublimating emotions by means of art.

As for Willie, she has given up art for dreams, and pleasant dreams at that. She has rid herself of a male child, of Edgar, and of all his rowdy friends, and her personality has opened up. Early in the film she developed an empathy with Pinky when the younger girl admired her sand painting. When Pinky tried to take her own life, Willie was the first one in the water to save her, and she followed Pinky to her hospital room. Obviously, Willie prefers Pinky to the male sibling whom Pinky helped destroy: she treats Pinky with tenderness in the final scenes.

As the film closes with Altman's camera panning away from the three women's house, we hear their voices as they conduct a day-to-day existence without men or threatening phallic symbols. In fact, in the film's final moments they have retreated into the womblike enclosure of the house behind the bar. Although they have apparently killed in order to achieve this peaceful existence, they do not seem to be haunted by guilt or disturbed by the fact that they will never know the love of the handsome prince. While the resolution of the dream may serve the proverbial function of guarding the dreamer's sleep, it may be the enemy of the dreamer's ultimate psychological growth. As Freud (1925a) reflected in a later addition to his dream theory, when the solution to a problem of life is attempted in a dream, the dream solves the problem in the form of an irrational childhood wish rather than in a constructive rational manner. It would be interesting to speculate about what forces turned a fairy tale into the modernist vision of sex roles that 3 *Women* represents. Altman has created a myth that speaks to cultural anxieties about the relations between the sexes as engagingly as it does to the secret wishes of the unconscious.

CHAPTER 10

Narcissism in the Cinema I: The Cinematic Autobiography

Early in Bob Fosse's film *All That Jazz* (1979), an aspiring actress (Deborah Geffner) tells director Joe Gideon (Roy Scheider): "I want so to be a movie star. Ever since I was a little kid, I wanted to see my face on the screen, forty feet wide." This comment is whispered into the ear of Gideon as she is in the process of seducing him in exchange for his casting her in his Broadway show. The exchange between them is a microcosmic glimpse of the narcissistic culture in which they and we live. Christopher Lasch (1979) has compellingly described this culture as one in which there is a worship of celebrity, a fascination and obsession with electronic images produced by the media, a ruthless pursuit of being "visible" and "recognized" despite the fact that no substantive content may exist beneath the image. Moreover, within the narcissistic society's corrupt value system, the supremacy and security of intimate personal relationships brings disillusionment as well as the exploitation of others for one's own ends.

One of the unusual characteristics of our self-absorbed contemporary culture is a pervasive kind of stage fright, an acute self-consciousness related to a fantasy of a ubiquitous audience (G. Gabbard 1979, 1983). As Lasch puts it, "All of us, actors and spectators alike, live surrounded by mirrors. In them, we seek reassurance of our capacity to captivate or impress others, anxiously searching out blemishes that might detract from the appearance that we intend to project" (1979, 2). This sense of always being "on," always performing, always trying to impress has led to an intense self-scrutiny and a rapidly increasing flow of confessional writing. Autobiographical and confessional statements now come not just from great writers and famous actors but from mere show business personalities who are far from being household names.

An even more recent phenomenon is the cinematic autobiography. The medium of film lends itself to narcissistic self-display even better than the novel or the play. What could be more exhibitionistic than to expose one's intimate and private self on the great silver screen and charge admission for people all over the world to bear witness to it? Fosse's *All That Jazz* and Woody Allen's *Stardust Memories* (1980) have successfully used the cinematic autobiography to depict the lives of two troubled artists. Bob Fosse directed and wrote *All That Jazz*, the portrayal of a self-destructive director-choreographer played by Roy Scheider. (Veteran screenwriter Robert Alan Arthur, who shares the film's writing credit with Fosse, died while *All That Jazz* was in production.) Even the sketchiest acquaintance with Fosse's own life reveals that the life of the film's protagonist, Joe Gideon, has striking parallels to Fosse's marriage with dancer Gwen Verdon, his work on the film *Lenny*, his near-fatal heart attack, and his own idiosyncratic contributions to musical comedy choreography, most notably the forward thrust of the female pelvis.

Woody Allen directed, wrote, and starred in *Stardust Memories*, a look at a few days in the life of Sandy Bates, a director struggling with life, love, success, and death while fighting those who condemn his new preference for making serious films instead of funny ones. Allen has denied that the film is directly autobiographical, but Pauline Kael (1980) has made the following observation: "Woody Allen calls himself Sandy Bates this time, but there is only the nearest wisp of a pretext that he is playing a character; this is the most undisguised of his dodgy mock-autobiographical fantasies." Andrew Sarris (1980), on the other hand, while hyperbolically calling *Stardust Memories* "the most mean-spirited and misanthropic film . . . in years and years from anyone anywhere," argues that the film is, in effect, not autobiographical enough because it omits any reference to the more sympathetic people who have cooperated with Allen on his films and because Allen, unlike Sandy Bates, does not appear at retrospectives of his films.

Both films owe an immense debt to Federico Fellini's 1963 masterpiece *8½*, as does Paul Mazursky's *Alex in Wonderland* (1971), which features Fellini himself in several scenes. Unabashedly autobiographical, Fellini's *8½* moves in and out of flashback and fantasy to explore the often funny, often tragic tensions between an artist's life and his work. Allen and Fosse have accepted a number of conventions from *8½* almost as if Fellini's film provided the obligatory framework on which an autobiographical movie must be constructed. All three films share the cataloging of lovers and wives, the caricaturing of critics and producers, the ceaseless searching for answers to grave problems, the idealizing of the protagonist's innocent youth, and the blurring of distinctions between illusion and reality. In one way or another, both *Stardust Memories* and *All That Jazz* appropriate the double ending of $8\frac{1}{2}$, in which Guido (Marcello Mastroianni), the surrogate Fellini, appears to die while at the same time participating in a fantasied procession of the people from his life, which culminates in a reconciliation with loved ones. We also should point out that all three films have made critics uncomfortable—each of them has received bitterly negative reviews from many quarters—and all three have provoked speculation about the psychology of their directors.

While writing and directing a movie about one's self may not be narcissistic in and of itself, the point we wish to emphasize is that both *All That Jazz* and *Stardust Memories* portray protagonists with severe narcissistic problems. These difficulties are presented differently in the two movies, and the vicissitudes of the protagonist's narcissism provide an absorbing experience for the viewer. We will systematically examine the narcissistic themes in both movies, comparing them and contrasting them with one another, and we will illustrate how both films reflect certain intrapsychic, interpersonal, and cultural phenomena.

Narcissistic Object Relations

Unlike the neurotics of nineteenth-century Viennese culture, narcissists are less likely to complain of symptoms and more likely to report difficulties in their interpersonal relationships. "The symptomatology of patients with narcissistic personality disturbances . . . tends to be ill defined, and the patient is in general not able to focus on its essential aspects, but he can recognize and describe the secondary complaints (such as work inhibitions or trends toward perverse sexual activities)," reports Heinz Kohut, who also describes "subtly experienced, yet pervasive feelings of emptiness and depression" as typical of the narcissistic personality (1971, 16). Otto Kernberg (1974) has identified the type as one who may be superficially smooth and effective in social situations but has serious disturbances in more intimate relationships. He may be extremely ambitious to the point of being grandiose, while at the same time he may feel inferior and extremely dependent on the applause and admiration of those around him to maintain his self-esteem. Furthermore, Kernberg states: "Along with feelings of boredom and emptiness, and continuous search for gratification of strivings for brilliance, wealth, power and beauty, there are serious deficiencies in [narcissists'] capacity to love and be concerned about others. This lack of capacity for empathic understanding of others comes as a surprise considering their superficially appropriate social adjustment. Chronic uncertainty and dissatisfaction about themselves, conscious or unconscious exploitiveness and ruthlessness towards others are also characteristic of these patients" (1974, 215).

Kernberg's words precisely describe Joe Gideon, the central character in *All That Jazz*. Gideon is a womanizing, chain-smoking, hard-drinking, pill-popping workaholic whose relationships with women are as loveless as they are exploitative. In one of the many fantasied conversations with Angelique, the Angel of Death (Jessica Lange), Gideon is asked if he believes in love. Gideon responds, "I believe in saying I love you. It helps you concentrate." And further, "It works," meaning he can manipulate the woman in question to obtain the desired results. In a later scene he is arguing with his girlfriend, Kate (Ann Reinking), about his infidelity. While Kate angrily expresses her jealousy and her love for Joe, Gideon approaches the interchange as though it were a scene in a play. Kate even coaches him on the reading of his lines to her while he utters stage directions for his statements as though sincerity were a quality that can be taught and affected. Similarly, when he engages in an otherwise serious confrontation with his ex-wife, the entire scene is choreographed, with Gideon making suggestions while his former wife works her frustrations into stylized gestures in the dance. When asked by his daughter why he does not get married, Gideon explains that he does not dislike anyone enough to inflict that form of torture on her.

Near the end of the film, when he lies close to death in the hospital, Gideon says to Kate that he really does love her. When Angelique questions his sincerity, he frankly acknowledges that he does not know if he meant it or not. He does not know "where the bullshit ends and the truth begins." In the elaborate fantasy production number before his death (plate 34), Gideon is introduced as a man who "allowed himself to be adored, but not loved." His success in show business, it is said, was matched by a dismal failure in his personal relationships. Even in his wake-up ritual each morning, he looks at himself in the mirror and says with a stylized gesture, "It's show time, folks." Life itself is theater where feelings are manufactured to "con" the "audience."

Fosse takes a split view of women in *All That Jazz*. On the one hand, the women around his protagonist are degraded, exploited sexual playthings, inspiring neither loyalty nor empathy. In contrast, the fantasied Angelique is portrayed as the ideal woman. Dressed in a virginal white wedding gown, she serves as Gideon's Horatio in his frequent internal dialogues. This splitting of

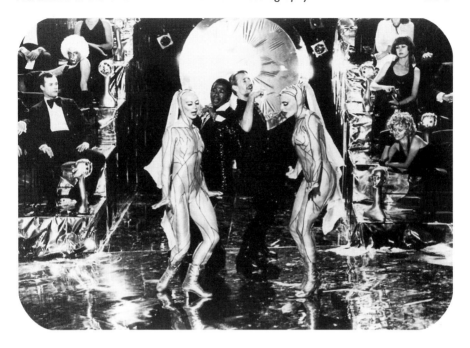

PLATE 33.   Bob Fosse's modernist, allegorical musical *All That Jazz* (1979). Columbia Pictures/Twentieth Century–Fox. The Museum of Modern Art/Film Stills Archive.

object representations is typical of the narcissistic personality, as Kernberg (1974) has pointed out. The wise, pure, understanding but seductive Angelique is the idealized representation of woman split off from the devalued sexual objects in external reality. By putting the scenes of Angelique in the setting of a dusty old attic, Fosse suggests that Angelique is an archaic internal object, that is, the good idealized mother who continues to haunt him and who is distinctly separate from the devalued bad maternal object representation. Appropriately, Angelique—like the Belle Dame Sans Merci—is also both lover and destroyer.

Gideon's devaluation of those about him does not know sexual distinction, however, as almost everyone in his world is viewed with contempt. This haughty disdain for others, so characteristic of the narcissistic personality, is strikingly revealed in his scene with the producers, composers, and writers of his Broadway show. Fosse makes these other characters into repulsive caricatures with no redeeming qualities. Similarly, in the initial read-through of the show, Gideon is definitively set off from the actors and other production

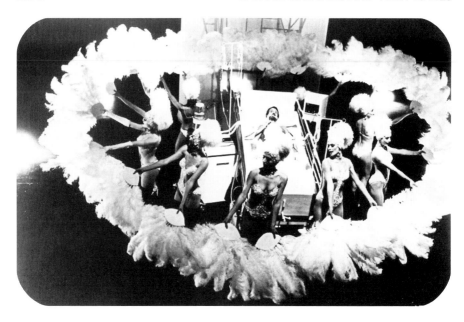

PLATE 34.   Joe Gideon (Roy Scheider) choreographs his own death in Bob Fosse's *All That Jazz* (1979). Columbia Pictures/Twentieth Century–Fox. The Museum of Modern Art/Film Stills Archive.

staff members. Apparently in the first throes of heart disease, Gideon's slightest gesture is greatly magnified by the sound track, while an entire roomful of people makes no sound whatever. When he is actually diagnosed as having heart disease and told that he must stay in the hospital, he contemptuously shouts, "What do doctors know?" He denies his condition and repeatedly disobeys the doctor's orders. Chronic and intense envy is often at the core of the narcissist. To avoid envying those around him, Gideon has to devalue the people with whom he comes in contact and to view them as having nothing to offer. The paradox is, of course, that he is then unable to have his needs met by other people.

Stardust Memories would seem to be based not only on *8½* but also on *Sullivan's Travels*, a 1941 American film written and directed by Preston Sturges. Surprisingly, Woody Allen has told Diane Jacobs (1982) that he saw Sullivan's Travels only after he had made *Stardust Memories* and Sturges's son sent him a copy. He was, of course, impressed at the "amazingly similar points" that the two films address (Jacobs 1982, 150). In *Sullivan's Travels*, Joel McCrea plays John L. Sullivan, a Hollywood director whose earliest films have been comedies with titles like *Hey Hey in the Hay Loft* and *Ants in*

Your Pants of 1939. However, at the outset of the film, he is in a struggle with the studio bosses, who seek to prevent him from making a serious film about human suffering called *Oh, Brother, Where Art Thou?* In particular, the opening scene of *Sullivan's Travels*, which begins with the final moments of Sullivan's film, strongly anticipates the beginning of *Stardust Memories*. However, in *Sullivan's Travels*, after some intense suffering of his own, Sullivan happily decides to return to making funny films. He also enjoys a traditionally romantic and wholesome relationship with a starlet played by Veronica Lake. Although some of the people he encounters wish to exploit him, in general Sullivan fits comfortably into his world. By comparison, we can see the extent to which the life and loves of Sandy Bates are involved with narcissistic problems.

The first scene in *Stardust Memories* shows significant differences between Allen's and Fosse's portrayals of narcissism. Allen's opening, which plays with both Bergmanesque and Felliniesque images, shows Bates sitting in a chillingly sterile railway coach among an assortment of misfits (plate 35). Another coach on a nearby track is filled with partying beautiful people, and Bates finds himself on the outside looking in. Hence we immediately see that Allen is much less defended against his envy and much more open to acknowledging that other people have good things that he lacks. Allen is more aware of shallowness in interpersonal relationships and much more inclined to poke fun at himself than is Fosse. In *Stardust Memories* a reporter even says that he is doing a piece on the shallow indifference of celebrities and would like to include Bates in the story. Later, Allen's protagonist participates in a brief and degrading sexual relationship with a female groupie, but he has an observer's distance about these affairs. He berates the groupie who wishes to go to bed with him by asking her if she really wants to engage in "mechanical sex with a stranger." When she responds that "empty sex is better than no sex," the film implies that he goes along with her to bed, anyway. The difference here is that Allen discourages the entire process and pokes fun at it, while Fosse seems deadly serious in his depiction of a strikingly similar scene. When the ambitious female dancer mentioned at the start of this chapter seduces Joe Gideon, Fosse uses nudity and romantic music to invite the audience to participate in the sensual pleasure of the encounter. Unlike Allen, Fosse asks the audience, at least its male members, to identify with the narcissistic pursuits of his protagonist.

Similarly, Allen is more inclined than Fosse to make a joke out of his character's pathological grandiosity. At several points in the movie he shows himself as a child, on one occasion putting on a cape (possibly a reference to the caped child who represented the young Guido in $8\frac{1}{2}$) and flying off like Superman. Later, we see the child performing magic tricks in a send-up of the posturing show business magician (Allen himself was deeply involved in magic as a child). The archaic grandiose self described by Kohut (1971) as central to the understanding of narcissism is here parodied in the embodiment of this self in a young boy with magical and superhuman powers. One of the clearest examples of Allen's ability to take comic distance from his own narcissism, and also one of the funniest lines in the movie, comes in response to a fan who asks Bates what he thinks of the criticism that his movies are narcissistic. Bates replies that if he were to associate himself with any figure from Greek mythology, it would be Zeus rather than Narcissus.

Although Fosse seems much more angry in his satirical attacks, Allen's protagonist shares some of Fosse's contempt for those around him. The multitudes of fans surrounding Sandy Bates at the Hotel Stardust are characterized by distorted facial features and inane chatter. Bates is portrayed as superior to all of his revolting and flawed admirers. Moreover, he feels him-

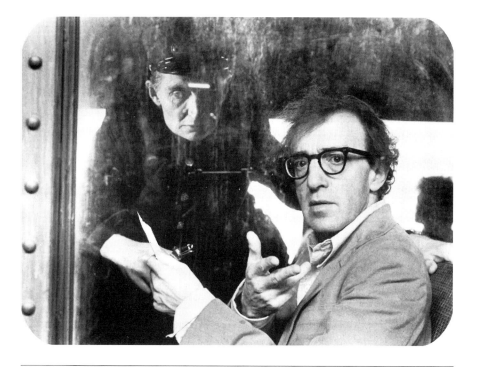

PLATE 35.   Woody Allen is on the wrong train (although both trains lead to the same place). *Stardust Memories* (1980). United Artists. The Museum of Modern Art/Film Stills Archive.

self a victim of the masses of people who want to use him or take something from him. On the one hand, Allen's Bates is committed to humanitarian concerns: he contributes to cancer research, committees to help Russian dissidents, and so forth. But it is his awareness of human suffering that makes so much of his success unsatisfying, and of course this awareness exists on a highly abstract level.

Sandy Bates shares Joe Gideon's problems with women, although, once again, Allen appears to have more compassion for his female characters than Fosse has for the women who pass through Gideon's life. Allen shows us a world where Bates's needs can never be met. He is in relentless pursuit of the perfect woman, although he is, by his own admission, "fatally attracted" to women for whom a sustained, stable relationship is impossible. As a result, his relationships with women begin with idealization, only to be followed by disillusionment. This dilemma, too, he approaches with humor. When he is asked if he really thinks that no such a thing as a perfect mate is possible or that good relationships do not depend on compromise, he replies that all good relationships are based on luck. Significantly, the film ends with Bates making what appears to be a sincere commitment to Isobel (Marie-Christine Barrault), the one woman in the film who shows the potential for a mature relationship. However, this scene turns out to be a film within a film, and as in *8½*, we are unsure to what extent it represents a satisfying end to the romantic problems that the film presents. Throughout most of *Stardust Memories*, Sandy is regularly reminded of how much he loved the hopelessly manic-depressive actress Dorrie (Charlotte Rampling).

The notion of celebrity is central to the culture of narcissism (Lasch 1979), and we will examine three different films in this context in chapter 11. In *All That Jazz*, Gideon wallows in the fringe benefits of his celebrity and enjoys it, but in *Stardust Memories*, Sandy Bates feels beleaguered by the multitudes of his fans as well as ill-served by the many people placed in his service by his financial success. When a policeman questions him about a gun for which he lacks a permit, Bates informs the policeman that an exception can be made in his case because he is a celebrity. The next scene reveals him sitting in a jail cell, showing Allen's ability to take an ironic distance from his sense of celebrity entitlement. Nevertheless, the many scenes in which Allen caricatures Sandy Bates's admirers seem to have upset many of his fans, perhaps because they construed these uncharitable portraits as personal attacks by Allen on them. Allen's treatment of his fans also prompted some of the most bitter attacks from critics and reviewers. In his conversation with Jacobs, Allen touched on the fan/celebrity question:

So many people were outraged that I dared to suggest an ambivalent, love/hate relationship between an audience and a celebrity; and then shortly after *Stardust Memories* opened, John Lennon was shot by the very guy who had asked him for his autograph earlier in the day. I feel that obtains. The guy who asks Sandy for his autograph on the boardwalk and says, "you're my favorite comedian" in the middle of the picture, later, in Sandy's fantasy, comes up and shoots him. This is what happens with celebrities—one day people love you, the next day they want to kill you. And the celebrity also feels that way toward the audience; because in the movie Sandy hallucinates that the guy shoots him; but in fact Sandy is the one who has the gun. So the celebrity imagines that the fan will do to him what in fact he wants to do to the fan. But people don't want to hear this—this is an unpleasant truth to dramatize. (Jacobs 1982, 147–48)

In spite of Allen's recognition of the troubling relationship between fan and celebrity, the celebrity phenomenon is primarily handled with irony throughout *Stardust Memories*. The movie focuses on the public's fascination with celebrity and how empty that obsession is, grounded as it is in fantasy. Real life and life in the movies seem to be indistinguishable; both are impressionistic flashes and images. In the film's final moments an old Jewish man says, "I don't understand. He makes a living doing this? I like melodramas and musicals."

The film's final scene finds Bates in an empty theater with an empty screen, again reflecting his own internal emptiness. The image is probably meant to emphasize the artist's ultimate isolation from the public, but it also may recall the sad clowns of silent cinema like Charlie Chaplin, who were often left alone at the ends of their films. As we have pointed out, Allen has not, in the final analysis, made a "serious" movie in the way that Fosse has. Allen pokes fun at himself throughout, and this humor distances him from self-indulgence and self-aggrandizement.

Midlife Crisis

Seen from the perspective of adult developmental phases, the protagonists in both *All That Jazz* and *Stardust Memories* find themselves facing midlife issues. As Kernberg (1980) has persuasively argued, the midlife crisis is largely a crisis of narcissism. One needs to come to terms with one's mortality, one's limitations, and one's inability to attain all that one wished to achieve in one's lifetime. One must mourn one's own death, mourn the death of loved ones, and overcome one's envy of the youth who have supplanted oneself. Individuals with narcissistic personalities typically experience a worsening of their narcissistic sufferings in midlife, becoming increasingly aware of their inability ever to satisfy themselves. As Kernberg describes it:

> The patient's relentless greed, his avid and yet destructive incorporation of what he envies, the consequent deterioration of his object representations, his wanting things because they are not his rather than because of their intrinsic value, all increase endless greed while impoverishing and destroying what he receives. This affects the narcissistic patient's relationship to his past and to the future. He longs for a new narcissistic refueling, but discovers that lasting satisfaction is never to be found; consequently he restlessly hopes for and yet fears the future. (1980, 136)

Furthermore, as the narcissistic individual reaches middle age he becomes envious of what he himself was in the past and has a profound sense of having lost what he once had.

Elliot Jaques (1965), in his classic study of the midlife crisis from a Kleinian perspective, points out that a shift characteristically occurs in artists and writers around the age of thirty-five to forty. While pre-midlife work tends to reflect an optimistic youthful idealism about the inherent goodness in man, the later, post-midlife work reflects acknowledgment of and resignation to the fact that hate and destructive forces exist as well. For Jaques, the successful resolution of the midlife crisis involves overcoming an early adult idealism built upon unconscious manic defenses against two inescapable aspects of human life: personal death and the existence of hate and destructive impulses within all of us. The depressive position must be worked through once again; that is, love and hate must be integrated into an ambivalent view of one's self and one's relationships.

In examining the narcissistic struggles of our two protagonists from the standpoint of the midlife crisis, considerable differences can be found. Allen's protagonist has dropped the youthful manic defenses and has become acutely aware of suffering and death. Allen himself has said that the movie is about "a filmmaker/comedian who's reached a point in his life where he just doesn't find anything amusing anymore and so he is overcome with depression" (Moss 1980, 43). Allen's character sees the suffering everywhere around him, epitomized by the death of his high school friend Nat Bernstein from amyotrophic lateral sclerosis. Moreover, as Allen himself acknowledged in his 1982 conversation with Jacobs, Bates has a sense of his own destructive potential. *Stardust Memories* includes a satirical sketch from one of the director's films in which Bates joins police and hunting dogs in pursuit of a monster representing his narcissistic rage and his potential destructiveness.

All around him, and the monster, are dead bodies. His pessimism about being helped is dramatized by an ineffectual analyst's attempts to deal with the monster.

Allen's protagonist is also represented as an artist who has gone through the kind of transition that Jaques describes. He is a comedian who has recently turned to more serious themes in his movies, much as Allen has done in real life. After a series of slight, gag-filled comedies such as *Take the Money and Run* (1969) and *Bananas* (1971), Allen's films gradually turned toward the bittersweet romance of *Annie Hall* (1977) and *Manhattan* (1979). His most serious film was *Interiors* (1978), a Chekhovian drama about the tensions between and within the members of an affluent New York family. Though not without humor, *Interiors* was much grimmer than his audience had come to expect. In *Stardust Memories*, Bates comments, "I don't want to make funny pictures anymore. I look around and all I see is human suffering. Didn't anyone else read that piece on the front page of the *Times* about how matter is decaying?" Even when extraterrestrial beings appear to Bates in one of his fantasies, the film again expresses an ambivalent attitude toward the changes in Bates's career when the spacemen inform him that they liked the early, funny movies best. Moments later, Bates faints after another fantasy in which his adoring fan shoots him.

Fosse's Joe Gideon faces midlife with much less openness. He continues the use of his youthful manic defenses to ward off depression, acknowledgment of death, and an acceptance of his own destructive potential. Jaques notes that some individuals attempt to avoid midlife crisis by strengthening manic defenses. "The compulsive attempts, in many men and women reaching middle age, to remain young, the hypochondriacal concern over health and appearance, the emergence of sexual promiscuity in order to prove youth and potency, the hollowness and lack of genuine enjoyment of life, and the frequency of religious concern are familiar patterns. They are attempts at a race against time. And in addition to the impoverishment of emotional life contained in the foregoing activities, real character deterioration is always possible" (1965, 511). So while Allen has seen beyond his manic defenses to the despair beneath, Fosse's protagonist is desperately involved in a flight of overactivity in an effort to maintain his manic defenses. In *All That Jazz*, we see Gideon dealing with the important midlife issue of his own mortality in a scene from a film he is making called *The Standup*. (Fosse made a similar film about the life of Lenny Bruce called *Lenny*. The film received some unfavorable reviews, and although it would receive a half-dozen Oscar nominations, like Gideon, Fosse underwent coronary bypass surgery shortly after its opening.) In the scene from *The Standup*, a comedian played by Cliff Gorman does a blackly humorous parody of Elisabeth Kübler-Ross's five stages of dying. The most memorable stage in Gorman's rendition is "denial." In fact, one of his doctors says of Gideon, "Everything he does is a denial of his condition." Hence, Gideon does not see himself as middle-aged, dying, and in need of treatment.

According to the Kleinian perspective, the manic relation to objects is characterized by a triad of feelings: control, triumph, and contempt (Segal 1964). These feelings serve the defensive function of warding off guilt, mourning, a sense of loss, and feelings of having depended on a valued object. This manic triad manifests itself in Gideon's response when his doctor informs him that his condition is serious. In his fantasy he stages an elaborate production number involving the doctors as characters. He is in control now that he is the director, no longer a passive victim of the medical treatment, but rather the active master of his own destiny. Moreover, he is able to deny his dependence on the doctors by imagining that he controls the entire proceedings. Contempt is present in his portrayal of them as know-nothing performers in a production number. Triumph is seen in his denial of his depressive feelings about what is happening to him and about the impending losses of those he values. His narcissistic injury is graphically portrayed as Gideon, watching a television critic assail *The Standup*, becomes pale and short of breath, finally collapsing with an apparent myocardial infarction.

Death

The extinction of consciousness through death is the ultimate narcissistic injury, and the terror of death is one reason the narcissist does not age well. In *All That Jazz* and *Stardust Memories*, both protagonists are deeply concerned with death. After staving off his anxieties about death with drugs, alcohol, hypersexuality, workaholism, and the manic defenses mentioned above, Gideon finally shows a touch of despair after open-heart surgery when he says to himself about his life, "I'd like to run the whole thing over again." In another of these many blurrings of the line between show business and life, Gideon ventilates his anger at God by plaintively asking, "What's the matter, don't you like musical comedy?" However, this brief glimpse of the despair underneath is rapidly sealed over by a massive denial of death. His death becomes a manic triumph where as director he stages one production number after another. His ex-wife, his girlfriend, and his daughter perform for him as he lies in bed, while his double sits in the director's chair in charge of the proceedings. This doppelgänger effect allows us to see that while part of Gideon experiences the passive helplessness of dying, another, split-off part omnipotently imagines itself to be in control of everything happening to him. In a cynical eulogy that is a parody of show business sincerity, O'Connor Flood (Ben Vereen) says that Gideon spent his life bullshitting until he did not know what was real and what was bullshit. The only reality for Gideon was death. When the production numbers have ended, and he breathes his last, he finds himself floating up a tunnel toward the outstretched arms of Angelique, who waits to greet him with death's embrace. Here Fosse has appropriated elements of the often-reported "near-death experience" (Gabbard, Twemlow, and Jones 1981) to say something about Gideon's (and perhaps Fosse's) view of death. Even death itself is viewed with manic defenses as a joyous reunion with the idealized, all-good, internal mother. Fosse further defends against imminent mortality through sexualization, when the seductive Angelique begins to disrobe as Gideon approaches death.

As in the running joke about Alvy Singer's obsession with death that was central in *Annie Hall*, Allen views death in a much more sober fashion, as the ultimate narcissistic injury. He sees it as the inevitable outgrowth of the inherent destructiveness in human beings. When he is told that the public adores him, he responds by saying, "Today they adore you; tomorrow it's one of these," and he makes a gesture of shooting himself in the head. Paradoxically, though, while Allen's Bates has more insight into the reality of his own personal death than Fosse's Gideon does, Allen treats it with more humor. Gideon's self-destructive life is humorlessly portrayed as a form of slow suicide. In contrast, Allen presents the self-destructive workaholic in the person of a comic character riding an exercycle who says that he had two heart attacks before he started exercycling and two after. When he finishes his exercycling, he lights up a cigarette (plate 36). Allen seems to be saying that death is relentlessly stalking us no matter what steps we take to prevent it. Whereas Gideon's death is real despite his manic attempts at denying it, Sandy Bates's death is simply a fantasy in *Stardust Memories*.

In Woody Allen's film a psychoanalyst indicates that Bates's problem is that he has dropped his defensive denial and sees too much reality. Gideon's problem may be the converse in that he does not see reality but continually uses manic defenses to avoid it. In a sense, both situations are tragic. Gideon's is tragic because the manic defenses prevent him from seeing his own destructiveness, whereas Bates's is tragic because he is aware of his depression but feels impotent to affect it in any way. Because of his severe narcissistic impairment, he cannot allow his love to overcome his sense of destructiveness and his consequent suffering.

We have discussed two contemporary cinematic autobiographies that present the narcissistic struggles of the protagonists. Whether Bob Fosse and Woody Allen are themselves suffering from narcissistic character pathology is unknown to us, although Fosse's treatment of his narcissistic protagonist seems much more an apologia than does Allen's self-consciously ironic treatment of his main character. Whereas there is little doubt that *All That Jazz* is autobiographical, *Stardust Memories* is a bit more complex. Allen has repeatedly denied that his films are autobiographical. In a 1992 interview on the CBS program *60 Minutes,* in answer to a direct question, he deadpanned, "These are fictional characters." Later, in a 1996 interview with John Lahr, he again made it clear that he was nothing like the nebbish he so often portrays in films like *Stardust Memories*. He insisted that he was a medal winner in track, a reasonably good baseball player, and a kid who could get dates if he wanted to. He lamented the fact that the public cannot seem to separate him from the protagonists that appear in his films: "I'm not that iconic figure at all. . . . I'm very different from that" (68).

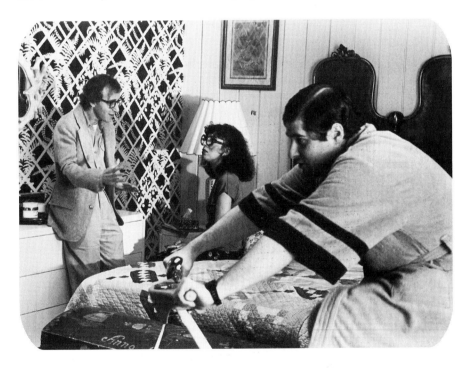

PLATE 36.   Absurdist therapy: Woody Allen with Anne de Salvo and Jaqui Safra in *Stardust Memories* (1980). United Artists. The Museum of Modern Art/Film Stills Archive.

Like most artists, Allen is uninterested in talking about the personal core of his art. Truffaut is alleged to have said that one repeatedly makes the same film, which is always about oneself, and Allen must surely recognize the inevitability of autobiography in cinematic art. As in a novel, a play, or any other creative work, the artist cannot avoid using himself and drawing from his own unconscious.

The plot thickens with *Deconstructing Harry*, Allen's 1997 film about Harry Block, a novelist who has made a wreck of his personal life while succeeding as an artist (see chapter 4). Throughout the film, Harry is seen betraying one woman after another, both by his sexual infidelity and by writing about them in his novels. The character is thoroughly despicable, and Allen had wanted to call the film "The Meanest Man in the World" at one point. He once again borrows liberally from Fellini's *8½*, most notably in the last scene of the film, where all of the characters in Harry's fiction and his life applaud him heartily as he parades before them. In another moment near the end of the film, Harry receives an award at his fictional alma mater and acknowledges that there is no sense in using disguise any more because the protagonists of his novels are him.

Whereas Fellini made no attempt to conceal that *8½* was an autobiographical film, Allen persists in denying that *Deconstructing Harry* is about him. In an interview with Martin Scorsese in the *New York Times Magazine* (Hirschberg 1997), Allen insisted that he wanted someone else to play the lead role because it was boring for him to do so. He went through a half-dozen people in quest of an actor who would take the role and finally decided to play it himself by default at the last minute. He resigned himself to the fact that audiences would think the movie was about him: "And there is no question: they'll think I am the character. But they think that on everything I do. I don't care. That is one of the curses or the blessings of what I do. That is why they come or why they stay away" (96).

Critics typically viewed *Deconstructing Harry* as his fantasy of revenge—an opportunity to get back at the media voices who relentlessly attacked him for his affair with Soon-Yi Previn and his breakup with Mia Farrow. In the film, Harry appears to be arguing that his art justifies whatever he does in his personal life. Greenberg (1998) thinks that Allen is crassly inviting the viewer into a guessing game about the point at which Harry leaves off and Woody begins. Rather than obsess about such ultimately unsolvable conundrums, Greenberg argues that Allen is essentially obsessing about himself and attempting to draw the audience into joining him, a further signifier of the narcissism inherent in Allen and in our celebrity culture.

In 1998, Barbara Kopple's documentary about Allen, *Wild Man Blues*, reached the theaters. The camera follows Allen and Soon-Yi Previn around Europe with his New Orleans–style jazz band, in which Allen plays clarinet. Although the protagonist of *this* film is ostensibly *not* a fictional character, he is utterly indistinguishable from the Allen persona on display in the films he wrote and directed. Amy Taubin (1998), in her review of the film, noted: "Once a camera is running (it doesn't matter to whom it belongs), Woody Allen plays Woody Allen. It's more than second nature to him. It's the only thing he can do" (67).

Trying to guess whether or not Allen *is* the characters he plays does not address the complexity of how an artist insinuates himself into the artistic product. In a dream, different aspects of the dreamer are commonly represented by different characters in the dream. Similarly, we would argue that in many of Allen's films, fragments of him appear in several different characters. For example, in *Crimes and Misdemeanors* (1991) the self-absorbed filmmaker played by Alan Alda probably has as much resonance with aspects of Allen himself as does the sensitive character that Allen actually portrays. The ophthalmologist portrayed by Martin Landau in the film also represents aspects of Allen himself. David Thomson made some penetrating observations about this connection:

> But in some grim contest with himself, Woody has found Landau as the only other actor around as unworthy of a lead role as himself. Landau's self-regard is unctuous and unwholesome. The thought of his affair with Ms. Huston is preposterous—indeed, the posed love matches in Allen films are often offered without the least conviction or spark. Obsessed with sex, he is terrified of looking at it. Landau's self-justification is humorless, clammy, and revolting. And when he tells his brother Jack (Jerry Orbach doing *Outlaw and Order*) 'I'm not going to let this neurotic woman destroy me!', we hear a line that was waiting to be traded back into Woody's real, ugly life with merciless ease. (1998, 19)

In *Hannah and Her Sisters* (1986), the brooding artist played by Max von Sydow undoubtedly has elements of Allen as well. And in *Husbands and Wives* (1992), the knockdown, drag-out fight between the Sidney Pollack character and his young girlfriend may mirror the messy aspects of Allen's own domestic life more completely than the harmony that infuses the marriage of the couple played in the film by Allen and Mia Farrow. It is significant that in all of these films Woody Allen appears as the more idealized version of himself while projecting his more unsavory qualities onto the characters played by other actors.

Like all artists, Allen's major subject is himself, even if his many acts of self-representation are highly mediated and constantly revised. Finding all or part of the real Woody Allen in his long list of films is always difficult because, paradoxically, Allen has chosen to act in so many of them, usually as characters who show a face to the audience that Allen most wants people to see. For this reason alone, *Deconstructing Harry*, in which Allen himself plays the film's most deeply flawed character, is a remarkable item in the Allen filmography.

CHAPTER 11

Narcissism in the Cinema II: The Celebrity

As we noted in chapter 10, fascination with celebrity is one of the dominant themes of our narcissistic culture. The cinematic medium, perhaps more than any other facet of modern society, has been instrumental in the creation of this infatuation with the rich and famous. Spinoffs from the phenomenon of the movie star—including the television personality, the rock star, the sports hero, the evening news anchorperson, and even the media-created political personality—are so thoroughly entrenched in contemporary popular culture that we may easily forget their origins: all of these versions of the celebrity owe a large debt to motion picture screen images, which have created or greatly enhanced their fascination for the public. An examination of narcissism in the cinema would be incomplete without an analysis of the notion of celebrity.

While the idea of celebrity is to a large extent the child of the twentieth century, it is simply the latest transformation of an archetypal figure as old as human culture itself—the hero. A quick glance at the earliest extant literary works—for example, the Gilgamesh epic and the works of Homer—reveals that an obsession with heroes was a fixture in the human psyche at the dawn of man's intellectual expression. As William James commented in 1902, when television was only the dream of a visionary inventor, "Mankind's common instinct for reality . . . has always held the world to be essentially a theatre for heroism" (1958, 281). Ernest Becker (1973) has persuasively argued that the problem of heroics is the central existential issue of human life. Unlike his fellow creatures in the animal kingdom, man lives with the terrible knowledge that amid all the ambiguities of life, one thing is certain: he will cease to exist at some point in the future. This unbearable certainty of extinction leads man to invent various immortality strategies. Religion is one. The heroic quest is another. Man longs for cosmic significance. He hungers to be "somebody," a hero who will be remembered and talked about long after he has gone to his grave.

Becker points out that narcissism is fundamental to the understanding of this human urge to heroism. From early childhood, the whole human organism demands to be the center of the universe, to be noted, admired, loved, praised, and even worshiped. In Becker's own words, this developmental phenomenon is "too all-absorbing and relentless to be an aberration, it expresses the heart of the creature: the desire to stand out, to be the one in creation. When you combine natural narcissism with the basic need for self-esteem, you create a creature who has to feel himself an object of primary value: first in the universe, representing in himself all of life" (1973, 3). As we grow and become socialized, the quest for heroism undergoes transformations that disguise it in one form or another; but, as Becker has observed, society creates hero systems that provide external validation for each individual who lays claim to his or her own heroic act: "Human heroics is a blind drivenness that burns people up; in passionate people, a screaming for glory as uncritical and reflective as the howling of a dog. In the more passive masses of mediocre men, it is disguised as they humbly and complainingly follow out the roles that society provides for their heroics and try to earn their promotions within the system: wearing the standard uniforms" (1973, 6).

Today our heroes are only rarely warriors, conquerors, or generals, and their achievements seldom equal the vanquishing of armies. The criteria for success have been redefined with the advent of the pervasive influence of the media. Lasch has characterized the change thus: "The good opinion of friends and neighbors, which formerly informed a man that he had lived a useful life, rested on appreciation of his accomplishments. Today men seek the kind of approval that applauds not their actions but their personal attributes. They wish to be not so much esteemed as admired. They crave not fame but the glamor and excitement of celebrity. They want to be envied rather than respected. Pride and acquisitiveness, the sins of an ascendant capitalism, have given way to vanity" (1979, 59). Today's hero is someone who has successfully manufactured a winning image that so appeals to the masses as to catapult him into a position of celebrity. The substance behind the image is of little concern either to the celebrities themselves or to those who worship them. Political campaigns, for example, are no longer issue-oriented but geared to the politicians' use of television to package an image worthy of the voters' confidence. During the 1984 presidential election, commentators observed repeatedly that voters often disagreed with Ronald Reagan on the issues that he supported, but they voted for him because of his appeal as a media personality. One wag even suggested that the only candidate who could have beaten Reagan in 1984 was Clint Eastwood, a comment that proved slightly prophetic in 1984 when Eastwood was overwhelmingly elected mayor of Carmel, California. Polls showed that many voters were impressed by Eastwood's charisma even more than by his politics. Bill Clinton's approval ratings increased dramatically in 1998 at the same time that he was being investigated for sexual dalliances with a young woman. A president's adherence to strict standards of moral behavior seemed to be of little concern to voters as long as the economy continued to thrive. Lasch makes the following observations:

> What a man does matters less than the fact that he has "made it." Whereas fame depends on the performance of notable deeds acclaimed in biography and works of history, celebrity—the reward of those who project a vivid or pleasing exterior or have otherwise attracted attention to themselves—is acclaimed in the news media, in gossip columns, on talk shows, and magazines devoted to "personalities." . . . Success in our society has to be ratified by publicity. The tycoon who lives in personal obscurity, the empire builder who controls the destinies of nations from behind the scenes, are vanishing types. Even non-elected officials, ostensibly preoccupied with questions of high policy, have to keep themselves constantly on view; all politics becomes a form of spectacle. It is well known that Madison Avenue packages politicians and markets them as if they were cereals or deodorants. (1979, 59–60)

Cinematic art has now developed the capacity to comment intelligently and critically on what the medium itself has created, as if Dr. Frankenstein had begun writing scholarly treatises on the adverse consequences of monster-building. Three films of the 1980s, *Zelig* (1983) and *The Purple Rose of Cairo* (1985), both written and directed by Woody Allen, and Martin Scorsese's *The King of Comedy* (1983), provide penetrating insights into the phenomenon of celebrity as well as the contribution of the electronic media themselves to the contemporary obsession with celebrity. However, the psychologically astute makers of these films have avoided implying that the problems developed de novo with the advent of movies and television. Rather, they treat the quest for heroism as a pervasive, preexisting human frailty that easily accommodated itself to the American media explosion.

The King of Comedy

Written by Paul D. Zimmerman and directed by Martin Scorsese, *The King of Comedy* points the camera at a most single-minded individual in contemporary Manhattan who bears the improbable name of Rupert Pupkin (Robert De Niro). Rupert is a thirty-four-year-old messenger who lives in his own special fantasy world. He writes and rehearses stand-up comedy routines in front of an imaginary audience in the privacy of his basement, where reality only occasionally intervenes when his mother demands that he quiet down. The principal idealized object that peoples his fantasy world is Jerry Langford (Jerry Lewis), a character based closely on Johnny Carson although the original script for the film, dating from the early 1970s, had been written for Dick Cavett (Frank and Krohn 1983). Rupert has a life-sized photograph of Langford (Lewis) at his talk show desk tacked to the wall next to an equally large photo of Liza Minnelli. He lives out his grandiose fantasies of glory and fame by sitting next to his Langford and Minnelli pictures while carrying on an imaginary dialogue with the famous host and affecting all the mannerisms of a regular guest on late-night talk shows.

Rupert Pupkin exemplifies what is perhaps Heinz Kohut's (1971, 1977) greatest contribution to our understanding of narcissism—that the regulation of self-esteem ranks with sexuality and aggression as one of the major forces in the human psyche. Rupert's fantasy life does not depend on aggressive or sexual conquests but rather on throngs of cheering fans worshiping him and on the idealized Langford begging him to take his place for six weeks while Langford vacations. He looks to acclaim and admiration as the panaceas for his anxiety and his internal emptiness.

The King of Comedy opens to the sound of Ray Charles singing an old torch song, "I'm gonna love you like nobody's loved you, come rain or come shine." We then see Rupert threading his way through a crowd of hungry autograph seekers outside the studio door through which Langford will soon pass. As Pupkin shoves his way to the front of the crowd, he strives to distinguish himself from his acquaintances in the odd subculture of autograph hounds, telling one repeatedly that acquiring the signatures of stars is "not my whole life." His flamboyant wardrobe is also much more elaborate than that of anyone else in the crowd, and he affects an air of superiority to the others. When he manages to work his way into Langford's car, he asks the renowned talk show host for a chance on his show. Barely able to tolerate Pupkin's unrelenting pleading, Langford tells him to call his office. Brimming with self-confidence, Rupert goes home and prepares a tape for Langford's assistant, now convinced that his wildest fantasies are about to be fulfilled.

He seeks out Rita (Diahnne Abbott), an idealized woman from his past, who now works as a bartender. He takes her to dinner and courts her with his "talent register," a book of autographs of the famous, many of whom he blithely insists are his personal friends. Even though Rita fails to find his book fascinating, Pupkin shows her page after page of signatures culminating with a page that bears his own scrawl. Otto Kernberg (1975) has noted how the narcissist, experiencing himself as fundamentally worthless, must attach himself to idealized objects in order to bask in the reflected glory of these objects. Rupert hopes to impress Rita by persuading her that the luster of the stars has rubbed off on him and that he lives in their shadows. He makes no effort to court her by selling her on his own qualities—only his association with those whose attributes are beyond question. Rita is singularly unimpressed by his name-dropping and is, ironically, more interested in Rupert himself. But Rupert seems unaware of his own charms and proceeds relentlessly to win her over in the only way that has meaning for him.

Rupert indulges in an elaborate fantasy about his meeting with Langford to discuss his tape. He imagines that Langford raves about his talent, proclaiming his envy for Rupert. In the fantasy, Jerry even invites him to his country house for the weekend. But when Rupert's tape is rejected by Langford's assistant (Shelley Hack), Rupert confuses fantasy with reality, eventually taking Rita on the train with him to Langford's house in the Hamptons, assuring her that he has been invited and that he and Langford are the best of friends.

The couple's ill-fated trip shows us the dark side of the celebrity's life. Early in the film the camera reveals Langford in his sumptuous Manhattan apartment, eating alone at a long table while three television sets play silently in the background. The emptiness of Langford's life recalls the widely publicized divorces of Johnny Carson, the personality that Langford most clearly suggests. In fact, after abandoning the original script for *The King of Comedy* written for Dick Cavett, Scorsese asked Carson to play the role. Carson refused, saying in effect that he was too accustomed to taping a show each night in one take and that he had no desire to enter into a process that required repeated shootings of the same scene: "If I wanted to make a film and repeat the same scene nineteen times, I would make it myself" (Frank and Krohn 1983). Some commentators subsequently praised Carson for his caution, arguing that *The King of Comedy* might inspire some fan to kidnap Carson, and some criticized Scorsese, whose earlier film *Taxi Driver* provided the fantasy that inspired John Hinckley to attempt the assassination of Ronald Reagan. However, it may also be that Carson understood Scorsese's intentions all too well and demurred at associating himself with a project that so thoroughly examined the nature of his celebrity status.

When Rupert and Rita arrive at Langford's country house, the audience witnesses again the emptiness and sterility of Langford's inner life, symbolized by the white-walled starkness of his home. Langford is called in from the golf course when they arrive, and he is uncompromising in his annoyance at this invasion of his privacy. He angrily explains to Rupert that he too has a life and that he resents this violation by the intruders. Rupert is blind to Langford's rage until Jerry is forced to tell him point-blank that when Rupert gained entrance to his limousine, Langford seemed to encourage him only in order to be rid of him. As Rupert leaves, he tells Langford how disappointed he is to find out what Jerry is really like. He tells him that he is going to work fifty times harder than Langford and become fifty times more famous. Langford's final comment to the intruder is, "Then you're going to have idiots like you plaguing your life."

Rupert responds to this devastating injury to his self-esteem with narcissistic rage, although Scorsese's oblique style of storytelling omits any scenes in which Pupkin's confident exterior is actually ruffled. Instead, we see Rupert plotting with another devoted autograph hunter, Masha (Sandra Bernhard), whose sense of reality is even more profoundly askew than his. They plan to kidnap Langford so that Rupert can blackmail the producers into allowing him to deliver the opening monologue on Jerry's show. After successfully carrying out his scheme, Rupert tells the FBI men who have been called in on the case that he will release Langford and surrender to their custody only after he has been allowed to watch the tape of his monologue in the presence of Rita at the bar where she works. Rupert's performance impresses Rita and the denizens of the saloon only slightly more than it does the FBI agents, one of whom says that he would also like to arrest the man who writes Rupert's material. Nevertheless, Rupert Pupkin has accomplished his goal, and he goes off to meet his fate cheerfully.

In Rupert's monologue (plate 37), he admits that he has kidnapped Jerry Langford in order to appear on his show. The audience laughs, not understanding that the man they are watching is not just another of the comedians who regularly attempt to amuse the television audience on Langford's program. They also laugh when he tells them that his rash act is worth it since it is better to be "king for a night than schmuck for a lifetime." The film ends with a newscaster intoning that the incident has made the name Rupert Pupkin a household word. His picture appears on the cover of *Time*, *Newsweek*, *Life*, *Rolling Stone*, and *People*, and he writes his best-selling autobiography while serving two years and nine months of a six-year prison sentence. In the open-ended conclusion to the film, Rupert is introduced as "the legendary, the inspirational, the one and only king of comedy, Rupert

Pupkin." The camera slowly zooms in on Rupert as he receives the audience's enthusiastic applause, his impassive face suggesting that he may already be aware of the ambiguous rewards of celebrity.

The publicity for *The King of Comedy* noted that Robert De Niro had prepared for the role of Rupert Pupkin by studying stand-up comedians in order to learn the secrets of their timing and delivery, just as he had learned to play the saxophone for Scorsese's *New York, New York* (1977). For the same director's *Raging Bull* (1980), De Niro had studied boxing and then gained forty pounds so that he could play the fighter Jake La Motta later in life. But the comedy routine that De Niro actually delivers in *The King of Comedy* does not rise much above the level of mediocrity established through the years by run-of-the-mill performers who fill up the schedule of "The Tonight Show." Scorsese has told interviewers that one of the elements of the film's first script that attracted him most was the monologue: because it is neither good nor bad, audiences have no way of evaluating the potential talent of Pupkin, who has, after all, scrupulously avoided performing in public until he

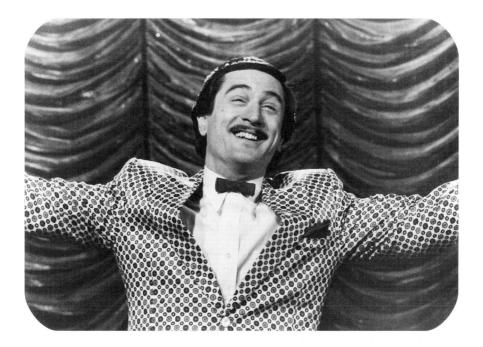

PLATE 37.   Rupert Pupkin (Robert De Niro) accepts the adulation of Jerry Langford's audience in *The King of Comedy* (1983). Twentieth Century–Fox. The Museum of Modern Art/Film Stills Archive.

reaches the big time on the Langford show (Henry 1983). Scorsese has intentionally left open the question, is Pupkin a truly funny comedian who merely
took an unconventional road to stardom, or is he just another desperate, va-
pid individual seeking the prize of celebrity? It would seem that he is just as
empty as Jerry Langford, who is in fact not portrayed as much of a comedian
either. Scorsese had taped Lewis performing a monologue for the beginning
of the film, but the director says that he excised it from the final print because it raised distracting questions about the relative merits of Pupkin and
Langford as comedians (Frank and Krohn 1983).

Scorsese and his screenwriter Zimmerman have made a film about how
our fascination with celebrity has led us to confuse genuine talent with a kind
of chutzpah or daring, which may be neurotic or even criminal. The increasingly sensationalistic world of American entertainment invites the blurring of
distinctions between what is legitimate and what is not, and the case of
Rupert Pupkin provocatively exposes this confusion. The crucial moment in
The King of Comedy may be the scene at Langford's country house in which
Rupert shows himself to be incapable of understanding Langford's question
about how he would feel if someone barged in on him the way Pupkin has in-
truded on Langford. The narcissistically disturbed individual's inability to
empathize with the feelings of others is beautifully illustrated here, as is
Pupkin's extreme idealization of Langford's life: Rupert cannot imagine how
anything in Langford's domain could be unpleasant, even when he himself
has caused the unpleasantness. Scorsese suggests that only someone as confused as Pupkin could envy someone like Langford.

However, Scorsese is working in a marketplace where subtle questions
about American attitudes are seldom associated with big box office. In *The
King of Comedy*, he has apparently sought to make two films: one for a naïve
or "right" audience, who may find De Niro's Pupkin to be as adept as any
other stand-up comedian presented by David Letterman or Jay Leno, and
who may assume that the film is another in a long series of American enter-
tainments about a little guy who beats the system. The other film that makes
up *The King of Comedy* is addressed to the ironic or "left" audience, who are
more acquainted with cinematic codes. Scorsese has asked this audience to
think more critically about America's television heroes, particularly in terms
of the issues that have been raised in this chapter. Even though *The King of
Comedy* was a box-office flop, Scorsese understands that he can be both an
artist and a commercially successful director if he makes his films in this way.
He achieved his greatest financial success with *Taxi Driver*, the twelfth-
largest-grossing film of 1976 (Steinberg 1980). Although most audiences and
even some critics lumped it with "street westerns" such as Michael Winner's

Death Wish, Robert B. Ray (1985) has shown that *Taxi Driver* reveals the psychosis that can lie beneath the unruffled exteriors of America's vigilante heroes. Naïve moviegoers in the film's audience may have perceived it as another glorification of violent revenge, but *Taxi Driver* represents a powerful attack upon "the belief in the continued applicability of western-style, individual solutions to contemporary complex problems" (Ray 1985, 351).

If we are right about Scorsese's dual intentions, we must not then be surprised that *The King of Comedy* has many moments of ambiguity. For one thing, episodes of fantasy are interwoven with episodes of reality. Since Scorsese does not use musical or cinematographical clichés to announce that the film is about to fade into a fantasy sequence, we are not even sure if the renown that Pupkin enjoys at the end of the film is in his head or in reality. Some critics have made the same observation about Scorsese's *Taxi Driver* (1976), in which the rise of Travis Bickle (De Niro again) to hero status at the film's end could be the fantasy of a man dying from gunshot wounds. Scorsese himself says that he likes "open endings" (Henry 1983).

If Scorsese and screenwriter Zimmerman did intend for the ending of *The King of Comedy* to be taken literally, they may be telling us that Rupert's narcissistic quest for heroism is no more or less absurd than society's need to make such personages into the objects of fascination and admiration. As Lasch puts it:

> The media have conferred a curious sort of legitimacy on antisocial acts merely by reporting them. . . . The criminal who murders or who kidnaps a celebrity takes on the glamor of his victim. The Manson gang with their murder of Sharon Tate and her friends, the Symbionese Liberation Army with its abduction of Patty Hearst, share with the presidential assassins and would-be assassins of recent years a similar psychology. Such people display, in exaggerated form, the prevailing obsession with celebrity and the determination to achieve it even at the cost of rational self-interest and personal safety. (1979, 84)

Rupert Pupkin can be viewed as a narcissistic Everyman. As Kernberg (1975) has written, the narcissist sees society divided into two groups consisting of famous celebrities on one side and mediocrities like himself on the other. The narcissist is "nobody" if he is not in the company of the great. The average or mediocre person is viewed contemptuously, as though he has no redeeming features and cannot lead a meaningful life. Rupert's efforts to link up with Langford are an attempt to confer greatness upon himself. Bob Fosse developed this same theme in his 1983 film *Star 80*, in which Paul Snider (Eric Roberts), filled with self-contempt and self-loathing, aspires to become "somebody" by exploiting his relationship with *Playboy*'s sweetheart Doro-thy Stratten in order to gain proximity to Hugh Hefner and the *Playboy* crowd. In hopes of gaining passage into the inner sanctum of the *Playboy* mansion, Snider cultivates an image through hours of rehearsal in front of a mirror and through excessive attention to his wardrobe. When both Hefner and his circle reject him, he reacts with murderous and suicidal narcissistic rage. If one is not a celebrity, one is an abject failure with no reason to live.

From analytic observations in a clinical context, Kohut (1977) described the narcissist's problem as an arrest of normal development of the self. Nar-cissistic patients typically form specific kinds of transferences in the consult-ing room. Two of these are (1) the *mirror transference* linked to an archaic, grandiose self that performs for mother, hoping to recapture the lost perfec-tion of infancy by winning her approval and thus an empathic validation of the self, and (2) the *idealizing transference* linked to an effort on the part of the undeveloped self to recapture the lost perfection by merging with an ide-alized parent image. While Rupert Pupkin certainly embodies the grandiose self's efforts to obtain mirroring validation from an audience of approving pa-rental figures, we also see how Jerry Langford functions as an idealized parent imago for Rupert's friend Masha. While Rupert is off at the studio conduct-ing negotiations for his appearance on Langford's show, Masha is reveling in her private audience with Langford, whom she has tied up in her dining room chair. As she undresses in front of him, she tells Jerry that she loves him, something that she has never even told her parents, who, she poignantly informs him, never loved her. She sings to him, "You're gonna love me like nobody's loved me, come rain or come shine." In this scene she pathetically reveals an important dynamic in the worship of celebrities, that is, the fan-tasy that the love between the celebrity and the follower would be of a pure and reparative nature, making up for the absence of love experienced as a child. Masha knows virtually nothing of the real Jerry Langford, but she does know that she loves him as she loves no one else. Langford is the object of an idealizing transference on Masha's part, and in her fantasy she can shore up her fragile self-esteem by merging with this all-loving and all-giving parent of her dreams through the act of making love.

Sandra Bernhard made her first film appearance as Masha in *The King of Comedy*, and it is a memorable one. When Langford, bound with several yards of masking tape, sits helplessly before a meal that Masha has prepared for him, she suddenly rakes her arm across the table and shoves the dishes to the floor so that she can recline on the table before him. The violence in her gesture momentarily suggests that the film may turn as violent as many of Scorsese's earlier films. However, even the gun that Masha had earlier trained on Langford turns out to be a toy, and he has no difficulty making his escape. Masha plays out her ambivalent relationship with Jerry in an earlier scene when she contemplates which color looks best on the talk show host while she dresses her prisoner in a sweater knitted especially for him. Masha has lost track of the difference between contemplating her idol on a television set and contemplating him as a hostage in her house.

In the throes of this idealizing and erotic transference confusion, Masha believes that she is successfully seducing Langford. While her idealization of Jerry is dependent on his ongoing love for her, Rupert's idealization is much more transparently a narcissistic exploitation of Jerry for his own self-aggrandizement. Rupert is only interested in Langford as a means of establishing himself as the King of Comedy. The transferential natures of both Rupert's and Masha's attachments to Langford make them unable to see that his real characteristics starkly contrast with the fantasied qualities that they attribute to him. In fact, Jerry Lewis plays Langford throughout the film as a character singularly lacking in personal charm.

Becker (1973) believes that the phenomenon of transference is a fascination with the fatality of the human condition. The essence of transference, as Becker sees it, is a taming of terror. Just as the infant deals with his helplessness by believing in his parents and ascribing to them an omnipotent control over fate, so does the adult connect himself with transference figures to deal with his anxiety over the seeming randomness of the universe. Becker notes: "The use of the transference object explains the urge to deification of the other, the constant placing of certain select persons on pedestals, the reading into them of extra powers: the more they have, the more rubs off on us. We participate in their immortality, and so we create immortals. . . . Man is always hungry . . . for material for his own immortalization" (1973, 148).

Celebrities represent immortality to their followers. How else can we understand the extraordinary mass grief reactions to the passing of idols such as John Lennon or Elvis Presley? The throngs of mourners are not so much crying for their heroes as for themselves. A bulwark against death has been ripped away, or as Becker comments, "The people apprehend at some dumb level of their personality: 'our locus of power to control life and death can *himself* die; therefore, our own immortality is in doubt'" (1973, 149). The movie star is preserved forever on celluloid, never to be erased from memory, captured in the zenith of his splendor and beauty, safe from the decaying effects of disease and age. Regardless of his own qualities, Jerry Langford provides meaning for Masha and for Rupert, just as the Reverend Jim Jones provided meaning for his followers in Guyana and Hitler provided meaning for his country in Nazi Germany. To find meaning, man must look outward for an externalized projection of what he lacks in himself. In one of Rupert's fantasies, he appears on the Langford show as a guest and is surprised when Jerry arranges for him to be married to Rita on his show. The justice of the peace who performs the ceremony thanks Rupert for giving meaning to everyone's lives as the King of Comedy marries his "Queen." The magistrate wishes them a successful reign as Rupert imagines himself bringing meaning to the lives of millions, just as Langford has brought meaning to his own life. His fans will live forever through their attachment to their immortal "King."

Zelig

Woody Allen brings a different perspective to the celebrity phenomenon in his 1983 film *Zelig*. Here we have another unprepossessing nebbish, Leonard Zelig, the film's protagonist. But whereas Rupert Pupkin sought fame and glory, Zelig desires nothing more than to be accepted by those around him. His chameleonlike ability to change his physical appearance and personality in order to blend in with his companions catapults him into celebrity in spite of himself. Allen works minor miracles with cinematographer Gordon Willis and editor Susan Morse in creating the ambience of newsreels and photographs from the 1920s and 1930s, the setting for the film (plate 38). The rise and fall of Leonard Zelig is charted almost entirely as a major news story of the Jazz Age and the early 1930s, an ingenious conceit that underscores the media's role in creating this unlikely celebrity. Throughout the film, Allen interjects comments on the Zelig phenomenon from real-life intellectuals Bruno Bettelheim, Saul Bellow, Susan Sontag, Irving Howe, and John Morton Blum. They speak with great authority as though they actually knew Zelig, a parody not only of the witnesses in Warren Beatty's 1981 film *Reds* but also of Allen's mock-documentary style in his first directorial effort, *Take the Money and Run* (1969).

When Zelig comes to the attention of a psychiatrist, Dr. Eudora Fletcher (Mia Farrow) (plate 39), she embarks on a heroic effort to cure him of his tendency to take on the characteristics of whomever he is with. His case receives extensive media attention, and various experts from the medical field expound their theories about his illness. Meanwhile, he is the object of the American public's intense fascination. A man interviewed in a barbershop paradoxically proclaims, "I wish I could be Leonard Zelig, the changing man, and be different people, and maybe someday my wishes would come true." Another man interviewed describes Zelig as "one of the finest gentlemen in the United States of America." The adulation and the envy hardly seem war-

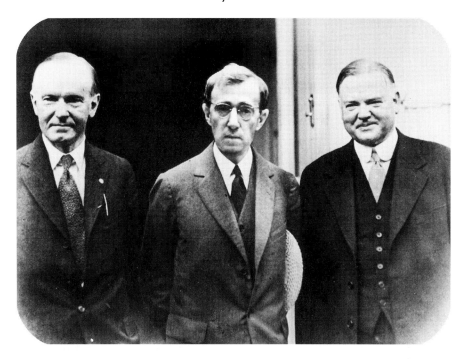

PLATE 38. Zelig (Woody Allen) becomes a Republican. *Zelig* (1983). Orion Pictures Company/Warner Brothers. The Museum of Modern Art/Film Stills Archive.

ranted given Zelig's real characteristics—he is a simple man who explains that he assumes the characteristics of others because "I want to be liked." Nevertheless, a dance called "The Chameleon" is created to celebrate him, and a movie of his life is made in Hollywood. Allen shows us a few scenes from the imagined movie, called "The Changing Man," an accurate parody of the B movies of the 1930s. "The Changing Man" is also a glamorous distortion of Zelig's real situation, a further comment by Allen on how movies encourage the public in their transference distortions.

Zelig's rise to celebrity status reflects the public's need to believe in someone. Society is fascinated by a man who has no self, no personality of his own. He is literally the projected image of themselves, a mirror that reflects back the person's own image. In one scene the film shows Zelig sitting alone, staring into space, as the narrator comments: "Though the shows and parties keep Zelig's sister and her lover rich and amused, Zelig's own existence is a nonexistence. Devoid of personality, his human qualities long since lost in the shuffle of life, he sits alone quietly staring into space, a cipher, a nonperson, a performing freak. He, who wanted only to fit in, to belong, to go unseen by his enemies, and be loved, neither fits in nor belongs, is supervised by enemies and remains uncared for."

As the plot develops, Zelig disappears following the murder of his sister, and everyone easily forgets him. The one exception is Dr. Fletcher, who launches an exhaustive search. When she finally discovers him, she has her cousin make a film of her work with Zelig because, as she explains, "I'm planning to make history." The film even questions the motives of Dr. Fletcher, who wants to exploit Zelig's freakish qualities to make herself famous. Moreover, Allen once again points out how the medium of film itself turns Dr. Fletcher and her bizarre patient into famous celebrities. In search of an understanding of the psychopathology of Leonard Zelig, Bruno Bettelheim is interviewed in one of the witness shots. Bettelheim makes the following comment: "The question of whether Zelig was a psychotic or merely neurotic was a question that was endlessly discussed among his doctors. Now I

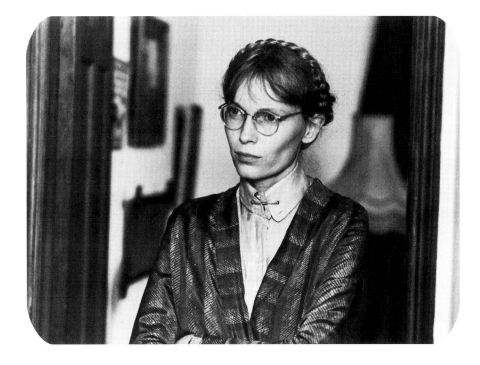

PLATE 39.   Mia Farrow as Dr. Eudora Fletcher, the savior and lover of Leonard Zelig in Woody Allen's *Zelig* (1983). Orion Pictures Company/Warner Brothers. The Museum of Modern Art/Film Stills Archive.

myself felt his feelings were really not all that different from the normal, what one would call the well-adjusted, normal person, only carried to an extreme degree, to an extreme extent. I myself felt that one could really think of him as the ultimate conformist." For Bettelheim, Zelig's celebrity is the outgrowth of his effort to conform himself to everyone around him. This situation is, of course, only slightly removed from the situation of the present-day politician, who tries to conform to every imaginable constituency in order to gain sufficient popularity to be elected. The real personality and the real beliefs may be as difficult to discern as the real identity of Leonard Zelig. (The fact that Allen was able to persuade people like Bettelheim, Bellow, and Sontag to participate in his project makes a strong statement in and of itself. The lure of being preserved on celluloid is tempting, even for the most prestigious and well established.)

A breakthrough in Dr. Fletcher's treatment of Zelig comes when she begins to emulate the qualities of the chameleon man herself. Zelig is acting like a psychiatrist, of course, since he is in the company of a psychiatrist. Recalling an earlier confession of Zelig's, she tells him that she has lied about having read *Moby-Dick* because she was with an erudite group of people and wished to impress them. She says to him, "I want so badly to be liked, to be like other people so I don't stand out." Zelig breaks down and says, "I'm nobody. I'm nothing." Indeed, Zelig is in reality nothing, serving the same function as an inkblot on a Rorschach card, that is, the role of a container into which people project aspects of themselves. In that regard he functions as an ideal celebrity, since he has little personality of his own to interfere with the transference feelings of his adoring public. As Dr. Fletcher's cure begins to take effect, however, he allows himself to disagree with others. He carries the cure too far and begins to disagree violently with another doctor about the weather, even to the point of striking the doctor with a rake. The narrator tells us matter-of-factly that Zelig has become "overopinionated."

When the cure is complete, Zelig is once again a hero because he has stopped being a chameleon. He now preaches to schoolchildren, "Be yourself." The masses who once loved him for being a chameleon with no personality of his own now love him for having stopped his "as if" transformations. It matters little what Zelig is or says; he is merely a repository for innumerable projections. He is not loved or adored for what he is, but only for what he represents to those who adore him. One of the witnesses, historian John Morton Blum, identified here as "author of *Interpreting Zelig*," says that Zelig is a man of symbolism—he was one thing to Marxists and another to the Catholics. The American people, in the throes of the depression, "found in him a symbol of possibility, of self-improvement and self-fulfillment. And of course, the Freudians had a ball—they could interpret him in any way they pleased. It was all symbolism. But there were no two intellectuals who agreed about what it meant." Elsewhere, the announcer tells us that to French intellectuals, Zelig was a symbol for everything.

As the saga continues, Zelig disappears after a series of exposés about his sordid past, which includes polygamy and the abandonment of women he impregnated. The public turns on him, and he is universally condemned, falling from his pedestal because he has not lived up to the public image of him. When he eventually turns up in Nazi Germany, Saul Bellow comments that his presence in that country made eminently good sense because "although he wanted to be loved, craved to be loved, there was also something in him that desired immersion in the masses, anonymity; and fascism offered Zelig that opportunity so that he could make something anonymous of himself." While Rupert Pupkin in *The King of Comedy* embodies the narcissistic quest for recognition and fame, the character of Zelig demonstrates another aspect of the narcissist's wish for approval, that is, the wish to blend in with those around him so that he feels a sense of acceptance. The approval of one's peers may be the ultimate desire of the narcissist, and he may do whatever is necessary, including distorting his personal beliefs, to gain approval. Lasch (1979) notes how conscious emulation of role models is superseded in the narcissistic character by an unconscious and automatic imitation of those around him, reflecting not a true search for a role model but rather the emptiness of the narcissist's reservoir of self-images. As his own identity is obliterated, the narcissist cannot identify with someone else without seeing the other person as an extension of himself and thereby obliterating the other person's identity as well. *Zelig* demonstrates the two-way process of narcissistic mirroring. While Leonard Zelig attempts to please others by becoming like them and gaining their approval, others see themselves in the character of Zelig and idealize what they see. By attaching themselves to this idealized parental imago projected onto Zelig, they feel their own self-esteem enhanced, just as Zelig feels enhanced by the approval of those with whom he blends. The process might be likened to a hall of mirrors in which each distortion is reflected back in a refracting series of constantly changing images.

As Dr. Fletcher is rescuing Zelig from Nazi Germany, he makes a dramatic escape from a squadron of Nazi fighters by flying upside down across the Atlantic. Zelig is once again an instant hero—his past philanderings seemingly forgotten and forgiven—and he is awarded the medal of valor. In another scathing satire on the inanity of the public's creation of celebrities, Allen has Zelig make the following comment in his acceptance speech: "It shows exactly what you can do if you're a total psychotic." In other words, the patient's psychiatric disorder makes him a hero and the object of worship and envy for the masses. Leonard Zelig, like Rupert Pupkin in the closing scene of *The King of Comedy*, is adored and idolized despite obvious and pathetic character flaws. Both Pupkin and Zelig are men who have "made it," an accomplishment that trivializes all of their many shortcomings.

The Purple Rose of Cairo

Two years after the appearance of *Zelig*, Woody Allen again explored the theme of celebrity in *The Purple Rose of Cairo*. It may be useful to conceptualize *Stardust Memories*, *Zelig*, *The Purple Rose of Cairo*, and his later film *Celebrity* as Allen's "celebrity tetralogy" since the filmmaker's attitude toward the phenomenon of celebrity undergoes an evolution in these four films. The contemptuous attitude toward celebrity worshipers that Allen conveys in *Stardust Memories* is transformed into empathic understanding by the time of *The Purple Rose of Cairo*. In *Purple Rose*, Allen recognizes that the fascination with celebrities serves an almost religious function in our secular society. It fulfills one of mankind's strongest psychological and spiritual needs and may be an essential antidote to the toxins associated with the vicissitudes of life. Moreover, *The Purple Rose of Cairo*, more than the other two parts of the trilogy, acknowledges the centrality of movies and movie stars in our construction of life-sustaining illusions. Allen himself regards *The Purple Rose of Cairo* as a favorite among his own films. It simultaneously operates on many different levels: as a comedy, a tragedy, a feminist commentary on sexual relationships, a quasi-religious existential statement, a psychological examination of the meaning of movies to the human psyche, an ironic and self-parodic commentary about the shallowness of movies and movie people, a simple love story, and a Pirandellian exploration of the nature of reality and illusion. As he did in *Zelig*, Allen returns to the Great Depression as the setting for his film, perhaps drawing some parallels between the financial bankruptcy of that era and the spiritual and psychological bankruptcy of our own.

Cecilia (Mia Farrow), the protagonist of *Purple Rose*, lives in an unbearable reality. She is married to an out-of-work slob named Monk (Danny Aiello) who beats her whenever the spirit moves him. She is stuck in a dead-end job in an era when people are lining up to jump out of windows rather than face their financial hardships. For Cecilia, the movies represent an alternative to this harsh reality. Relationships are easy in the movies. Boy meets girl; boy falls in love with girl; and boy and girl live happily ever after. Sexual anxieties do not exist in the movies because there is a fade-out after the first kiss. At one point in the film, a woman in a movie house comments that her middle-aged husband comes to the movies because he is a student of human personality. She goes on to emphasize that he has trouble with real-life human beings, but he is much more successful in relating to celluloid characters.

After losing her job and walking out on her adulterous husband, Cecilia sits in the darkened movie theater for one showing after another of *The Purple Rose of Cairo*, a film-within-a-film that transports her from her desperate situation in New Jersey to a romantic adventure on another continent. She becomes particularly fascinated with the handsome and naïve hero of the film, Tom Baxter (Jeff Daniels). After multiple viewings, the heroine's fantasy becomes reality: Tom Baxter comes off the screen and into the movie house to sweep Cecilia off her feet. Without a moment's hesitation, she flees with him through a back alley as he attempts to escape from the cinematic world of fantasy into the stark reality of Cecilia's world.

The stranger-in-a-strange-land theme of *The Purple Rose of Cairo* is as irresistible to audiences as it is to filmmakers. Many films have been made about a visitor from another world, or another dimension, who arrives on earth as an incorruptible innocent, unfamiliar with the ways of real people. This visitor may be a mermaid, an extraterrestrial, a foreigner, or, in the case of *The Purple Rose of Cairo*, a celluloid character who exists only on the screen. The following films appeared in just the few years preceding the release of *The Purple Rose of Cairo*: John Carpenter's *Starman*, Steven Spielberg's *E.T.*, Ron Howard's *Splash*, Paul Mazursky's *Moscow on the Hudson*, and John Sayles's *The Brother from Another Planet*. The prototype of this story of innocence among the corrupt is, of course, the Christ story. Woody Allen is obviously aware of this parallel as he pans to a shot of a crucifix when Tom Baxter visits a church on his tour of Cecilia's world. Indeed, it is in the church that Cecilia's husband confronts Tom and challenges him to fisticuffs (plate 40). Tom gets the better of his opponent as long as the fighting is fair. But when he offers to shake Monk's hand and apologizes for the pain he has inflicted, Cecilia's husband knees him in the groin. Tom crumples to the ground, complaining in disbelief that his rival is not engaging in fair fighting.

Tom Baxter only knows the principles of fair play: deceit and dishonesty are alien to him. When he wanders innocently into a bordello, he is on unfamiliar ground. As the prostitutes surround him and listen intently, he speaks to them about the wonders of childbirth and the mysteries of existence. So taken with this inspirational young man, the ladies offer to service him for free. He thanks them for their offer but turns them down in deference to his love and loyalty for Cecilia. The denizens of the brothel are duly impressed,

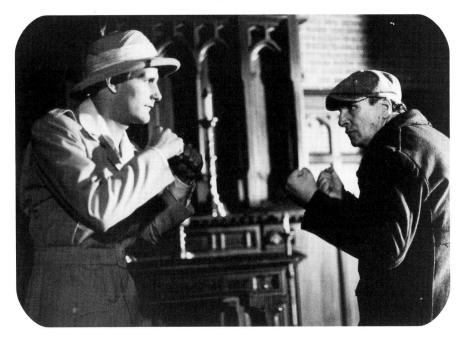

PLATE 40.   Different styles of combat: Jeff Daniels and Danny Aiello in *The Purple Rose of Cairo* (1985). Orion Pictures Corporation. The Museum of Modern Art/Film Stills Archive.

and one expresses a wish that there might be other men like Tom in the "real" world.

The parallels with Christ and the plethora of Christ figures in literature and film are obvious. Perhaps our strongest psychological need is for the illusion that somewhere, whether it be in a stable in Bethlehem or on the great silver screen, there exists an individual with transcendent, near-perfect qualities. The most salient feature of the movie hero is that he is not like us. He is unfettered by human selfishness and greed, by the baser instincts characteristic of the dark side of man. Hence, in the midst of perhaps the blackest era of American history—the Great Depression—Allen illustrates how film idols provided hope that a transcendent realm existed where a young man and young woman would meet, fall in love, and dance around the room in stunning fashion to the accompaniment of "Cheek to Cheek."

George Bernard Shaw once observed: "There are two tragedies in life. One is not to get your heart's desire. The other is to get it." Cecilia would undoubtedly agree. When her movie idol descends from the heavens to profess his love for her, more problems are created than solved. Tom is unable to function in a world where stage money is not accepted as currency, where cars do not start just because one sits behind the wheel, and where people do not behave as though they are the inventions of screenwriters. Moreover, Gil Shepherd (also played by Jeff Daniels), the actor who portrays Tom Baxter in the film within the film, appears on the scene. The producers of the movie are livid at Tom's departure from the screen and have enlisted Shepherd's assistance in persuading Tom to return. Gil pursues Cecilia in an intensive effort to court her away from Tom (plate 41). If he can win Cecilia's heart, he can save his career from ruin by forcing Tom back into the film. As we get to know Gil, we are stunned to find that the transcendently flawless Tom Baxter is a creation of an actor who is not fit to wear Tom's pith helmet, let alone his halo. Gil Shepherd is a man of extraordinary vanity. Like Monk, he is a man of the real world, who exploits Cecilia according to his own needs, with little regard for the impact of his exploitation of her.

The film's climax occurs when the heroine must choose between Tom and Gil in the empty movie theater while the characters on the screen look on. Reality and fantasy have reversed themselves. The action is now taking place in the darkened house, while the audience consists of a group of actors peering out from the movie screen. Gil seems aware of the strange state of affairs and comments, "I know this only happens in the movies, but I love you." Faced with an agonizing decision, Cecilia chooses Gil and says to Tom, "I have to choose the real world." A hard-bitten actress warns her from the screen, "You're throwing away perfection." Cecilia would have been wise to listen to this prophetess of doom. After Tom returns to the screen, Gil slips off to Hollywood without even a word of explanation. To Cecilia's horror, she discovers that she has made the wrong choice and is once again taken advantage of by a callous and self-serving man of the real world. She is left with a reality that is too grim to face, so she returns to the movie theater and immerses herself in yet another escapist fantasy: that of dancing with Fred Astaire. The film ends as it began, with the camera glued to Cecilia's face, her eyes transfixed with an almost beatific glow as she worships in her cinematic sanctuary.

As he does in *Stardust Memories* and *Zelig*, Allen again illustrates the folly of celebrity worship. We all know that Tom Baxter does not exist independently of the actor playing him. While Tom may be a virtuous and loyal Boy Scout, he turns out to be the creation of a narcissistic and insensitive boor who exploits and victimizes our heroine. However, while our sympathies lie primarily with the celebrity protagonists of *Stardust Memories* and *Zelig*, in *The Purple Rose of Cairo* our hearts are with the celebrity worshiper. We empathize with her predicament and with her psychological need to believe in

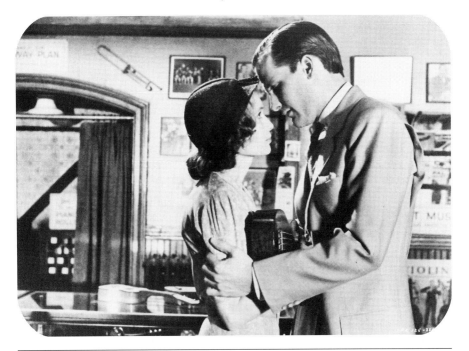

PLATE 41. Mia Farrow with the real thing (Jeff Daniels) in *The Purple Rose of Cairo* (1985). Orion Pictures Corporation. The Museum of Modern Art/Film Stills Archive.

Tom Baxter and Gil Shepherd. One way that Allen plays on our sympathies is to demonstrate our own vulnerability to believing in the illusions that movies offer. Like Cecilia, we find ourselves believing and hoping that Gil and Cecilia will go off into the sunset at the end of the film to live happily ever after. Even though we know rationally that such an outcome would never realistically come to pass, we are willing to suspend our disbelief to collude with the filmmaker's illusion. After we are jolted by the harsh reality of Gil's departure, we must accept that we are vulnerable to the same escapist fantasies as Cecilia.

Allen also helps us understand Cecilia's need to believe in Tom Baxter. As with Masha and Rupert's transference to Jerry Langford, Cecilia's transference to Tom represents the only available means of alleviating her despair. Just as the analysand may perceive his analyst as having idealized characteristics that bear little resemblance to the normal human flaws of the analyst's true personality, so Cecilia perceives Gil Shepherd. By the ingenious device of splitting the fictional character and the actor into two different people, Allen provides us with a graphic example of the difference between transference and reality. Tom is the idealized transference creation, while his counterpart, Gil, represents the nonfictional man behind the transference. When Cecilia looks at Gil, all she can see is Tom. Never mind that Gil's real attributes in no way resemble those of his doppelgänger, Tom. Cecilia is blind to the vanity of Gil because she needs the transcendent, Christlike qualities of Tom to tame the terror of her existence.

Tom Baxter is for Cecilia what Jerry Langford is for Masha in *The King of Comedy*. Both manifest idealizing transferences to their respective male celebrities. Each woman is made whole simply by standing close to her illustrious heroes and basking in the reflected glory. Kohut (1971) originally described this form of transference as typical of patients suffering from narcissistic personality disorder. However, in his posthumously published third book (Kohut 1984), he revised his thinking because of his increasing awareness of the ubiquity of such transference phenomena. He came to realize that even the healthiest person has a normal narcissistic need for idealized selfobjects in his environment. They are as necessary for psychological survival as oxygen is for physical survival. Cecilia's idealization of Tom is then a matter of survival. After reeling from the devastating blows to her self-esteem inflicted by her husband and her boss, Cecilia could enter the movie theater and revel in a buoyant sense of well-being because of her connection with this transference figure. When her self-esteem plummets after she realizes that Gil Shepherd has deceived her, she rapidly restores a cohesive sense of self by returning to the movies and sitting in the shadow of Fred Astaire and Ginger Rogers.

In film after film, Woody Allen sends this message: there is no special luster to celebrities. They are far more similar to us than they are different from us. Despite his sobering vision of the folly of celebrity worship, Allen's worldview has evolved to the point in *The Purple Rose of Cairo* where he realizes that Cecilia would probably have been better off living in her fantasy than opting for the reality of the vain, self-serving Gil. Perhaps the movies represent an opportunity for us to fulfill in a harmless way the need for fantasy and illusion that is intimately linked to our primal terror associated with the meaninglessness of existence.

Although *The Purple Rose of Cairo*, like *Zelig*, appears to be a film about a particular period in American history, the themes of the films reverberate with images of our contemporary culture. Near the end of *Zelig*, Irving Howe appears as a witness and makes the following observation: "It was absurd in a way. He had this curious quirk, this strange characteristic, and for a time everyone loved him. Then people stopped loving him; then he did this stunt with the airplane; and then everyone loved him again. And that was what the twenties were all about. And if you think about it, has America changed that much? I don't think so."

Ironically, the fourth feature in the celebrity tetralogy, *Celebrity* (1998), focuses less on the celebrity phenomenon than do the three earlier films. Kenneth Branagh, executing a Woody Allen imitation that would be humorous in a five-minute skit but becomes grating in a film that lasts longer than two hours, plays journalist Lee Simon, who writes profiles on the rich and famous but devotes most of his energies to the desperate pursuit of beautiful women. A failed novelist who is also trying to sell a screenplay, Simon goes from one empty relationship to another with a narcissistic pattern of initial idealization followed by loss of interest. In some ways another Allen surrogate, Judy Davis plays Robin Simon, the ex-wife of the Branagh character. Like Branagh, Davis frequently stammers and effects other mannerisms associated with Woody Allen. Although initially thrown for a loop when her husband abandons her, Robin is eventually saved by Tony Gardella (Joe Mantegna), who seems so perfect a lover that Robin is briefly convinced that their relationship must be doomed.

In one of the most compelling scenes in the film, Lee Simon tries to discuss his screenplay with teen idol Brandon Darrow (Leonardo DiCaprio) while the star is destroying his hotel room, terrorizing his girlfriend, and narrowly avoiding arrest. Darrow nevertheless finds time to take Simon under his wing and treats him to a limo ride, a boxing match, and group sex. Although clearly pleased to be part of the fast-lane life of a superstar, Simon is almost completely out of his element, at one point broaching the subject of his screenplay while Darrow is busy copulating with his girlfriend.

Even more so than in *The Purple Rose of Cairo*, Allen seems to have come to terms with the need for celebrities, their obvious shallowness notwithstanding. He still manages to poke fun at the emptiness and absurdity associated with celebrity, as when Robin visits Tony's family while they discuss a hot celebrity's visit to one of the kids' schools. They explain to the matriarch of the family that this particular celebrity was taken hostage and has become famous. The grandmother looks puzzled about the celebrity status, pointing out that all he did was get captured. At the end of the film, however, when Robin has become a minor celebrity who appears on television interviewing slightly less minor celebrities, an elderly woman approaches Robin to tell her how much she loves her program. After a brief conversation, the woman says, "God bless you" to Robin, who returns the blessing with utter sincerity. Compare the tone of this encounter with how Allen's characters treat the grotesques who are drawn to his celebrity allure in films such as *Annie Hall* and *Stardust Memories*.

Ultimately, however, Allen does not really extend his view of celebrity in this fourth film of the tetralogy. He continues to be ambivalent, suggesting on the one hand that being a celebrity is satisfying, while insisting on the other that a mutually loving relationship is the true source of satisfaction. The Branagh character's pursuit of perfect romance and his efforts to ride the coattails of celebrities leave him in abject despair at the end of the film, while the Davis character seems to have found fulfillment with her husband, her career, and her worshipful fans. Thus Allen sends mixed signals about what it means to be a celebrity. In his review of the film, J. Hoberman (1998) wrote: "But what exactly is Woody's complaint? If anything, the world of *Celebrity* is what his movies have always been. Allen is no stranger to self absorption. Nor, beginning with the Marshall McCluhan gag in Annie Hall, has any film-maker made more of the celeb cameo. The horror, I suppose, comes from his imagining himself being on the outside looking in" (117).

As we suggested in Chapter 10, Allen may have once again split himself in half as he projects different aspects of himself into characters. Branagh's schlemiel may be the disavowed version of Allen's self, especially the neurotic pursuer of young women. Judy Davis's Robin may represent more of Allen's current view of himself as someone who has settled into a fulfilling marriage. Although Allen consistently invites the audience to gaze at celebrity actors playing celebrities—not to mention "real" celebrities such as Donald Trump and Mary Jo Buttafuoco playing themselves—he ultimately seems most interested in venerating familiar notions of happiness and self-realization. But like *The Purple Rose of Cairo* and *Zelig*, *Celebrity* suggests once again that our need to idealize the famous has remained a constant throughout the twentieth century.

Indeed, we have not changed that much since the 1920s and 1930s. We live in an age where thousands of screaming teenagers worship rock stars who spit blood and blow up Oldsmobiles on stage, where daredevils scale skyscrapers in defiance of the law but in full view of television cameras, and where ordinary citizens forsake their privacy and rough each other up in order to appear on television talk shows. Many of these people are admired because they have not settled for the mediocrity of the masses, for being "nobody." They have made something of themselves through their own idiosyncratic version of the American dream. *The King of Comedy* and *Zelig* depict two such protagonists who emerge from anonymity into celebrity. The irresistible folly of their rise to stardom, like the irresistible folly of Cecilia's attraction to her movie idol, touches something profound and human in all of us as we sit in the darkened movie theater, knowing that our own existence is shortened with each unrelenting tick of the clock. Lahr (1996) comments on

Allen's prolific creation of films over the last thirty years: "To a man like Allen, who is hyperaware of his finiteness, the medium of film offers certain exquisite properties. Movies not only stop time and kill time—they preserve time" (74).

CHAPTER 12

Alien and Melanie Klein's Night Music

A*lien*, Ridley Scott's hugely successful science fiction film of 1979, is at some moments so horrific that it might more appropriately be classified a horror film. Indeed, *Alien* may share with John Carpenter's *Halloween* (1978) the dubious distinction of having brought the graphic violence of marginal or "cult" movies such as *The Texas Chainsaw Massacre* and *Night of the Living Dead* to mainstream audiences. Regardless of its genre, however, the success of Scott's film—it was the fourth largest grossing film of 1979 (Steinberg 1980)—may not depend entirely on its fascination with grisly death. Large numbers of ticket-buyers do not go to theaters simply to gaze at bleeding intestines, even if that appears to be the lesson that many in the film business have learned from *Alien*. Clearly, the film is more skillfully made than the rash of monster and mad-slasher movies of the 1980s and 1990s; but *Alien* also draws much of its power from its possibly unintentional evocation of infantile anxieties best described in psychoanalytic terms by Melanie Klein. As Noël Carroll (1981) pointed out prior to his apostasy (see chapter 7), psychoanalysis "is more or less the *lingua franca* of the horror film and thus the privileged critical tool for discussing the genre" (16). Particularly useful are Klein's theories on part-objects, introjection, and projection. If Klein is right, none of us ever completely overcome the angst of our earliest childhood imaginings. More so than most films of its kind, *Alien* skillfully evokes these early but imperfectly repressed anxieties about nurturing figures that can turn against us, about our own aggressive tendencies that can punish us from within or without, and about our tenuous relationship to bodies with no discernible beginning or end.

Many horror and science fiction films besides *Alien* can be understood in terms of Klein's work, most obviously her account of how the infant uses introjective-projective mechanisms to deal with primitive annihilation anxieties, including derivatives of the death instinct and of early oral aggressive drives. In *The Exorcist* (1973), as well as in its sequels and imitations, the Devil or some other possessing spirit moves back and forth among child and adult victims in ways consistent with this fantasy. This evil spirit is analogous to the bad, persecutory object, which is alternately projected and re-introjected.

Other films have played upon a child's ambivalence toward his or her love objects in somewhat different ways. For example, in a B movie from 1953 called *Invaders from Mars*, a boy witnesses the gradual takeover of his community by alien forces. His own parents are the first to be transformed. One day they return home visibly unchanged but exhibiting the conventional affectless behavior of alien-inhabited humans in science fiction films. The child is portrayed as well-behaved and affectionate, but he is abused by his possessed parents even when he attempts to demonstrate his love for them. The boy learns that the infected members of his community can be identified by means of a small wound at the back of the neck, clearly the site of penetration by the Martian invaders. Eventually, the boy seeks help from a pair of parent surrogates—his female teacher and an archetype of the 1950s, an oracular space scientist. The boy explains to them that his real parents are "wonderful" and would never behave so unpleasantly unless they were changed by aliens. When the boy encounters the aliens themselves, their leader appears as a large head inside a transparent sphere. Attached to the head are phalluslike tentacles, which undulate slowly within the globe. This nightmare combination of parental betrayal and disembodied part-objects in fact turns out to be the child's dream at the film's conclusion. By comparison, Tobe Hooper's 1986 remake of *Invaders from Mars* contains several in-jokes for science fiction film buffs but shows scant understanding of the original. Unlike Philip Kaufman's 1978 remake of *Invasion of the Body Snatchers*, Hooper's film makes no attempt to update the odd combination of infantile anxieties and anti-Communist hysteria that created an especially fertile soil for science fiction films in the 1950s. Kaufman, by moving the action of his film to San Francisco, changed the McCarthyist politics of the original *Invasion of the Body Snatchers* into an amusing satire of 1970s hedonism and human potential platitudes. The film did not, however, dilute any of the power that the original derived from depicting the paranoid states in which the characters constantly find themselves. Hooper's remake of *Invaders from*

Mars, on the other hand, keeps its tongue in its cheek throughout, poking appropriate fun at the original's plot but also frittering away the film's potential power by joking with the child's terror. Even in a summer of weak competition from undistinguished action films, the 1986 version of *Invaders from Mars* quickly vanished from theaters.

Film scholars have identified the original *Invaders from Mars* and a number of other American films from the 1950s with the reactionary politics of the McCarthy era. The first *Invasion of the Body Snatchers*, the most commonly cited example of this trend, can also be considered from both a political and a Kleinian perspective. The belief that communists could and would project themselves into a loved one and overnight transform him or her into a soulless and hostile creature finds its metaphors in the same science fiction conventions that touch on the childhood anxieties identified by Klein. One film that played on the generalized xenophobia of the McCarthy period was *The Thing*, directed by Christian Nyby in 1951. The creature from outer space—part plant, part animal—manifests itself in unusual ways and threatens to break into the protected domain of the intrepid heroes. Central to Klein's understanding of infantile development is the tendency to split off the "bad" or aggressive aspects of the self and project them into objects in the environment, thus producing paranoid anxiety about external attack within the infant. This concept operates in audiences' responses to *The Thing* as well as to virtually any film about destructive creatures trying to break into the fragile safety of our immediate surroundings. (A Kleinian analyst would have much to say about the "monsters from the id" that Walter Pidgeon unconsciously projects in *Forbidden Planet*.) John Carpenter's 1982 remake of *The Thing* takes us even deeper into a uniquely Kleinian world where evil forces are introjected by people and even transformed into grotesque combinations of human body parts. The suspense in this film derives from the paranoid tension concerning whether the invader from space is inside or outside the members of the team of Arctic scientists.

The protagonists in all of these films contend with a similar dilemma: they cannot be sure if their family members, colleagues, and loved ones are who they say they are. In both versions of *Invasion of the Body Snatchers*, no one can be trusted, because familiar bodies have been transformed into pod people. The police and even the psychiatrist in the film cannot be counted on since they have become part of "them." In *The Exorcist*, Regan (Linda Blair) has the same body but is no longer the same person. Similarly, in George Romero's *Night of the Living Dead* (1968), when an injured and helpless little girl is left alone in the basement with her father's corpse, she is later discovered to be making a meal out of her father, having been transformed into a flesh-eating zombie. In Carpenter's *The Thing*, the protagonist (Kurt Russell) must resort to a blood test to determine which members of the Arctic crew are "really themselves" and which have been invaded by the alien force and taken over from inside.

Part of the horror in these films lies in their obsession with the notion of the double—the idea that a good person can be transformed into an alter ego or doppelgänger of an unrelentingly evil nature. The protagonists then must assume a hypervigilant stance toward all their familiar friends and acquaintances to discern which of them can be trusted and which must be destroyed. In clinical psychiatry, a rare nosologic entity, known as Capgras's syndrome (Lehmann 1980), describes just this state of affairs. Persons afflicted with this syndrome are consumed with a variant of paranoia in which they believe that friends or family in their environment are actually impostors. The person affected with Capgras's syndrome may point out minute differences between the impostor and the actual person. While Capgras's syndrome represents an extreme at one end of the continuum, the cinematic theme of the double in horror films is chilling to the audience because it touches on a normal developmental experience that is universal. As infants mature, they experience the mother as alternately good and bad, depending on the extent to which she is satisfying their needs. The transformation of the good, loving mother into the bad, persecuting mother is clearly a source of intense anxiety for the infant. This developmental moment, in which mother is split into a good mother and a bad mother, may well be perceived in the infant's mind as a transformation similar to the one portrayed in the horror films that we have described. Hence, many of the most effective horror films replay the Kleinian theme involving the transformation of a good object into an identically appearing evil object, which Klein would understand as a projection of the split-off bad self. This motif achieved a tasteless if inevitable fulfillment in the 1984 Christmas release *Silent Night, Deadly Night*, in which Santa Claus is transformed into an ax murderer. When the television commercials advertising this film created a grassroots protest movement, it was withdrawn from many theaters. Parents made it clear that Santa Claus was one good object that would not be taken over from within by evil forces.

No science fiction or horror film, however, has evoked the full range of Kleinian anxieties so thoroughly as *Alien*. It may be more than an interesting coincidence that approximately midway through the film, Captain Dallas (Tom Skerritt) of the star ship *Nostromo* is relaxing in "the shuttle," listening to the second movement of Mozart's "Eine Kleine Nachtmusik." This lovely serenade is especially disarming because it is the only music in the film that is not part of the background score, and because its courtly associations are jarringly inappropriate to the grim, automated world of the space vessel. A number of explanations can be offered for the presence of this music in *Alien*. First, it is in the shuttle—a small ship attached to the enormous hulk of the *Nostromo*—that Ripley (Sigourney Weaver) makes her escape back to Earth and away from the dangers of outer space: we should not be surprised that earlier in the story it is shown to be a place where a character might find solace from the troubling events taking place in the rest of the ship. Also, since *Alien* is part of the grand tradition of technically sophisticated space adventures that began with Stanley Kubrick's *2001: A Space Odyssey* (1968), it is possible that the film's makers are paying tribute to the earlier film; *2001* was remarkable for its association of classical music with spaceships, and in its final scenes it placed an astronaut in a drawing room from the late eighteenth century, the era of Mozart.

The use of a few measures of "Eine Kleine Nachtmusik" also reminds us that the action of the film takes place in the eternal night of space and that the film is full of nightmare imagery and, of course, nightmarish content. But the ironic fact that this nightmare movie begins with people waking up and ends with one going to sleep is paralleled by the inconsistency of Mozart's sublime night music with the tones of horror struck throughout the entire film. The title "Eine Kleine Nachtmusik" implies an evening's entertainment, and *Alien* is an entertainment that deals with the stuff of nightmare. The infantile anxieties described by Melanie Klein pervade the entertainment.

Alien was one of the first films to make full use of the new technologies, which greatly expanded the film's impact on its audience: 70-mm projection equipment and six-track Dolby sound have made *Alien* an overwhelming experience. The audiences who flocked to the film in the summer of 1979 did not object to a plot that awkwardly sent characters off by themselves to be done in by the monster. Nor were they scared away by the scenes of explicit violence, which unnerved the film's more squeamish critics. Most likely they were attracted by those scenes that compellingly touched their most primal terrors. As Freud (1920) pointed out, there is a compulsion to repeat those traumatic events that were passively experienced in an effort to gain mastery over them. People line up to see movies like *Alien* in order to reencounter powerful unconscious anxieties while retaining a sense that they have some active control the second time around. Moreover, the movie provides an aesthetic distance so that audience members know that the terror on the screen is not actually happening to them, and they can experience relief along with their fright. The successful reactivation of primitive universal fears also depends on the director's handling of his subject matter, and we should point out certain technical achievements of Ridley Scott and his coworkers that serve to present these infantile experiences in an effective and affecting manner.

Alien owes a debt to its two major predecessors, *2001* and *Star Wars* (1977). Whether we see humans fighting machines, monsters, or other humans, all three films show a fascination with highly refined technology and how it creates a new kind of explorer/hero. Like *2001*, *Alien* alludes to a computer-oriented power structure in which human considerations can become secondary. But like *Star Wars*, *Alien* shows us a future in which technology lacks the antiseptic sheen covering the great inventions of *2001*. In *Star Wars* and *Alien*, gadgets can show their age and even break, although, as Miller and Sprich (1981) have written, *Star Wars* may have achieved its overwhelming success by speaking to a culture that has difficulty finding meaning in an increasingly technological society. Set in a world that is even more technologically complex than our own, *Star Wars* strongly affirms that meaning can be brought to our lives.

In *Alien*, director Ridley Scott has rejected the technological fairy world of *Star Wars* and created instead an entirely new vision of the future in which urban and rural blue-collar workers haggle about their shares of company wages while rusty chains and leaky pipes clutter the spaceship's untended corridors. This setting sharply contrasts to the innumerable science fiction films in which citizens of spacious, spotless cities stroll about in Hellenic revival gowns. (Some science fiction films were still adopting this approach to design as late as 1976—for example, *Logan's Run*—but the look already had been parodied by Woody Allen in 1973 in *Sleeper*.) The motley crew of the *Nostromo* in *Alien* is the predecessor of the grimy working-class population of the lunar mining village in *Outland* (1981). Scott developed this vision even further with the fully realized chaos of twenty-first century Los Angeles in his next film, *Blade Runner* (1982).

The future that *Alien* creates is not just the dehumanizing computer culture of *2001* in which humans must outwit their machines in order to climb to the next rung in the evolutionary ladder. As a revisionist science fiction film, *Alien* creates a genuine dystopia in which urban decay and frustration have expanded into outer space and in which a sinister "company" blithely declares its employees expendable at the whim of its "weapons division." The film transcends the idealism that generated the paranoid films of the post-Watergate years, such as Alan Pakula's *The Parallax View* (1974) and Sydney Pollack's *Three Days of the Condor* (1975). The conspiracies in those films create waves of indignation in their characters because of a belief that political conspiracies at the highest level do not take place in the West. But in *Alien*, the consummate cynicism of the characters and their world is voiced by Captain Dallas, who says, "I don't trust anybody." The crew of the

Nostromo is primarily made up of malcontents who do their unpleasant work purely for money and who show absolutely no ideals about family, country, or company. The only real human feelings in the film are directed by Ripley toward her cat.

The social and political setting of *Alien*, which has been extensively eluci-dated by Harvey Greenberg (1983), is an especially effective background for the nightmare action of the film. Just as there is no place in the ship in which to hide from the monster, there is no familiar, consoling institution to give meaning to the persecution of the characters. Even in *Outland*, Sean Connery had a wife and child to keep in mind when he went out to preserve his self-respect *High Noon*–style against the forces of evil, and *Blade Runner* ends with the hero escaping into a vernal paradise with his android lover.

Furthermore, Scott has used a number of cinematic devices to create a powerful sense of foreboding and anxiety. For one thing, he has frequently made the actors' dialogue incoherent. Even the characters themselves delib-erately obscure their words: when Ripley goes to the lower deck to check on repair work undertaken by Brett (Harry Dean Stanton) and Parker (Yaphet Kotto), she has to shout over the noise of steam escaping from a valve. As soon as she leaves, Parker laughingly turns off the steam. Parker is much like the director himself, who does not care if everyone's exact words are under-stood.

The sound of the film (which won a British academy award for Derrick Leather, Jim Shields, and Bill Rowe) is also confusing, especially in the multitrack Dolby version. At many moments it is difficult to distinguish be-tween which sounds are part of Jerry Goldsmith's atonal score and which are actual sounds on the ship. Furthermore, sounds frequently come from iso-lated corners of the stereophonic system, and, of course, one never knows when that corner is the one from which the alien will make its terrifying ap-pearance.

Scott also has intensified the film's effects by using close-ups where we would expect establishing shots. Filmmakers have always used this technique for the creation of suspense, but Scott's technological expertise and styli-zation set him apart from conventional directors. For example, in the scene in which Brett goes looking for Jones, Ripley's cat, the audience never really sees much of the remote part of the ship in which Brett finds himself. In-stead, Scott gives us suffocatingly tight close-ups of Brett's face and vertigi-nous tracking shots of the leaky heights of the ship rather than of the floor-level environs, which could conceal a lurking alien. We never see the expected establishing shots, and consequently we never have the least idea of what objects could do the concealing. Much the same effect is achieved toward the end of the film when Scott's camera closes in on Ripley's face, even though we are much more concerned about the proximity of the monster.

Most notably, Scott and his cinematographer, Derek Vanlint, never give us the opportunity to examine carefully the fully grown monster, which dominates the action of the film's last half. Although the camera often lingers on the beast's fingers or teeth, the entire alien is glimpsed only briefly, sometimes in a shot with such bright backlighting that the monster in the foreground is obscured. Scott has learned from Joseph Conrad that what we do not know can be more horrifying than what we know all too well. (Conrad's short story "The Duellists" was the source of Scott's first film; the novel *Nostromo* gave its name to the ship in *Alien*, and Conrad's theme of the double dominates *Blade Runner*.) Just as the horrors that Kurtz inflicts on the natives in *Heart of Darkness* are more disturbing for never being revealed, so the monster that we never quite see is all the more terrifying.

The movie opens within the womblike confines of the mother ship. The camera pans the inside of the craft in some detail and finally comes to rest on the sleeping bodies of the seven crew members. As we examine the spaceship's interior, we hear unformed and atonal noises, reminiscent of intrauterine existence, which are not readily identifiable but are eerily familiar. We then see the diaper-clad crew begin to wake up from their frozen sleep state (plate 42). From this symbolic birth at the beginning, the movie goes on to create a world much like Klein's view of the infant's early months of life. The cinematographic technique of omitting establishing shots contributes to a spatial disorientation, which may well represent the infant's early cognitive experience. Furthermore, we hear heartbeats and breathing throughout the film, echoes of the first few months of life when the mother's heartbeat and breathing are essential to the infant's sensory world.

Klein indicates that the infant turns all of his libidinal desires and all his destructiveness onto his mother's body. Hanna Segal, an articulate interpreter of Klein's writings, has observed that the infant's desires involve objects imagined to be inside the mother's body, including "fantasies of scooping out and possessing all of its contents, particularly . . . her babies" (1964, 7). This fantasy is portrayed early in *Alien* when the crew investigates the abandoned spacecraft on the remote planet. The inner lining of the ship is remarkably similar in appearance to the inside of a body (plate 43). The resemblance to the fantasied mother is all the more compelling because of the presence of egglike forms lying deep in the ship's hold. When Kane (John Hurt) disturbs one of these eggs, he realizes the fulfillment of the scooping-out fantasy as well as its punishment when the alien leaps out of an egg and attaches itself to his face.

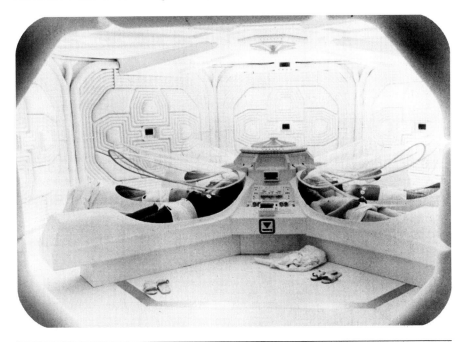

PLATE 42. The crew of the *Nostromo* wakes up at the behest of "Mother," the ship's computer in Ridley Scott's *Alien* (1979). Twentieth Century–Fox. The Museum of Modern Art/Film Stills Archive.

When Kane is returned to the *Nostromo*, diagnostic studies reveal that it is impossible to remove the creature from his face. One X-ray study reveals that the monster has extended an appendage down his throat and is keeping him alive. This situation can be understood in terms of the vicissitudes of early infantile development. The ego undergoes splitting and projects that part of itself containing the aggressive instinct, or the death instinct in Kleinian terms, into the original external object, the mother's breast. The infant then feels that the breast is bad, resulting in feelings of persecution. The terrifying but life-sustaining creature in *Alien* represents the bad, persecuting breast: it is the recipient of the first projection of the child's internal aggressive drives, while at the same time it performs the traditional nourishing function.

Once the infant has projected his aggression into the mother's breast, he then lives in terror that the persecutory object will get inside him and destroy both him and his good internalized objects. Segal (1964) describes this fear as the leading anxiety in the paranoid-schizoid position, a normal phase in the first several months of infantile development. The terror of annihilation ac-

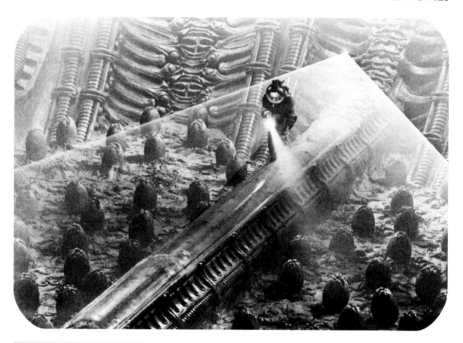

PLATE 43.   Kane (John Hurt) explores the maternal body of a derelict ship in *Alien* (1979). Twentieth Century–Fox. The Museum of Modern Art/Film Stills Archive.

companying this phase of development leads to the evolution of defense mechanisms, principally the use of introjection and projection:

> The ego strives to introject the good and to project the bad. This, however, is not the only use of introjection and projection. There are situations in which the good is projected, in order to keep it safe from what is felt to be overwhelming badness inside, and situations in which persecutors are introjected and even identified with in an attempt to gain control of them. The permanent feature is that in situations of anxiety the split is widened and projection and introjection are used in order to keep persecutory and ideal objects as far as possible from one another, while keeping both of them under control. The situation may fluctuate rapidly, and persecutors may be felt now outside, giving the feeling of external threat, now inside, producing fears of a hypochondriacal nature. (Segal 1964, 26–27)

These defensive operations are graphically demonstrated in *Alien* when Kane is discovered to be free of the adhesive creature and is apparently back to his normal state of health. After sitting down to eat with his fellow crew members, he is destroyed from within when the alien ruptures his chest wall and escapes into the ship. To translate this sequence into the language of the paranoid-schizoid position, Kane introjected the bad persecutory object with the unconscious fantasy of gaining control over it. The dinner scene is characterized by much unnatural laughter, a kind of manic denial based on the fantasy that the persecutor has been annihilated. The dinner is disrupted by Kane's hypochondriacal concern about something within his body. The bad object is then re-projected—literally, when the alien rips through his chest wall—and is once again the source of persecutory anxiety as it disappears into the spacecraft's corridors.

At this point, Scott's carefully crafted nightmare ambience can be seen as part of the persecutory anxiety that afflicts the remaining crew members, who are never sure where the alien, the projected bad object, is hiding and when it will strike. Captain Dallas's unwillingness to trust anyone is just one of the many manifestations of paranoia that strike all but two characters in the film. The first of these two is Ash (Ian Holm), the science officer, who turns out to be an android. The second is the ship's computer, appropriately bearing the name "Mother." This maternal object also turns out to be bad when it reveals that it is in collusion with the company and is programmed to bring back the alien at all costs, even if the crew must be sacrificed for its capture. Just before the ship's destruction, Ripley gives the computer an order, which it does not acknowledge. In a rage, Ripley screams, "You bitch!" and smashes one of the computer's monitors.

Ripley's rage reflects the terror associated with the realization that she is living in a paranoid-schizoid world. It is a world devoid of good maternal objects. Nor are there any whole or ambivalently perceived mature objects in this chilling setting. The alien represents a thoroughly bad part-object, unrelenting in its evil and destructive nature. Ash, in commenting on this quality, expresses his admiration for the "purity" of the monster's devotion to the malevolent destruction of life. This ambience of part-objects, so typical of the paranoid-schizoid position, is heightened by the camera's tendency to show only part of the alien's anatomy at any one time. Here we see another version of the familiar Kleinian Capgras theme, as developed in films such as *Invasion of the Body Snatchers*, *The Exorcist*, and John Carpenter's *The Thing*. The crew naïvely trusted Ash, a science officer, to make judgments regarding the appropriate handling of the alien. They are shocked to learn that Ash is not who they thought he was. Rather, he is an android impostor with malevolent intentions. Moreover, "Mother," the ship's computer, is itself an evil force bent on their destruction rather than on their survival and safe return to Earth.

To intensify the paranoid anxieties even further, the film shows all father figures being destroyed or, in the case of the robot Ash, working in tandem with the evil maternal computer. There is no rescuing father in this grim world of infantile terror. Contrary to the viewer's expectations, Captain Dallas, whom we assume to be the hero and the father figure of the ship, is killed relatively early in the movie, running counter to the convention of the science fiction or horror film. With the strong father figure now out of the picture, the crew has lost both its first and second command officers, leaving the strategy against the monster to be devised by two women, two childlike male figures, and the robot Ash.

The role of Ash in the movie leads us to another dimension of Klein's account of early infantile fantasies. Segal (1964) notes that the "infant's first dawning perception of the parental intercourse is of an oral nature, and the mother is conceived of as incorporating the father's penis in intercourse. Thus, one of the riches of mother's body is this incorporated penis" (4). The mother, then, becomes a more terrifying object because of the infant's fantasy that she contains a penis in addition to the breast. These fantasies lead to anxiety about the "phallic mother," who is capable of destructive penetration, and to confusion about the equivalence between penis and breast. Indeed, the notion of the phallic mother is central both to children's stories and fairy tales and to a number of successful horror movies. The most obvious example of the fairy tale is the Halloween witch who rides with a broomstick between her legs. Movies such as Alfred Hitchcock's *Psycho* and Brian De Palma's *Dressed to Kill* portray female murderers who stab their subjects with sharp objects and who are later discovered to be men dressed as women. These terrifying figures resonate with the infantile concern that mother may possess a hidden phallus.

When Ash goes berserk in his confrontation with Ripley, he rolls up a girlie magazine and attempts to cram the phallic object down Ripley's throat, hence replicating the infantile terror that the mother's penis will be offered instead of the breast. Moreover, the monster itself is strikingly phallic, with its awesome tail, its long, tubular head, and its inner set of teeth, which extend and destructively penetrate its victims. The condensation of these oral and phallic elements is further illustrated by the fact that the monster also eats at least one of its victims.

The movie ends by fulfilling the audience's wish to master its infantile anxieties. Through an ingenious strategy, Ripley manages to overcome a considerable number of obstacles and extrude the monster from the shuttle, eventually blasting it out into space. Literally, Ripley has rid herself of badness via projection and then destroyed the projected badness. The film's last shot shows Ripley entering a blissful sleep with her cat, as though the extrusion of the all-bad part-object has allowed for an all-good world of symbiotic bliss to replace it. Hence, the audience can vicariously experience not only mastery of the paranoid anxieties associated with the persecutory object but also the achievement of the nonambivalent, blissful union with the all-good mother as the outcome of such mastery.

The special power of *Alien* is strikingly demonstrated by comparing it to the 1986 sequel, *Aliens*, which also was a great commercial success. With his producer and then-wife, Gale Ann Hurd, director James Cameron infused *Aliens* with the same energy and imagination that he brought to his first major film, *The Terminator* (1984). In many ways a careful homage to the original, *Aliens* continually finds ingenious ways of inflating the plot, settings, politics, technology, and special effects of Scott's film. Cameron and Hurd are members of a new generation of commercially savvy and technically accomplished filmmakers who know exactly how to appeal to every segment of the audience. Their work is intelligent but not intellectual, involving but not challenging, startling but not unnerving, and is thoroughly enjoyable if not entirely admirable. (Cameron struck gold with this combination in 1997 with *Titanic*.) In contrast to the comic book hyperbole of the sequel, Scott's *Alien* now seems like a pensive, scrupulously drawn chamber film.

In their most remarked upon departure from the original, Cameron and Hurd masculinized women in ways that were soon to be commonplace in Hollywood films. Not only is Ripley (Sigourney Weaver again) braver, tougher, smarter, and more resourceful than all the men in the film, so is at least one female marine. But Ripley also excels in virtues traditionally associated with women: she is the only character able to communicate with a nine-year-old girl (Carrie Henn), who is the only survivor of an alien attack on a distant planet and the kind of innocent but streetwise child that exists only in Hollywood. After promising to fulfill all the maternal needs of the little girl, Ripley saves her life by fighting to the death with another supermother, the alien queen bee. To further heighten the tension, the film has Ripley rescuing the child while the planet's nuclear destruction is seconds away.

Although *Aliens* quotes from the original in many ways, the movie has excised almost all the Kleinianisms that made the first film so fiendishly effective. The change was probably intentional. Cameron and Hurd may have understood what made *Alien* successful, but they surely understand that most blockbuster hits do not stray as far from Hollywood's paradigms as does Scott's film. Whereas *Alien* did away with all reassuring father figures rather quickly, none are needed when the sequel's Ripley is the ideal mother and a better protector than the most attentive father. Furthermore, the romance that was so thoroughly missing from *Alien* has been provided, not just in the sequel's gushy evocation of mother love but also in the sexually charged conversations between Ripley and a soft-spoken marine (Michael Biehn), who is cut from a sensitive, caring Alan Alda mold. Even the political paranoia of the original has been transformed: the horror of *Alien* was enhanced by the gradual realization that no institution could provide solace when the "company" was revealed to be as malevolent as anything lurking on the ship; a similar vision of an evil military-industrial complex is presented in the sequel, but its agent (Paul Reiser) is portrayed as just another movie bad guy, no match for the indomitable Ripley. *Aliens* ends on a deeply reassuring note as a man, a woman, and a child enter peaceful hypersleep, a postnuclear family returning to the bosom of Mother Earth. Audiences familiar with the original might have expected a baby monster to burst out of Carrie Henn's chest after she had been rescued from the aliens. This perverse touch might have been consistent with the introjection-projection motifs of the original, but it would have been completely inconsistent with the upbeat spirit of the sequel.

If the first sequel moved away from the claustrophobic, almost chamber film qualities of *Alien*, the next two films in the series opened up numerous connections with more topical concerns. Specifically, the sequels activated concerns about abortion and AIDS that are only vaguely suggested in the original. And as Tom Doherty (1996) has suggested, each new film in the series has added a new level of intertextual relations to other kinds of films. Just as *Aliens* bore many resemblances to the return-to-Vietnam films that flourished during the Reagan years, *Alien³* (1992) brought in genre conventions from the prison film, and *Alien: Resurrection* (1997) added large helpings of the maternal melodrama to the mix. As we point out in chapter 13, the fourth film in the tetralogy, *Alien: Resurrection*, plays on the conflicted image that Sigourney Weaver has acquired since her first star turn in *Alien*. In fact, the entire series has taken up the issue of the "phallic" woman, who both titillates and horrifies the typical male in the audience at the same time that she both supports and undermines various feminisms circulating in late-twentieth-century American culture. The fourth film is also typical of all the sequels in that it elaborately restages all the important scenes of the first film in new situations, often with a generous amount of irony. We could certainly argue, however, that for better or worse none of the sequels seem at all interested in developing the Kleinian themes of the original.

The plot of the original *Alien* is simple: a monster is at large and must be destroyed. But as we have shown, the film has developed a complex method of telling the story and has connected it—intentionally or otherwise—with the audience's long-forgotten but still powerful anxieties. We have not argued that the film coherently works out a one-to-one correlation between its plot and these anxieties. Rather, we have shown how images of these fantasies emerge variously in much the same way that images appear in primary-process thought and how these images strongly suggest the infantile fantasies identified by Melanie Klein. Consequently, *Alien* taps into the dark, unconscious anxieties of the audience and produces a reaction that spectators might not quite understand, just as they are not quite able to understand much of the dialogue in the film. Clearly, the preverbal ambience of the paranoid-schizoid position is not dependent on a clear understanding of language. In more ways than one, the audience of *Alien* is kept profoundly in the dark.

CHAPTER 13

"Phallic" Women in the Contemporary Cinema

The critic Georgia Brown (1990) has observed that if the old formula for terror in movies was a woman alone pursued by a berserk man, the new formula is a harmless man terrorized by a crazed woman. Brown characterizes the 1990 film *Misery*—in which an immobilized James Caan is at the mercy of a powerful and overlooming Kathy Bates—as "*Rear Window* with James Stewart in the same room with Raymond Burr in drag." On the one hand, the violent phallic woman in *Misery* can be understood as one more manifestation of the "backlash" against the various feminisms of the recent past (Faludi 1991). Women who stray from traditional female roles—or pervert these roles as Bates's character does in *Misery*—are increasingly likely to take monstrous forms in Hollywood movies. So long as women's assumption of power is widely regarded as aberrant, America's entertainment industries will continue to capitalize on collective fantasies that are widely forbidden and hence profitably displaced into the narrative of a film. On the other hand, Hollywood has produced a dazzling variety of phallic women in recent years, many of whom are presented sympathetically and some of whom operate in narratives that do not speak directly to feminist issues, pro or con. Regardless of how popular cinema presents phallic women, psychoanalysis provides a means for understanding the developmental, political, and cultural forces that lie behind this trend. Specifically, we would argue that psychoanalytically derived techniques of dream interpretation can be read into a cultural criticism of Hollywood's commodified fantasies. The omnipresent image of the phallic woman in recent cinema is surely an overdetermined phenomenon, one that speaks to a variety of anxieties and fantasies, some more clearly articulated than others. An especially complex example of the phenomenon occurs in a handful of recent films that revolve around the discovery that a woman does *not* possess the phallus.

Our argument begins where so much of contemporary film theory starts—with Laura Mulvey's extraordinarily influential article "Visual Pleasure and Narrative Cinema" (1975). As we have argued in chapter 7, Mulvey's theory of the cinematic punishment and fetishization of women as a means of assuaging the castration anxiety of the male viewer is only a partial account of gendered and nongendered pleasure at the cinema. More specifically, the possibility that a woman may *not* be castrated—that she may in fact possess a penis—has been identified as an even more fundamental fear than castration anxiety (Lurie 1981–82; Modleski 1988). While a number of films from the eighties and nineties have foregrounded women with phallic qualities, this chapter will address two of them, *Sea of Love* (1990) and *Working Girl* (1988), that are more concerned with male anxiety about the *possibility* that a woman may possess a penis, or something very much like it.

The Phallic Mother

Freud wrote that the fantasy of a maternal phallus is a fundamental and therefore universal aspect of normal development. An extensive elaboration of this theme appears in his notorious psychobiographical study of Leonardo da Vinci (Freud 1910). Freud seized on the symbolic meaning of a screen memory from Leonardo's childhood in which the artist remembered a large bird's tail being inserted into his mouth while he was an infant in a crib. Relying on a secondary text that mistranslated "nibio" as "vulture" instead of "kite," Freud searched for mythological correlates of this childhood fantasy. Noting that the vulture-headed Egyptian mother goddess Mut was typically represented as having both an erect male organ and breasts, Freud suggested that the male child must naturally assume that women possess a penis like his own. For Freud, mythology was preserving a primitive fantasy of the mother's body that reflected a universal developmental period in the male child.

In subsequent writings, Freud used the fantasy of the female phallus as the centerpiece of his explanation of fetishism (1927, 1940). The male's castration anxiety leads him to regard the fetish with a peculiar form of intrapsychic splitting in which the fetish is both a denial and a confirmation that women are castrated. In subsequent elaborations on perversions by Bak

(1968) and Stoller (1975), the fantasy of the woman with a phallus continued to play a key role in the pathogenesis of other forms of sexual deviation. Bak, for example, even went so far as to state, "In all perversions the dramatized or ritualized denial of castration is acted out through the regressive revival of the fantasy of the maternal or female phallus" (1968, 16). Stoller linked the fantasy to transvestitism, in which a man dresses as a woman in an effort to give substance to the unconscious fantasy that women do indeed possess a penis.

This myth of the phallic mother, however, has other functions besides relieving the male child's castration anxiety by reassuring him that women are just like he is. Beneath the genital imagery resides an omnipotent pregenital phallic mother born out of the male child's fear of a castrating, penetrating, all-powerful mother who may take advantage of his vulnerability (Brunswick 1940; Chasseguet-Smirgel 1964; Eigen 1974). Perhaps the most obvious example of the phallic mother's centrality is the ubiquitous image of the witch on her broomstick with facial hair and pointed hat. By 1945, Geza Roheim had already traced the phallic mother theme to legends about witches in European folklore. Roheim also pointed out the association of mythological witches with cows or milk that is ruined or poisoned. In 1986, Nancy Kulish wrote, "The phallic mother is really the oral mother, then, the witch who attacks the source of milk and embodies the infant's aggression against the mother" (394). This equation of penis and breast is clearly present in the Leonardo screen memory. As Freud (1910) noted, the active situation of the infant suckling at the breast is transformed in Leonardo's memory into a passive version in which the phallus/breast is thrust into the infant's mouth as he passively receives it.

For Kleinian theorists, the infant combines breast and penis by assuming that father's penis is contained in mother. In her lucid introduction to Klein's work, Hanna Segal (1964) comments that "the infant's first dawning perception of the parental intercourse is of an oral nature, and the mother is conceived of as incorporating the father's penis in intercourse" (4). The male child may further fantasize that mother has orally castrated father and thereby augmented her own power with that of the paternal penis (Eigen 1974). In this view, the phallic mother is *both* castrating and penetrating.

Derivatives of Leonardo's screen memory are ubiquitous in dominant American cinema. In chapter 12 we noted that in *Alien* (1979) and in James Cameron and Gale Ann Hurd's 1986 sequel, *Aliens*, a maternal monster functions simultaneously as a bad, persecuting breast and as a phallic destroyer. At one point in the first film, a character is kept alive by a phallic-like extrusion that the creature has inserted down his throat, an almost literal representation of the phallus/breast described by Leonardo. A more recent, more displaced example of this type of conflation appears in *Misery*, in which Annie (Kathy Bates) has been trained as a nurse, thus allowing her to nurture James Caan whenever she is not smashing his ankles with a sledgehammer, shooting him with a gun, or poking a hypodermic needle into his arm.

The character of Annie in *Misery* is an especially good example of a phallic mother, but she is not typical of the new breed of phallic women *without* maternal qualities who regularly populate American films. In the 1940s and 1950s, a commonplace of film noir was the decidedly nonmaternal woman who deploys a gun or a knife to demonstrate her assumption of male prerogatives (Kaplan 1989). In a film such as *Johnny Guitar* (1954), this tradition of the gun-toting female gargoyle borders on parody. Many films in the eighties and nineties have appeared in which women keep guns and knives under their skirts—or somewhere below the waist—and actually shoot men in the genitals. Significantly, these women are inevitably marked as sexually desirable and frequently placed in stark relief against more conventionally maternal women. The character played by Sharon Stone in *Total Recall* (1990) conceals both a gun and a knife along the lower reaches of her body, and at one point her entire frame takes on the same kind of murderous, phallic intensity that the replicant enacted by Daryl Hannah displayed in *Blade Runner* (1982). Seductive women have guns literally strapped to their inner thighs in *License to Kill* (1989), *Desperate Hours* (1990), and *King of New York* (1990). In *Sudden Impact* (1983) and *Last Rites* (1988), avenging women shoot bullets into the genitals of their male victims. Significantly, the female perpetrators in the latter two films go unpunished within the respective narratives. As in the emerging genre of rape-revenge films, of which the purest example may be *Ms. 45* (1981) and of which the best-known example may be *Thelma and Louise* (1991), Hollywood has succeeded in making phallic women both titillating and unthreatening by providing them with victims who deserve castration or death (Lehman 1992). Variations of this maneuver dominated many of the most popular films of the 1990s, including *Thelma and Louise* as well as *Sleeping with the Enemy*, *The Silence of the Lambs*, *Terminator II*, *A Rage in Harlem*, *Lethal Weapon III*, *Batman Returns*, *The Long Kiss Goodbye*, *G.I. Jane*, and even the art house hit *La Femme Nikita*.

Sea of Love

In the last few years, uncertainty about women's phallicness has become a trope in American films—sexy but aggressive women may or may not conceal a gun, a knife, or some kind of phallus. *Fatal Attraction* (1987) became widely popular at least in part by suggesting that an assertive woman may ultimately resort to the use of a knife to achieve her goals. This film epitomizes the splitting of powerful women into maternal and nonmaternal types, with the mother (Anne Archer) eventually blowing a hole in the body of the non-mother (Glenn Close). A film that surely represents a twist on the myths in *Fatal Attraction*, and was probably bought by the studio as an attempt to capitalize on its success, is *Sea of Love*.

In *Sea of Love*'s opening scenes, the audience sees a naked male buttocks engaged in rhythmic pelvic motions on a bed while the 1950s' rhythm-and-blues hit *Sea of Love* plays in the background. As the camera pans up to the figure's head, it becomes clear that the man is terror-stricken and vulnerable. Seconds later, a handgun is discharged into his head. While the gender of the murderer is unknown, the phallic symbolism of the revolver is not in question. The case is assigned to down-and-out, alcoholic policeman Frank Keller (Al Pacino). Frank is depressed and psychologically castrated at least in part because his ex-wife discarded him for a fellow cop. His impotent rage at this rejection leads him into a half-hearted physical assault on his wife's current husband, to whom he later apologizes.

After the killer strikes for the second time, Frank engages in some conventional *policier* bonding with Sherman (John Goodman), a policeman from another New York City borough. After discovering that each victim had sought female companions by running a poem in the personals column of a singles' magazine, the police set a trap by placing a similarly structured ad themselves. Each of several women who answer the ad meets Frank in a restaurant where he poses as a lonely man working as a printer. The subtext of this scam as the search for a phallic woman is only partially repressed. When one of the respondents senses that Frank is lying about his profession, she exclaims, "If you're a printer, I've got a dick." As she storms away from the table, Frank shouts after her, "I didn't doubt it for a minute, baby." Rehashing their evening's work, Sherman asks Frank, "Could you go for a girl with a dick?" Frank replies, "It depends on her personality."

Frank finds the girl with the right personality in Helen Cruger (Ellen Barkin). Although she leaves no fingerprints to establish her guilt, Helen quickly becomes the prime suspect—both for the police and for the audience—after she flamboyantly rejects Frank at the restaurant. Nevertheless, she soon becomes the policeman's lover after a chance meeting at a delicatessen. Indeed, the film is especially interesting as a kind of return of what is repressed in the personals—there is an unacknowledged equivalence between seeking a lover and stalking a victim, an unsettling element in contemporary (especially urban) romance that most American films deny. *Sea of Love* puts it back on our plate by creating a situation in which the woman is just as likely to be Frank's lover as his killer. Ellen Barkin plays the part of Helen with a carefully calculated degree of ambiguity. Audiences are just as likely to associate her mannerisms with a sexy but harmlessly aggressive woman as with a serial killer. In fact, Barkin's screen persona possesses sufficient menace that in her next film, Walter Hill's *Johnny Handsome* (1990), she was cast as a particularly nasty version of the cold-blooded, castrating mankiller. As if to further her phallic reputation, Barkin subsequently appeared in Blake Edwards's *Switch* (1991), in which she played a man who has come back from the dead in the body of a woman.

In *Sea of Love*, Helen becomes romantically involved with Frank shortly after their initial encounter. Helen's phallic dimensions are depicted in the tension of the question whether or not she is the killer as well as in her predatory approach to finding sex partners. While Frank has not had a date since his divorce and is still stuck on his wife, even phoning her in the middle of the night, Helen goes through one casual relationship after another. Significantly, in their first love scene, the nude Helen embraces Frank from behind, engaging in a kind of humping motion not at all typical of Hollywood sexuality. Frank does not register dread at her phallic nature, however, until he discovers a gun in her purse that she carries into his bathroom at the very moment when she decides to have sex with him. He reacts with fear, verging on panic, as he runs around the room, desperately seeking a way of defending himself against a seemingly imminent attack. When Helen emerges from the bathroom, Frank frisks her, police fashion. The camera provides a below-the-neck two-shot to show that he has searched her genital region. The tension is relieved when we discover that the gun is a harmless starter pistol. Why she carries such an item is never explained. Nor does the film offer a reason why she carries a toy gun toward the end of the film when Frank thrusts his hand up her skirt in search of further phallic treasures. (In addition, the film never explains the significance of the song that gives the film its title and that plays in the background when the first victims are dispatched.) A more aroused and less suspecting Frank also inspects Helen's crotch toward the middle of the film when she arrives wearing nothing but a raincoat. Although he again inserts his hand into the coat at her genitals, on this occasion he is not inspecting her for a literal weapon. The second policeman, Sherman, meanwhile, is furious when he discovers that Frank has become involved with a prime suspect in the case. Sherman invokes appropriate imagery to express his exasperation when he asks Frank what he anticipates testifying in court: "What do you say to the judge, 'First I whipped it out, then she whipped it out'?"

The mystery about Helen and her imagined phallus, however, should have ended halfway through the film when the audience discovers that she has a daughter. Once inserted into the realm of conventional, childbearing sexuality, women in dominant American myth seldom possess negative phallic qualities. Even Linda Hamilton in *Terminator II*, knowing that a computer expert will eventually cause a nuclear holocaust, breaks down and cries rather than murder him in front of his child; her biceps and assault weapons notwithstanding, she is still a mother. Although Helen's exculpatory motherhood is established early, *Sea of Love* does not reveal the identity of the killer until the final moments when Helen's ex-husband bursts into Frank's apartment: Helen's rejected mate has been systematically stalking and killing his ex-wife's lovers. Male and female audience members are reassured that the instrument of phallic destruction is associated with the appropriate gender and that Helen is simply a vulnerable, often nurturing sexpot who has helped restore Frank's potency. In this regard, *Sea of Love* works against Mulvey's original hypothesis. While scenes occur in which Barkin's body is fetishized for the male spectator, *denial* of castration is not the primary purpose at these moments. Rather, the film repeatedly demonstrates that the female figure is indeed castrated.

The discovery of Helen's lack of a phallus is especially important for a number of reasons, not the least of which is the film's view of equivalence between penis and gun. Helen also becomes a legitimate sex partner in a scenario that activates homoerotic overtones in the relationship between Frank and Sherman. As Robin Wood (1986) has argued, "buddy films" such as *Butch Cassidy and the Sundance Kid*, *Midnight Cowboy*, and *Thunderbolt and Lightfoot* must work hard to deny the unmistakably homoerotic elements when two men have more intense feelings for each other than for any of the women in the narrative. Frank's pursuit of Helen and particularly his discovery that she has no penis serve to relieve a good deal of the tension created by the "buddy" portion of *Sea of Love* in that they establish Frank's erotic interests as clearly heterosexual. In a similar manner, the depiction of Helen as unequivocally female functions as a counterpoint to the phallic-aggressive male-male conflicts between a husband and an ex-husband and ultimately between a lover and an ex-husband.

Working Girl

A list of films with phallic women—or more specifically, with women who conceal guns and knives—would primarily include gangster movies, films noir, or their contemporary equivalent. *Total Recall* is a good example of how film noir conventions have seeped into science fiction, with an even better example being *Blade Runner*. One might not expect to find a phallic woman—or a potentially phallic woman like *Sea of Love's* Helen Cruger—in the romantic comedy *Working Girl*. But Hollywood has always had a gift for exchanging material from one genre to another.

Mike Nichols's *Working Girl* opens with an elaborate helicopter shot of the Statue of Liberty. The Lady in the Harbor is certainly an overdetermined symbol of American values, but for Nichols it hardly signifies the dropout utopianism of *Catch-22* (1970) or the anticorporate paranoia of *Silkwood* (1983), two films that he directed in earlier eras. Actually, the Statue of Liberty functions as a kind of double for Tess (Melanie Griffith), the statuesque overachiever from Staten Island who bluffs her way into the corporate elite and becomes an American success story. This doubling is especially important in terms of body shape. At the climax of *Working Girl*, Tess tells her duplicitous, upper-class boss, Catherine (Sigourney Weaver), "Get your bony ass out of here." The line is repeated twice, and audiences have consistently greeted it with the film's biggest laugh. The suggestion that Catherine has a "bony ass" draws attention toward Catherine/Weaver's body and away from Tess/Griffith's. In fact, some significance can be found in the fact that Tess possesses a softer, more maternal derrière.

In this sense, the film is especially typical of Hollywood in writing its most important questions—here, ones of social class—across the bodies of women. The first woman whose body the film invites us to inspect is the Statue of Liberty. In the opening shot of the film, the camera begins with a close-up of Liberty's face, circles around to the back of her head, and then draws away so that we see her enormous derrière, modestly draped though it may be. According to an only partially facetious book by Paul Fussell (1983, 51–54), working-class people in the United States, historically, have eaten themselves to a higher social level. The spare tire around a construction worker's middle says, "I've got mine." Melanie Griffith had put on a little weight after the birth of a child just before she started shooting *Working Girl*. She was trimmer in *Something Wild* (1987), released a year earlier. Rather than concealing this extra flesh, *Working Girl* makes the most out of it. In fact, Griffith's zaftig thighs, buttocks, and breasts are repeatedly fetishized throughout the film, beginning when she first sits down at her desk and allows her miniskirt to ride up while she changes her shoes. In this fashion, the film takes sides with the cherubic working classes, who are also associated with the generously proportioned Statue of Liberty. *Working Girl* portrays its aristocrats as much less angelic, even to the point of privileging Melanie

Griffith's body over Sigourney Weaver's in spite of the fact that Weaver might be considered more attractive, at least according to the standards of feminine beauty currently prescribed by American advertising.

During the first hour of the movie, Tess is victimized by her cheating boy-friend (Alec Baldwin), the chauvinistic men she works for, and a predatory yuppie in a stretch limo. In a sense, Catherine comes on the scene as one more phallic victimizer who "screws over" Tess. In spite of the film's many attempts to establish itself as a feminist document, *Working Girl* regularly judges Catherine by sexist standards (Greenberg 1989). As Tess's boss, she is stigmatized as a woman in a man's job. She tells dirty jokes (specifically, ones involving anal penetration) with the guys at a cocktail party. And she aggressively steals Tess's money-making idea and appropriates it as her own. Catherine's habit of dressing like a man is underlined in a comment by her fiancé, Jack (Harrison Ford), when he first meets Tess. Immediately attracted to Tess, Jack tells her that she "dresses like a woman instead of how she thinks a man would dress if he were a woman."

Like Griffith, Weaver is displayed several times in lingerie, but only when she is wearing an ungainly cast on her leg. She is undressed to show not only that she has phallic qualities but that her phallus (the leg cast) is enormous and ridiculous. This is especially evident when Catherine attempts to seduce Jack toward the end of the film; although she tries to conceal her cast with an afghan, Jack immediately unveils the stiff white appendage when he walks into her bedroom. Although the scene has an obvious comic intent, it bears some resemblance to Al Pacino's deadly serious attempts to find a pistol or a penis beneath Ellen Barkin's skirts. The phallic character of Catherine's cast is further established when Jack knocks on it to determine the extent of its rigidity or, shall we say, its boniness. In this scene Jack is not at all aroused by a woman with a huge erection, lingerie or no lingerie. In fact, he seems almost frantic to find a way out of Catherine's apartment. Appropriately, Catherine receives her comeuppance from a benevolent patriarch (Philip Bosco), who repeats the charge that she remove her bony ass. In a moment imbued with more pathos than may have been intended, Catherine hobbles out of the narrative on her crutches, her phallic power revealed to have been temporary and highly contingent.

The term *bone*, used three times in connection with Sigourney Weaver's body, may have more than one meaning. Weaver herself has regularly played phallic if sympathetic women, most memorably in the *Alien* and *Ghost-busters* films. Significantly, Weaver's phallicism in the first *Alien* (1979) and the first *Ghostbusters* (1984) slides dramatically toward maternal power in the corresponding sequels. In *Ghostbusters II* (1989), Weaver is primarily concerned with protecting her infant child, and in *Aliens* (1986) the climax features the "battle of all mothers," with the huge phallic monster, the queen of the alien creatures, squared off against the powerful and resourceful Ripley (Weaver). But a plot twist in *Alien: Resurrection* (1997), the fourth film in the series, reveals the radical contradictions in the maternal aspects of Weaver's movie persona. Although she plays a nurturing role with the android played by Winona Ryder, Weaver/Ripley must ultimately come to terms with her hideous offspring, the bizarre result of alien DNA being mixed with her own. In the end, the mother kills her own monster/child. The ambiguity of Weaver's screen persona is part of the is-she-or-isn't-she dynamics of *Working Girl*, not unlike the similar questions in *Sea of Love* that are based to a great extent on Ellen Barkin's ambiguous persona. Both Weaver and Barkin have become texts unto themselves into which a certain amount of phallic strength or menace has been written. Few other actresses could have successfully brought the proper balance of qualities into either *Working Girl* or *Sea of Love.*

Psychoanalysis and Gender Confusion

The enormous popularity of movies involving cross-dressing and ambiguous gender attest to the universal need to master anxieties related to genital differences. Some of these films, such as Alfred Hitchcock's *Psycho* (1960) and Brian De Palma's *Dressed to Kill* (1980), fall into the horror genre. No doubt the terrifying figures presented in those films—female murderers who stab their subjects with sharp objects and who later are discovered to be men dressed as women—resonate with infantile concerns that mother may possess a hidden phallus. To that extent they offer experiences of active mastery over passively experienced trauma.

Of course, comic films regularly invite laughter at the spectacle of a man dressed as a woman. Popular American films, such as *Some Like It Hot* (1959), *Victor/Victoria* (1982), *Tootsie* (1982), and *Crocodile Dundee* (1986), have used this device with great success. Cross-dressing has been a staple of Western literature at least since Thetis dressed Achilles as the daughter of Lycomedes to keep her son out of the Trojan War. The tradition is best-known in Shakespeare's comedies. In all of those works, audiences derive pleasure from knowing more than the characters about the true nature of the disguised character's genitals.

Psychoanalytic reconstructions in the treatment of adult patients and developmental studies of children demonstrate that the young child has a good deal of curiosity, not to mention anxiety, about the characteristics of the opposite-sex parent's genitals. Narratives that exploit this anxiety tap into an important developmental moment in the unconscious of the audience—namely, when the child suddenly discovers that the opposite-sex parent has different genitals. In this manner the passively experienced infantile anxieties, curiosity, and discoveries are all relived by the audience vicariously at a safe distance. When one is viewing the film, however, the trauma is reversed—the audience knows the secret and is not surprised, while the characters in the film (or play) are traumatized by the discovery. Much of the humor in contemporary films stems from a similar moment of discovery—when Crocodile Dundee, for example, discovers that the woman with whom he is about to go home is a man. A more striking instance occurs at the climax of *Tootsie*, when Dustin Hoffman removes his wig on camera, and each of the principal characters in the movie reacts with shock when they see that the famous soap opera actress is actually a man.

Whether or not the clearing up of gender confusion in these films is ideologically neutral is a difficult question. While questioning bourgeois notions of gender and sexuality is potentially subversive, these same norms are powerfully reaffirmed by the film's end. As Studlar (1989) has pointed out, even "cult" films like *The Rocky Horror Picture Show* (1975) and *Pink Flamingos* (1972) do little to undermine the dominance of patriarchy in sexual hierarchies. For all their celebration of disorienting sexuality, these films invariably associate women with perversion and men with dominance. In the last decade or so, American films have found ways of recuperating women who cross gender boundaries so long as these transgressions are tightly circumscribed (Straayer 1992).

A discussion of the phallic woman would not be complete without reference to male masochism. Men seek out prostitutes in the dominatrix role because the wish of some men to be forced into submission—and even penetrated by a dildo—is a common and powerful fantasy. Movies that portray threatening women who castrate and penetrate men may consciously or unconsciously gratify the secret wishes of certain male audience members.

New Directions in Female Phallicism

Throughout the 1990s the American cinema has regularly presented women with phallic qualities, especially qualities that can in some way be redeemed within the narrative. That is, Hollywood continually finds new ways to arm women without upsetting more fundamental gender images. In *The Silence of the Lambs* and *Sleeping with the Enemy*—the two most successful films during the early months of 1991—the heroines take up weapons only when their lives are at stake and the film has thoroughly stigmatized their male victims. The phallic elements of Linda Hamilton are similarly contained in *Terminator II*, the most popular film of the summer of 1991. In *V. I. Warshawski*, Kathleen Turner deploys her martial arts skills almost entirely to protect her surrogate daughter, even going so far as to kill the child's natural but infanticidal mother. The climactic moment in *A Rage in Harlem*, in which Robin Givens uses a gun on the villain only in order to save the life of virtuous Forest Whitaker, suggests that the project of forgiving sexy female shooters may be colorblind. In what was surely the most widely discussed film of 1991, the protagonists of *Thelma and Louise*—neither of whom has children—do not survive their few transgressive days as gender outlaws. The widely diverse readings of *Thelma and Louise* seem to bear out the fundamental thesis of "cultural studies" that popular narratives are not so much texts inscribed with meaning as they are sites where readers create meaning. We would simply observe that the film ends with a hyperbolic display of male phallic power before which the women give up their lives, if not their souls. Although the male spectator at *Thelma and Louise* can participate in a pregendered or nongendered identification with the heroines, he leaves the theater knowing that their threat to patriarchy has ended in the final whiteout over the Grand Canyon.

Although Carolyn Polhemus (Greta Scacchi) in Alan J. Pakula's *Presumed Innocent* (1990) never picks up a weapon, she fits many of the categories developed throughout this chapter. Amelia Jones (1991) has revealed a number of similarities between the women in *Presumed Innocent* and those in *Fatal Attraction*. Just as Alex (Glenn Close) in the earlier film constantly engaged in perversions of motherhood, Carolyn in *Presumed Innocent* has had a tubal ligation. This information is not uncovered until the autopsy after Carolyn is brutally murdered. By renouncing all things maternal, Carolyn was able to rise quickly within the highly competitive district attorney's office, deploying her sexuality for pleasure but more often for higher position. Throughout the film, several suggestions are made that the woman was "bad news" and that her death was in some way a fitting retribution for her assumption of phallic power. One of Carolyn's conquests is Rusty Sabich (Harrison Ford), eventually charged with her murder. But as in *Fatal Attraction*, the audience ultimately learns that the highly sexed career woman was killed by the wife of the man with whom she was having an affair. When Sabich discovers that his wife, Barbara (Bonnie Bedelia), has murdered Carolyn by repeatedly striking her with a hammer, he keeps the information to himself, proclaiming in a voice-over that "I couldn't take his mother from my son." Jones (1991) has remarked upon the curiously awkward wording of this phrase in which the woman is grammatically if not completely objectified (313). The idea that some kind of family harmony has been restored after the nonmaternal phallic woman has been eliminated is an invention of the film. As Jones points out, Scott Turow's novel on which the film is based ends with the couple separated, the murder having become too great an obstacle to their marriage. Once again, Hollywood has recuperated a maternal phallic woman at the expense of a transgressively nonmaternal one.

The trend of the testosterone-driven woman may have reached a nadir of sorts in another film directed by Ridley Scott, *G.I. Jane*, which appeared in 1997. Demi Moore, pumped up courtesy of her personal trainer, appears as a Navy lieutenant who is a pawn of politicians embroiled in a conflict over the appropriate role of women in the military. She is subjected to extraordinarily brutal and sadistic Navy Seal training. As the only woman, she is repeatedly humiliated and mocked by her fellow sailors. At the film's climax, she engages in fisticuffs with the monstrous Master Chief (Viggo Mortensen) in front of her cheering comrades. After both G.I. Jane and the Master Chief have gotten in their share of licks and both are thoroughly bloodied, G.I. Jane asserts her defiance by shouting at her opponent, "Suck my dick!" The cheering of her male peers in response to that line suggests that she has finally become "one of the guys."

As in *Thelma and Louise*, Ridley Scott's intentions here are not entirely clear because of the implausibility of *G.I. Jane*'s basic premise. Is Scott really championing the cause of equality for women in the military? Or is he simply indulging in a male fantasy of what it would be like if an attractive woman were subjected to the rigors of Navy Seal training? Scott's brand of feminism constantly dances along the border of parody.

At least a few words should be said about *Basic Instinct*, the most popular film of the first half of 1992. Like *Sea of Love*, which it resembles in myriad ways, *Basic Instinct* features a woman (Sharon Stone) who is strongly marked as sexually desirable and who may or may not be guilty of killing men, in this case with an ice pick. The film begins when a man is murdered by an unidentified blonde woman with whom he is having sex. One of the policemen working on the case (Michael Douglas), like Al Pacino in *Sea of Love*, is a troubled alcoholic who has difficulty communicating with women but who nevertheless becomes sexually involved with the prime suspect in the murder case. Another obvious similarity between *Sea of Love* and *Basic Instinct* is the homoerotically charged relationship between the protagonist and his best buddy on the police force. George Dzundza, the one actor in Hollywood who may be effectively interchangeable with John Goodman, actually meets Michael Douglas in a gay bar shortly before one of the climaxes in *Basic Instinct*. Sharon Stone, like Ellen Barkin, has played mankillers in the past, and like *Sea of Love*, as well as *Fatal Attraction, Basic Instinct* dwells on the similarities between an intelligent, sexy, in-control woman and a murderous psychopath. Whether or not the Sharon Stone character possesses a phallus is an especially interesting question in *Basic Instinct*. The film goes to some lengths to show that Stone does not put on underwear beneath her minidress just before she departs for the police station to be questioned. As if to prove her innocence during her questioning, Stone briefly opens her legs to display her vulva and to confound a roomful of male cops sitting opposite her. Although she clearly does not have a phallus with its usual power, she establishes a great deal of power by showing what she does have. She effectively uses her vagina as if it were a phallus. And in the paranoid, misogynist ideology of the film, Stone's ability to manipulate men and maintain complete control at almost every moment is tantamount to having a phallus. Furthermore, as in *Sea of Love*, the revelation of the female protagonist's sexual organs makes her a sanctioned sexual partner for the hero in a narrative driven largely by homophobia. The sexuality of Stone's character, however, is entirely devoid of a childbearing element. She even expresses contempt for "rug rats" at a crucial moment near the end. This unrecuperable side of her sexuality is an important element in the film's notoriously ambiguous ending.

Male anxiety over the phallic woman is a common subject in American cinema, at least in part because it is a universal theme in the male unconscious. If we can conceptualize popular movies as in some ways analogous to the dreams of a culture, we can find valid analogies for the dream work in how Hollywood manipulates drives, images, and anxieties—all the residue of people's lives that affects them on some profound level. Male anxiety about women can be displaced first into a number of culturally specific narrative possibilities. Two surprise hits of 1990, *Pretty Woman* and *Ghost*, create beautiful, lively women who are nevertheless entirely dependent on their men, and in the case of Demi Moore in *Ghost*, dependent on her man even after he dies. Another, darker version of this displacement is the nightmare image of the castrating monster, like Glenn Close with her knife in *Fatal Attraction* and Kathy Bates with her panoply of weapons in *Misery*. These films represent a double displacement because they first displace generalized male fears into cinematic narrative and then displace the specific fear of a female phallus into knives, guns, and sledgehammers. A thematic reading of films from a specific historical moment can be understood psychoanalytically as reflecting—and perhaps reinforcing—anxieties that are generally repressed throughout the culture. This kind of reading can lead to clarification even in borderline cases such as *Working Girl* and *Sea of Love*. In both films, the fear of the phallic woman spills into narratives in which, on many levels, the women do not in fact possess the phallus.

Epilogue

$\mathbf{F}$ilmmakers appear to be just as fascinated by psychiatry as psychiatrists are by movies. Psychiatrists and psychiatric matters have been regular subjects in films at least since 1904, and many writers have probed the mysteries of the cinema with psychoanalytically informed methodologies. Unlike other books about the interaction of movies and minds, this work has dealt with the relationship from both sides.

In Part One we discussed some of the ways in which movies have stereotyped psychiatrists and appropriated them to serve the mechanical needs of plot and genre as well as the cinematic mythology of the day. In surveying more than 450 American films, we have found only a handful that have not indulged in radically simplified or stylized portrayals of psychiatry, and, most often, these films eventually turn from the examination of psychotherapeutic interactions toward familiar cinematic clichés. For example, *Spellbound, One Flew Over the Cuckoo's Nest,* and *Ordinary People* have little in common, but all three begin with themes relating to mental illness and ultimately end with highly conventionalized depictions of the psychiatrist saved by a lover, the clinical victimization of a Christlike hero, or the climactic drama of a cathartic cure.

Psychiatrists are paradoxical figures for filmmakers. On the one hand, their work is extremely difficult to understand and has the potential to bring exciting action to a deadly halt. On the other hand, if psychiatrists are not observed too closely, they can conveniently provide the perfect forum for exposition and character development. They also can supply the legitimization of sexual themes, the rationalist contrast to supernatural "truths," the secular salvation of troubled souls, the romantic interest for misunderstood individuals, the convincing explanation for mysterious behavior, the commonsense solution for domestic crises, and the repressive opposition to free-spirited heroes. In addition, the unsettling message of psychoanalysis—that we are not fully conscious of the motivations that direct our lives—has always been at odds with its image as a beneficent means to self-help, thus leaving its portrayal open to polar opposites.

Few professions, ethnic groups, or social classes have been immune from a similar process of cinematic stereotyping, but psychiatrists may be unique for having occupied both the highest and lowest levels of prestige in their motion picture incarnations. We have charted these changes from the quacks of the early years through the secular saints of the Golden Age (1957–63), through the fools and criminals of the 1960s and 1970s, and finally to the more variegated group of movie psychiatrists in the 1980s and 1990s. In all of these periods, however, the needs of cinematic genres are almost always paramount; if they are not devalued beyond all reason, psychiatrists are usually idealized to an equally extreme degree. The need to see others as heroic and idealized—the celebrity phenomenon we described in chapter 11—is highly relevant in this context. Most movies demand idealized heroes because audiences demand them. These exaggerated figures give audiences hope, helping each of them weather his or her own existential storms, if only for two hours in a darkened theater.

We have found that very few filmmakers have broken out of narrow generic conventions and put cinematic psychiatrists to imaginative uses. In particular, Woody Allen and Paul Mazursky have understood that mixtures of positive and negative traits are much more typical of human beings than heroism or villainy, and they have directed films in which psychiatry provides the means for examining this ambiguity. Their psychiatrists are seldom the Olympian healers of the Golden Age or the ridiculous figures of the late 1960s but rather the inhabitants of a world where difficult choices characterize human reality. Ironic comedy and gentle satire usually dominate the works of these directors, largely as a turning away from both the gravely serious social realism of the Golden Age and the chic nihilism of the 1960s and 1970s.

In Part Two, we discussed a number of films that can be better understood through the application of critical techniques derived from psychoanalysis. In the two chapters (10 and 11) on narcissism in the cinema, we examined the manifestation of cultural patterns that dominate the themes of five recent films. Psychoanalytic methodologies can open up these works and lead to a larger view of contemporary American culture. After considering intrapsychic and cultural interactions in the adult world, we turned to the earliest experiences in the development of the child. A strikingly different methodology gives us insight into Ridley Scott's *Alien* and the genre of horror/science fiction films. Our reading of that film is designed to offer reasons for the primitive origins of horror film conventions as well as for the enduring appeal of these films. Similarly, we have relied on other theories of development to understand the many films that endow female characters with "phallic" qualities. Finally, we hope that we have demonstrated how a knowledge of the dream work is essential to an understanding of Robert Altman's otherwise puzzling *3 Women*. Taken as a whole, Part Two of this book is meant as a brief introduction to the immense potential of psychoanalysis as a tool in film criticism. As psychoanalytic approaches to film study become more prevalent, it may soon be argued that cinema, more than fiction, poetry, or drama, is ideally suited to the kinds of analysis that Freud and his followers applied to the arts as well as to individuals and cultures. Moreover, the richness and complexity of the human psyche brought to light through psychoanalytic approaches illustrate the inadequacy of the one-dimensional stereotypical portraits of psychiatrists described in Part One. It is disconcerting to practitioners of depth psychology to see movies paint such superficial portraits.

While it may be true that filmmakers and psychoanalysts are mutually intrigued by each other, it is also true that they share a tendency toward mutual outrage. Filmmakers often react with incredulity or even ridicule at what analysts "read into" their movies, and therapists are appalled at the film industry's portrayal of their therapeutic activities. Both sides feel misunderstood. The psychiatrist's reaction calls to mind the frequent response of the therapist who sees his or her videotaped interview of a patient for the first time. Typically, the therapist gasps in disbelief, "Do I look like *that*?" or "I can't believe I said that" or "That's not what I meant." Clearly, how psychiatrists imagine themselves clashes with what is recorded by the camera's dispassionate eye. While the cinematic medium has an immense narcissistic appeal, its power to inflict narcissistic injury is equally strong. It may well be that those who choose to be psychotherapists are attracted to the privacy of the procedure, by which they are insulated from prying eyes and criticism from others who would judge their work. The filmmaker's intrusion into the privacy of the consulting room may therefore be viewed as an extraordinary violation. The well-known reluctance of psychotherapists to tape their work undoubtedly is related to more than an altruistic concern over the preservation of patient confidentiality. Most therapists, one suspects, worry that their technique is lacking in some respect and would fail to hold up to scrutiny by peers.

Beyond the anxiety about the quality of one's work, however, a sense may exist among psychiatrists that the mere depiction of psychotherapy is almost obscene. Christian Metz (1982) notes that a peculiar kind of voyeurism is involved in the cinematic experience. What specifically defines this voyeuristic form is the absence of the object seen, which is not only contrary to true voyeurism as a clinical phenomenon but also in contrast to the theater, where the object is actually present on stage. In this sense, cinematic voyeurism is experienced as more unauthorized and more forbidden than its theatrical counterpart, where the actors fully sanction the audience's desire to look at them. Metz argues that this differentiation establishes a stronger link to the primal scene in the cinematic audience than in the theatrical one. Thus, both the lure and the repugnance intrinsic to cinematic portrayals of psychiatric treatment may resonate with more primitive concerns about what is acceptable to see or show.

The double-edged power of the cinema both to enhance and to devastate one's self-esteem is evident in the response of real-life therapists who have appeared in films. Dr. Penelope Russianoff, who played a role in Paul Mazursky's *An Unmarried Woman*, is quite candid about her response to the filmed experience (personal communication, 1984). She was not nearly as bothered by her portrayal in the movie as a possible lesbian as she was by a few bad reviews. Six years after the movie, she still could quote from them. Even though she was not an actress, the criticisms may have stung because the film showed her at work as a psychotherapist. One can empathize with her reaction since it is difficult to divorce her performances as actress and therapist. An unusually tall woman, she was accustomed to people staring at her on the street. After the film, she said that she was never sure if people were staring because she was tall or because she was in the movie. A few strangers spoke to her about the film, and some seemed incapable of separating her real character from the one they saw on the screen. These experiences, plus the few bad reviews, eventually sent her back for a brief refueling visit to her own therapist. Despite the emotional toll, she longed to do more acting. She was disappointed when no subsequent film offers came, and she acknowledges that she would have liked to play the role of Dr. Berger in *Ordinary People*, a film that she believes her performance in *An Unmarried Woman* helped make possible.

When Dr. Dean Brooks of the Oregon State Hospital in Salem was approached about playing a psychiatrist in *One Flew Over the Cuckoo's Nest*, he had a number of misgivings. Although he knew that the film was only entertainment and not a documentary, he found it difficult to detach himself from the fact that it was being made in his hospital. He thought to himself, "Oh my God, my professional career is on the line. People will think that the hospital is really this way" (personal communication, 1985). Before he would agree to the in-hospital filming, he secured a commitment from producers Saul Zaentz and Michael Douglas that the movie would in no way denigrate patients. During the first half of the filming, Brooks continued to go through internal struggles about his participation. He reports that he was finally able to overcome these misgivings when he accepted that it was just a movie and decided to have fun. He commented that the movie actually hired eighty-nine patients, some of whom were paid more than he was. He described an extraordinary camaraderie between the cast and crew of the production and the hospital's patients, which he felt had a positive effect on many patients.

Ten years after the filming, Dr. Brooks was convinced that *One Flew Over the Cuckoo's Nest* had no deleterious effect on his professional career. He also said that the hospital was in no way hurt. Initially, however, he experienced a number of criticisms from colleagues who felt that the film was "venal" or that it had "set psychiatry back twenty-five years." He defends his participation, pointing out that the view of the movie as a negative portrayal of psychiatry is a narrow one. He believes that Ken Kesey was writing about institutions in general rather than about mental hospitals in particular and that the film opened people's eyes to a number of concerns about institutions. Like Dr. Russianoff, he caught the acting bug as a result of *Cuckoo's Nest*, and he went on to act in another film, *Three Warriors*, which was never released theatrically but has appeared on cable television. He said that he never seriously considered leaving psychiatry to become an actor, but he unabashedly acknowledged that he loved being in front of the camera and enjoyed the celebrity that went with the experience. Donald Muhich, who has appeared in Paul Mazursky's *Bob and Carol and Ted and Alice*, *Blume in Love*, *Willie and Phil*, and *Down and Out in Beverly Hills*, had acted even before he become a psychiatrist (personal communication, 1985). As a high school student in Minnesota, Muhich had been offered a scholarship to study acting at Northwestern University, a major proving ground for aspiring young actors. Although he eventually chose to accept an academic scholarship instead, Dr. Muhich has always kept his hand in as a producer and screenwriter as well as an actor. In addition to appearing in Mazursky's films, Muhich has participated in the writing of at least ten of the director's movies, and he has produced a number of documentaries on his own. In 1970 he helped develop a short-lived television series, *Matt Lincoln*, which brought *Ben Casey* star Vince Edwards back to television medicine, this time as a community psychiatrist. Muhich says that he terminated his brief career in commercial television when the producers of the struggling program brought in writers "to give the show heart."

The long and continuing association between Muhich and Mazursky began in the 1960s when Mazursky was writing jokes for Danny Kaye as well as the screenplay for Hy Averback's *I Love You, Alice B. Toklas* (1968). As Mazursky himself once acknowledged on the Johnny Carson show, he went to Muhich for treatment, knowing that the psychiatrist had a private practice in Beverly Hills primarily for creative people. Shortly afterward, when Mazursky learned that he would be allowed to direct *Bob and Carol and Ted and Alice*, he called Muhich and said, "I'm going to direct my first film. Come on out and we'll have a party!" Mazursky knew that Muhich had a good deal of acting experience and cast him for his knowledge of the performing arts as well as for his familiarity with the practice of psychiatry. In fact, Muhich has had a good deal of control over his appearances in Mazursky's films, and he continues to correspond with the director concerning all aspects of Mazursky's work. In both *Bob and Carol and Ted and Alice* and *Blume in Love*, Muhich worked closely with the director to achieve what he calls "the fine line between satire and realism." For example, the tight close-up in *Bob and Carol* that shows Muhich pinching his own cheek while listening to Dyan Cannon was suggested by the psychiatrist as a means for capturing the slightly irreverent tone that he and the director intended. Muhich says that he never set out to represent the profession as it really is and certainly not to glorify it. He believes that psychiatrists often claim more expertise than they are entitled to and that some chipping away at their image may not be an unworthy pursuit. He was amused by the number of mental health professionals who found his scene with Dyan Cannon to be an accurate presentation of psychotherapy, but he also admits that he stopped getting referrals from other psychiatrists after the film was released. Clearly, Muhich has derived immense pleasure from working with movie stars and filmmakers, and he recalls his acting experience in the movies as great fun.

The accounts from these three mental health professionals illustrate both the exhilaration of performance and the personal and professional vulnerability intrinsic to cinematic exposure. In the final analysis, the power of the cinema is probably multidetermined. The prospect of being preserved on celluloid is an immortality strategy that ensures one of surviving beyond the limitations of human mortality. The siren call of celebrity has a magnetic attraction that few of us can resist. Another determinant may be related to the Janus-faced dimension in all of us involving exhibitionism and scopophilia. While the actor in the movies may be sublimating exhibitionism, the psychotherapist in the privacy of his office sublimates his voyeuristic interests. While seemingly disparate in this respect, psychiatry and the cinema are both capable of offering a compelling glimpse into the human psyche. It is, of course, this point of convergence that will keep these two unlikely companions inextricably bound for years to come.

A Filmography for the Depiction of Psychiatry in the American Cinema

This list is by no means complete, omitting numerous low-budget films of the horror and sex genres and most made-for-TV movies. In addition, a number of relevant films undoubtedly were not uncovered in our research. We have listed a handful of films by European directors that we consider especially important. Directors are identified immediately after a film's date, and the summary refers primarily to how each film characterizes psychiatrists or psychiatry.

The Accused (1949) William Dieterle. Loretta Young is psychology professor who commits murder for the right reasons.

Ace Ventura, Pet Detective (1994) Tom Shadyac. Fourteen years after his stint as a psychiatrist in *Dressed to Kill*, David Margulies again dons a white coat and deadpans his way through an over-the-top scene with Jim Carrey.

After the Thin Man (1936) W. S. Van Dyke. George Zucco plays crackpot with Coke-bottle glasses who accuses nice young man (James Stewart) of being crazy. When Stewart turns out in fact to be quite mad, Zucco says, "Good heavens, I was right. The man is crazy."

Agnes of God (1985) Norman Jewison. Jane Fonda has personal problems, and she smokes too much, but her concern for patient (Meg Tilly) strongly recalls *Ordinary People*'s Judd Hirsch. Since the film suggests with leaden ambiguity that a nun may have been impregnated by an angel, Fonda may also be another rationalist who cannot appreciate The Unknown.

Airplane II: The Sequel (1982) Ken Finkleman. Testifying in court, John
    Vernon is asked to give his impression of the defendant. His reply: "I'm
    sorry, I don't do impressions. My expertise is in psychiatry."

Alice's Restaurant (1969) Arthur Penn. Arlo's immortal words at the draft
    board: "Shrink, I wanna kill."

The Amazing Dr. Clitterhouse (1938) Anatole Litvak. Absurd psychiatrist
    testifies in court against Edward G. Robinson but only creates confu-
    sion.

Amos and Andrew (1993) E. Max Frye. Bob Balaban is called in to talk
    sense to kidnapper over telephone. Long after the would-be patient has
    left, shrink continues talking, mostly about his childhood.

Anatomy of a Murder (1959) Otto Preminger. Fresh-faced Orson Bean is
    not exactly an oracular psychiatrist, but his presence plays against Vien-
    nese stereotypes.

Angel Heart (1987) Alan Parker. Morphine addict Michael Higgins once
    took bribe to falsify medical records. Killer detective (Mickey Rourke)
    shoots him in the eye.

Angel on My Shoulder (1946) Archie Mayo. In a plot similar to *Here Comes
    Mr. Jordan*, Paul Muni is crime boss whom Satan chooses to put into
    the body of a respected judge. Psychiatrist friend figures that some-
    thing is wrong, but judge's girlfriend (Anne Baxter) believes in her man
    (and eventually in mobster as he reforms) and lectures psychiatrist on
    the limits of his profession.

Annie Hall (1977) Woody Allen. The eternal analysand's guide to life.

Another Woman (1988) Woody Allen. Repressed academic heroine (Gena
    Rowlands) overhears analytic sessions in adjoining apartment. For
    better or worse, the film makes no attempt to undermine the analyst's
    competence.

Antz (1998) Eric Darnell and Tim Johnson. In this animated feature, the
    voice of Woody Allen inhabits an ant in analysis with a fellow ant,
    whose voice is supplied by Paul Mazursky. He has come to analysis be-
    cause he is struggling with being the middle child of 5 million.

Armageddon (1998) Roland Emmerich. A rough-and-ready team of oil drill-
    ers flies into space and saves the world from destruction, but the psy-
    chologist who tests the team members declares them all to be unfit.

The Arrangement (1969) Elia Kazan. Analyst Harold Gould is one of several
    ineffectual characters involved in Kirk Douglas's midlife crisis.

Arsenic and Old Lace (1944) Frank Capra. In Capraland, only a psychia-
    trist would be so foolish as to think that these lovable eccentrics ought
    to be locked up.

Article 99 (1992) Howard Deutch. Kathy Baker is a beleaguered psychiatrist in a crowded VA hospital. She has little success with her chronic patients but has time for a "quickie" with a surgeon.

As Good as It Gets (1997) James Brooks. Lawrence Kasdan in a cameo as a psychiatrist with solid professional boundaries.

Attack of the 50 Ft. Woman (1993) Christopher Guest. Frances Fisher is entirely supportive of her patient (Daryl Hannah), even when Hannah is too large for the consulting room.

Austin Powers: International Man of Mystery (1997) Jay Roach. Carrie Fisher leads group therapy session in which Dr. Evil (Mike Myers) tries to convince his son to follow in his footsteps. When the son says he wants to become a dentist, the father says, "Yes, but an evil dentist."

The Bachelor and the Bobby Soxer (1947) Irving Reis. Court psychiatrist (Ray Collins) is a bit pontifical, but he gracefully solves the romantic problems of his two nieces (Myrna Loy and Shirley Temple).

Bad Dreams (1988) Andrew Fleming. After fourteen years in a coma, heroine wakes up in contemporary hospital in the care of two psychiatrists, a young attractive one (Bruce Abbott), who falls in love with her, and an older one (Harris Yulin), who turns out to be a mad scientist feeding her hallucinogenic drugs.

Bad Timing: A Sensual Obsession (British; 1980) Nicholas Roeg. Theresa Russell drives Art Garfunkel, an American psychiatrist in Vienna, to distraction, to sodomy, and, finally, almost to necrophilia.

Basic Instinct (1992) Paul Verhoeven. Let's see . . . Jeanne Tripplehorn, the police psychologist having an affair with a patient, turns out to be bisexual and maybe even a murderer. Troubled cop Michael Douglas yells at a roomful of grotesque shrinks, "You're all full of shit!"

Batman Forever (1995) Joel Schumacher. Nicole Kidman portrays your typical femme fatale forensic psychologist.

The Beast from 20,000 Fathoms (1953) Eugene Lourie. Very unsympathetic psychiatrist tries to convince hero that he did not actually see a "rhedosaurus."

Bedlam (1946) Mark Robson. Boris Karloff, no less, is the sinister and cruel warden at the eighteenth-century institution to which courageous Anna Lee is committed.

Bedroom Eyes (1986) William Fruet. Voyeur hero is charged with murder, but he is protected by his beautiful psychiatrist (Dayle Haddon), who eventually marries him.

Bedtime for Bonzo (1951) Frederick de Cordova. Amiable as ever, psychology professor Ronald Reagan proves his nurture-over-nature theories, instilling morality into a chimp.

Bedtime Story (1964) Ralph Levy. Con man David Niven poses as a Swiss psychiatrist in order to bilk Shirley Jones.

The Believers (1987) John Schlesinger. Therapist leading man (Martin Sheen) never quite overcomes the power of a voodoo cult.

The Bell Jar (1979) Larry Peerce. Anne Jackson tries valiantly, but film grimly argues that no one as sensitive as Sylvia Plath (Marilyn Hassett) can survive in this world.

Benny and Joon (1993) Jeremiah Chechik. Schizophrenic teenagers (Johnny Depp and Mary Stuart Masterson) are too cute to be institutionalized, but black female psychiatrist is credible.

Bewitched (1945) Arch Oboler. Edmund Gwenn cures Phyllis Thaxter of schizophrenia.

Beyond Therapy (1987) Robert Altman. Heavy-handed farce with Tom Conti and Glenda Jackson playing therapists who are much, much crazier than their crazy patients.

Big Wednesday (1978) John Milius. A spaced-out surfer puts on a gay act to convince the psychiatrist for the Army that he ought to be exempted from the draft.

Bill and Ted's Excellent Adventure (1989) Stephen Herek. Two adolescent ne'er-do-wells travel through time to bring back historical figures for a presentation for their history class. Among their finds is Sigmund Freud (pronounced "frood"), who dazzles the class with a theatrical display of abreaction and catharsis.

Bird (1988) Clint Eastwood. Hospital psychiatrist wants to administer ECT to jazz genius Charlie Parker (Forest Whitaker), even though Parker's wife (Diane Venora) argues that the treatment will destroy his creativity. Doctor: "If it was my own brother, I would shock him." Wife: "What does your brother do for a living?" Doctor: "I don't have a brother."

Birdy (1985) Alan Parker. A double whammy on John Harkins: in his misguided treatment of bird-obsessed Vietnam vet (Matthew Modine), he exhibits worst stereotypes of psychiatry and the military.

The Black Cat (1934) Edgar G. Ulmer. Possessed Hungarian psychiatrist (Bela Lugosi) takes revenge on his old enemy (Boris Karloff) by skinning him alive.

Blind Alley (1939) Charles Vidor. Ralph Bellamy plays first godlike psychiatrist in an American film.

Blindfold (1966) Philip Dunne. "Dr. Bluebeard" Rock Hudson has trouble with women, but his powers of detection are beyond reproach.

Bliss (1997) Lance Young. Terence Stamp is a sex therapist who treats frigidity with a "hands-on" technique.

The Bliss of Mrs. Blossom (1968) Joe McGrath. Bob Monkhouse is no help to Richard Attenborough, whose symptoms are actually caused by the man secretly kept in the attic by his wife (Shirley MacLaine).

Bluebeard's Eighth Wife (1938) Ernst Lubitsch. Stereotypical sanitarium director Professor Urganzeff (Lawrence Grant) appears briefly. Stock market fluctuations drive one of his patients to crow like a rooster.

Blue Sky (1994) Tony Richardson. Corrupt military psychiatrist (Gary Bullock) commits Tommy Lee Jones so that the lecherous Powers Boothe can spend more time with Jones's wife (Jessica Lange).

Blume in Love (1973) Paul Mazursky. Real-life psychiatrist Donald F. Muhich sees George Segal through marital crisis.

Bob and Carol and Ted and Alice (1969) Paul Mazursky. Muhich again, this time assuming stone-faced neutrality in psychotherapy with Dyan Cannon.

The Boomerang (1925) Louis Gasnier. High jinks and romance among the staff at a sanitarium. First American movie to use the word *psychoanalyst.*

The Boston Strangler (1968) Richard Fleischer. Police inspector (Henry Fonda) knows how to handle killer with a split personality (Tony Curtis) much better than psychiatrist (Austin Willis).

The Boy Who Could Fly (1986) Nick Castle. Understanding therapist (Louise Fletcher) tells teenage heroine that it's OK to believe that her boyfriend can fly. (He can.)

Brainstorm (1965) William Conrad. Jeffrey Hunter tries to get away with murder by feigning insanity. Female therapist (Viveca Lindfors) appears to believe that Hunter is faking, using an almost seductive charm to entice him into submitting to her tests. She ultimately testifies in court that he is insane, which turns out to be the correct diagnosis.

Bridal Suite (1939) William Thiele. When he forgets for the second time that he has a date to get married, Robert Young goes to Switzerland to see the famous Dr. Grauer (Walter Connolly) and ends up marrying the doctor's daughter (Annabella).

Bringing Up Baby (1938) Howard Hawks. Fritz Feld perfects the stereotype of the officious Viennese quack.

Bronco Billy (1980) Clint Eastwood. Woodrow Parfrey plays Dr. Canterbury, a buffoon-like asylum director who wears a pair of six-shooters over his white coat.

Bulletproof Heart (1994) Mark Malone. A drunken psychiatrist appears briefly in a party scene.

The Butcher's Wife (1991) Terry Hughes. Jeff Daniels is an informal neighborhood psychiatrist practicing in Greenwich Village. After one session with a clairvoyant patient (Demi Moore), he finds himself falling in love with her despite his skepticism about her psychic powers.

Butterfield 8 (1960) Daniel Mann. Audiences know that call girl Liz Taylor is in love when she goes to see her Viennese-accented psychiatrist to tell him that she no longer needs him. But because this Golden Ager cares about her, he warns that love does not solve all problems and that she is welcome to return.

The Cabinet of Caligari (1962) Roger Kay. Dan O'Herlihy is benevolent healer, but disturbed patient Glynis Johns perceives him otherwise.

The Cabinet of Dr. Caligari (German; 1919) Robert Wiene. Expressionist masterpiece takes place in the mind of a mental patient who fantasizes that his psychiatrist is a malevolent mountebank sending a somnambulist (Conrad Veidt) on missions of murder.

The Caine Mutiny (1954) Edward Dmytryk. Pompous Whit Bissell is ultimately vindicated when he testifies that Captain Queeg (Humphrey Bogart) is not insane in spite of his ball bearings.

Calling Dr. Death (1943) Reginald LeBorg. Analyst loses control under hypnosis, leading to profound doubts about his own status as a rational professional and human.

Call Me Bwana (1963) Gordon Douglas. Brief gag when Bob Hope flies past window of psychiatrist, who then lies down on couch and begins talking about his childhood.

Captain Newman, M.D. (1963) David Miller. Gregory Peck can heal his patients, but he cannot change the world.

Captive Wild Woman (1943) Edward Dmytryk. Geneticist/psychiatrist engaging in experiments in "racial improvement" becomes typical mad scientist.

Carefree (1938) Mark Sandrich. Fred Astaire sings, dances, and hypnotizes his way into Ginger Rogers's heart.

The Caretakers (1963) Hall Bartlett. Compassionate Robert Stack overcomes tough head nurse Joan Crawford and brings enlightened new order to a West Coast mental institution.

The Case of Becky (1921) Psychoanalytically oriented "nerve specialist" saves daughter from evil hypnotist.

Casual Sex? (1988) Genevieve Robert. Solemn-faced psychologist kisses heroine (Victoria Jackson) at singles weekend but walks away saying that he is unable to develop any serious passion for her.

Cat People (1942) Jacques Tourneur. Simone Simon, who can actually turn into a panther, goes to suave, English psychiatrist (Tom Conway) who does not believe her. He substitutes seduction for therapy and pays with his life.

Caught (1949) Max Ophuls. Eccentric millionaire (Robert Ryan) marries fortune-hunting woman (Barbara Bel Geddes) largely to spite his officious analyst (Art Smith).

Celebrity (1998) Woody Allen. Protagonist Kenneth Branagh attends his high school reunion, realizes that he has wasted his life, and begins to talk to himself about what is in store for him. An analyst classmate overhears him and comments that "these are not my office hours," even though Branagh is clearly not speaking to him. Those in need of help seek the advice of fortune tellers and prostitutes in this film.

Chafed Elbows (1967) Robert Downey. Although his psychiatrist warns against it, protagonist marries his mother and lives happily ever after.

The Chamber (1996) James Foley. Female psychiatrist interviews death-row inmate (Gene Hackman) and declares him to be out of touch with reality.

Chances Are (1989) Emile Ardolino. Cybil Shepherd's analyst is irrelevant in her decision to make love to a 23-year-old boy who claims to be (and is) the reincarnation of her dead husband.

The Chapman Report (1962) George Cukor. Andrew Duggan, a thinly disguised Alfred Kinsey, is all business in this solemn sexploitation film.

Charlie Chan in Honolulu (1938) H. Bruce Humberstone. George Zucco starts out as a suspect but eventually helps Detective Chan find the real murderer.

Chattahoochee (1990) Mick Jackson. Conventional snake pit institution is transformed after Korean War vet (Gary Oldman) fights his way out.

A Child Is Waiting (1963) John Cassavetes. Though untrained, Judy Garland is better at helping retarded children than professional Burt Lancaster.

Children of Loneliness (1939) Richard C. Kahn. Pompous psychiatrist narrates two pseudodocumentary accounts of homosexual "deviance."

Child's Play (1988) Tom Holland. When a child reports (accurately) that his doll talks like a gangster, he is placed in an exceptionally dingy snake pit. Appropriately, the hapless rationalist foil who treats the child is shocked to death in the ECT room by the evil doll.

A Clockwork Orange (1971) Stanley Kubrick. Whatever crimes Malcolm McDowell has committed, he surely does not deserve what the Skinnerian social engineers do to him.

Coast to Coast (1980) Joseph Sargent. Michael Lerner pays the price for conspiring with husband of free-spirited Dyan Cannon in effort to have her committed.

The Cobweb (1955) Vincente Minnelli. Melodrama among the troubled staff at a plush psychiatric hospital in the Midwest.

Cold Feet (1984) Bruce van Dusen. Slightly eccentric psychiatrist (Marcia Jean Kurtz) gives good advice in several sessions with romantically troubled heroine (Marissa Chibas).

Color of Night (1994) Richard Rush. Bruce Willis announces to curious group therapy patients that he is both a "behaviorist" and a "psychoanalyst."

Coming Apart (1969) Milton Moses Ginsberg. Rip Torn sets up hidden camera in his apartment to record himself doing just what title says.

Communion (1989) Philippe Mora. Not at all a rationalist foil, Frances Sternhagen holds group meetings in her home for people who have been given rectal probes by aliens. She's no crackpot either—we see the hero on the aliens' operating table.

Compulsion (1959) Richard Fleischer. Psychiatric testimony in fictionalized story of Leopold and Loeb murder case is presented with an even hand; slightly caricatured psychiatrists make valid distinctions between legal and medical concepts of insanity. But mental illness ultimately becomes irrelevant when Orson Welles as Clarence Darrow phrases the issues in terms of liberal humanist caritas.

Condemned Women (1938) Lew Landers. Prison psychologist (Louis Hayward) falls in love with inmate (Linda Wilson) and helps clear her of false charges.

Conflict (1945) Curtis Bernhardt. Sidney Greenstreet is omniscient psychologist using powers of detection to expose murderous scheme of Humphrey Bogart.

Conspiracy Theory (1997) Richard Donner. Patrick Stewart plays an evil psychiatrist who practices mind control (borrowed from *The Manchurian Candidate*) to create assassins out of ordinary citizens like cab driver Mel Gibson.

Coogan's Bluff (1968) Don Siegel. Tough-minded Clint Eastwood straightens out Susan Clark, a psychobabble-spouting parole officer.

The Couch (1962) Owen Crump. Grant Williams is a psychotic killer stalking both his psychiatrist (Onslow Stevens) and his pretty niece (Shirley Knight).

The Couch Trip (1987) Michael Ritchie. Not only does con man Dan Aykroyd succeed triumphantly in masquerading as a shrink; the two psychiatrists he replaces end up institutionalized.

Cracking Up (1983) Jerry Lewis. Herb Edelman provides Jerry Lewis with an occasion to set up vignettes about life's absurdities. Parody of *Ordinary People* at conclusion. Rereleased in 1985 as *Smorgasbord.*

Crazy People (1990) Tony Bill. As in *The Dream Team,* a sympathetic institutional psychiatrist (Mercedes Ruehl) is in conflict with her authoritarian supervisor, but writing advertisements is much more therapeutic than any form of treatment.

Crime Doctor (1943) Michael Gordon. After an amnesia attack, a mob boss (Warner Baxter) becomes a criminal psychologist with special talents for solving crimes. Itself based on a radio series, the film was followed by six sequels.

Crimes of Passion (1984) Ken Russell. Actors in close-up speak directly into camera at group therapy session with unseen, unheard therapist.

The Criminal Hypnotist (1909) D. W. Griffith. Hypnotist uses his psychological powers for evil purposes.

Critical Condition (1987) Michael Apted. Desperate to escape prison, small-time con man (Richard Pryor) feigns insanity, but sour-faced female psychiatrist is not impressed.

The Crush (1993) Alan Shapiro. A fourteen-year-old bad seed murderer/stalker (Alicia Silverstone) dupes a well-meaning hospital psychiatrist who believes she is making progress when she is actually plotting to make him her next victim.

Dark Delusion (1947) Willis Goldbeck. Last of the Dr. Kildare movies, this time without Dr. Kildare. Dr. Tom Coalt (James Craig) uses narcosynthesis to help Dr. Gillespie (Lionel Barrymore) cure young girl's schizophrenia.

The Dark Mirror (1946) Robert Siodmak. With the help of Rorschach and free association tests, Lew Ayres solves the crime and wins himself a bride.

The Dark Past (1948) Rudolph Maté. Lee J. Cobb is oracular in faithful remake of *Blind Alley* (1939).

Dark Waters (1944) André de Toth. Franchot Tone is heroic doctor/detective/psychiatrist who helps Merle Oberon overcome villains trying to drive her crazy.

Daughters of Satan (1972) Hollingsworth Morse. Witches do not respond well to therapy.

David and Lisa (1962) Frank Perry. The title pair are lovable but seriously disturbed patients, and Howard da Silva's portrayal of the psychiatrist is wise and compassionate yet vulnerable.

Day of the Nightmare (1965) John Bushelman. Psychiatrist is killed by his transvestite son in retread of *Psycho*.

Dead Again (1991) Kenneth Branagh. In an uncharacteristically restrained performance, Robin Williams appears as a former psychiatrist (sex with patients), now a bitter but observant misanthrope who provides ultimately irrelevant advice to detective hero.

Dead Bang (1989) John Schlesinger. Extraordinarily wimpy psychologist flies out of control with countertransference when tough cop Don Johnson tells him that he resembles, of all people, Woody Allen. Psychologist is prepared to tell police superintendent that Johnson is unfit, but after hero threatens shrink and his family, Johnson is back on the force.

Dead Heat on a Merry-Go-Round (1966) Bernard Girard. Con man James Coburn seduces prison psychologist (Marian Moses) into arranging for his parole.

Dead Man Out (1989) Richard Pearce. Black prison psychologist (Danny Glover) struggles heroically to find the trace of humanity in doomed inmate (Ruben Blades).

Dead of Night (British; 1946) Alberto Cavalcanti, Basil Dearden, Robert Hamer, and Charles Crichton. Best example of a film in which an absurdly rational psychiatrist consistently denies the reality of otherworldly phenomena.

Dead of Winter (1987) Arthur Penn. Evil psychiatrist in wheelchair kidnaps, mutilates, and otherwise terrorizes Mary Steenburgen as part of an elaborate blackmail scheme.

The Dead Pool (1988) Buddy Van Horn. Although he is not caricatured, shrink confesses to Dirty Harry (Clint Eastwood) that he released a schizophrenic serial killer because he was not "a danger to society."

Death Becomes Her (1992) Robert Zemeckis. Black female psychiatrist is typically inconsequential as heroines pursue narcissistic and impossible cures for aging.

Death in the Air (1937) Elmer Clifton. John Elliott examines the survivor of a plane crash and determines that a psychotic ex–World War I flying ace, "Pilot X," has been shooting down airplanes during peacetime.

Death Wish II (1982) Michael Winner. Unlike heroic vigilante Charles Bronson, prison psychologist does not know his right from his left.

Deconstructing Harry (1997) Woody Allen. Even though she's in the middle of a session with a patient, Kirstie Alley keeps flying into a rage because she has just learned that her novelist husband, played by Allen, has been sleeping with her patients.

Deep Throat (1972) Gerard Damiano. Harry Rheems spends a good deal of time having sex with his nurses, but he also has enough expertise to discover that Linda Lovelace's clitoris is in her throat.

The Deer Hunter (1978) Michael Cimino. Army psychiatrist fails to appreciate Christopher Walken's sufferings.

The Demon Seed (1977) J. Lee Thompson. This may be the first film in which a female psychiatrist (Julie Christie) is shown to have a spouse (Fritz Weaver). As the film begins, however, he is in the act of ending their marriage, and she is soon raped by a supercomputer of his devising.

Desire (1936) Frank Borzage, produced by Ernst Lubitsch. Marlene Dietrich easily outwits "nerve specialist," played here by Alan Mowbray, who would later play a similarly inept psychiatrist in Lubitsch's *That Uncertain Feeling* (1941).

The Detective (1968) Gordon Douglas. Pompous Lloyd Bochner conceals evidence sought by detective Frank Sinatra.

Dial 1119 (1950) Gerald Mayer. Sam Levene dies in a heroic attempt to reason with an escaped psychotic killer (Marshall Thompson).

Diary of a Mad Housewife (1970) Frank Perry. Upside-down psychiatrist urges Carrie Snodgress to be traditional wife and mother to intolerable husband and children. (Psychiatrist scenes are only in version of film shown on television.)

Dishonored Lady (1947) Robert Stevenson. Omniscient psychiatrist (Morris Carnovsky) clears Hedy Lamarr of murder charge.

Disturbing Behavior (1998) David Nutter. The rowdy students at a suburban high school are being transformed into Stepford kids by a "neuropharmacologist" (Bruce Greenwood). When two students investigate his background, they find a snake pit straight out of *Marat/Sade*.

Doctor Doolittle (1998) Betty Thomas. Rationalist foil psychiatrist (Paul Giamatti) treats Dr. Doolittle (Eddie Murphy) because he talks to animals, but the audience learns that the shrink was last in his medical school class and has a pink tutu in his closet.

Doctors' Wives (1971) George Schaefer. Gene Hackman discovers that his wife is having a lesbian affair.

Don Juan DeMarco (1995) Jeremy Leven. Marlon Brando plays a weighty, aging psychiatrist who finds himself transformed by his delusional but passionate patient (Johnny Depp).

Donnie Brasco (1997) Mike Newell. Risking his life to work undercover, FBI agent Johnny Depp has no time for buffoon (Zach Grenier) telling him that he and his wife should schedule "intimacy days."

Down and Out in Beverly Hills (1986) Paul Mazursky. Donald F. Muhich continues his work with Mazursky by appearing as a delicately earnest psychiatrist attempting to treat the family dog.

Dracula (1931) Tod Browning. Unlike the wise Professor Van Helsing (Edward Van Sloan), sanitarium director Dr. Seward (Herbert Bunston) cannot see that Count Dracula is one of the Undead.

Dracula: Dead and Loving It (1995) Mel Brooks. As in *High Anxiety*, Harvey Korman is the director of a bizarre sanitarium.

Dracula's Daughter (1936) Lambert Hillyer. Heroic psychiatrist (Otto Kruger) defends Dr. Van Helsing against charges that he has killed Count Dracula and then joins the older psychiatrist in tracking down more vampires.

The Dream Team (1989) Howard Zieff. Sympathetic doc who opposes his institutional superiors takes his patients off their medication and accompanies them to sporting events. The film's plot ultimately revolves around their attempts to save him.

Dressed to Kill (1980) Brian De Palma. Michael Caine as the first homicidal transvestite psychiatrist in the American cinema.

Dr. Dippy's Sanitarium (1906) The psychiatrist makes his inauspicious debut on the American screen.

Dr. Jekyll and Ms. Hyde (1995) David Price. Harvey Fierstein's therapist (Julie Cobb) is astonished to learn that her gay patient is turned on by Sean Young. In fact, Young is the Ms. Hyde of Tim Daly's Dr. Jekyll.

Drop Dead Fred (1991) Ate de Jong. Phoebe Cates is taken to see Dr. Ryland, an authority on the "imaginary friend syndrome." Unfortunately, this rationalist foil fails to see that the companions are real.

Duet for One (1986) Andrei Konchalovsky. Terminally ill Julie Andrews
suffers so nobly and speaks so articulately that her therapist (Max von
Sydow) declares, "I am no longer your doctor," and becomes her companion during her last days.

Edward Scissorhands (1990) Tim Burton. Psychiatrist evaluates lethal-
handed adolescent hero for court but overlooks the obvious symbolism
in the boy's sexual development.

The End (1978) Burt Reynolds. Carl Reiner drops dead immediately after
inspiring Burt Reynolds with the joy of life.

End of the Road (1970) Aram Avakian. Although James Earl Jones's clinic is
probably meant to be a metaphor, the patients in this institution are
encouraged to have intercourse with chickens, and illegal abortions result in death.

The Entity (1983) Sidney J. Furie. If this film did not argue that invisible
demon rapists really do exist, everything Ron Silver does for Barbara
Hershey would make perfect sense.

Equus (1977) Sidney Lumet. Despairing Richard Burton cures psychotic
boy (Peter Firth) but envies him for his bizarre horse religion.

The Evening Star (1996) Bill Paxton sleeps with his elderly patient (Shirley
MacLaine), who is a dead ringer for his mother.

Everybody's Baby (1939) Malcolm St. Clair. Fathers spend the entire film
trying to expose a quack psychologist (Reginald Denny), whose book
urges mothers not to let anyone hold their babies.

Everyone Says I Love You (1997) Woody Allen. How else could Woody Allen find his way to Julia Roberts's bed except by learning how to excite
her sexually from a child who has eavesdropped on Roberts with her
psychiatrist?

The Evil (1978) Gus Trikonis. Richard Crenna rents haunted house for his
clinic, but the previous inhabitants object.

The Exorcist (1973) William Friedkin. Psychiatry is no match for The
Devil.

Exorcist II: The Heretic (1977) John Boorman. Especially when the psychiatrist is female (Louise Fletcher).

Exorcist III (1990) William Peter Blatty. Or a chain-smoking wimp who is
in fact destroyed by Satan.

Face to Face (Swedish; 1976) Ingmar Bergman. Female psychiatrist unravels into psychosis.

Faithful (1996) Paul Mazursky. Mazursky himself is a therapist with a gam-
bling addiction. His hit man patient (Chazz Palminteri) gets free therapy in exchange for tips from a bookie.

PSYCHIATRY AND THE CINEMA, SECOND EDITION

Fearless (1993) Peter Weir. John Turturro is hired to help Jeff Bridges, who seems to have entered a euphoric state after surviving an airline crash. Eventually the airline psychologist drifts out of the picture, and Bridges is "saved" by his wife (Isabella Rossellini).

Fear Strikes Out (1957) Robert Mulligan. Faceless Adam Williams cures baseball player Jimmy Piersall (Anthony Perkins). The film treats psychiatry so reverentially that even electroconvulsive therapy becomes benign.

Female Perversions (1997) Susan Streitfeld. In a narrative inspired by Louise Kaplan's book of the same title, a female psychiatrist (Karen Silas) enters into a lesbian affair with power-hungry lawyer (Tilda Swinton) but breaks it off when she realizes that Swinton can't love.

The Fifth Floor (1980) Howard Avedis. Low-budget imitation of *Cuckoo's Nest* touches usual bases—a staff much sicker than patients uses ECT for punishment.

Final Analysis (1992) Phil Joanou. Richard Gere tells Kim Basinger that he cannot have sex with her because she is the sister of his patient. Quick cut to the two in bed making love. Quick cut again: Gere tells a colleague that he checked the AMA ethics code, and there is no prohibition against sex with a patient's sibling. Whew!

A Fine Madness (1966) Irvin Kershner. Motley crew of psychiatrists (Patrick O'Neal, Colleen Dewhurst, Clive Revill) lobotomize free-spirited poet (Sean Connery) but cannot tame him.

The First Wives' Club (1996) Diane Keaton's husband is having an affair with their marriage therapist.

Fixed by George (1920) Lee Moran and Eddie Lyons. When rich patient becomes infatuated with her psychiatrist (Eddie Lyons), he decides not to tell her that he's married for fear of losing a large fee.

The Flame Within (1935) Edmund Goulding. Ann Harding as first female psychiatrist to lose her heart to a patient, in this case, Louis Hayward.

Fourteen Hours (1951) Henry Hathaway. Lovable cop (Paul Douglas) finally succeeds in coaxing suicidal Richard Basehart off ledge after two ineffectual psychiatrists fail.

Frances (1982) Graeme Clifford. Lane Smith can barely control himself during Jessica Lange's outbursts, and she pays dearly for her insolence.

Free Love (1930) Hobart Henley. Psychiatrist gives woman bad but expensive advice about her marriage.

Freud (1962) John Huston. Montgomery Clift is miscast, but the film comes very close to hagiography.

From Beyond (1986) Stuart Gordon. Beautiful, audacious female psychiatrist (Barbara Crampton) develops a passion for sadomasochistic sex after experimenting in the fourth dimension. A jealous female competitor, not so beautiful and unconventional, wants to punish her with ECT.

From the Terrace (1960) Mark Robson. Joanne Woodward's psychiatrist lover (Patrick O'Neal) is not very sympathetic, but then neither is anyone else in this melodrama.

The Front Page (1931) Lewis Milestone. Viennese quack hands gun to convicted murderer as part of examination. Remade in 1940 as *His Girl Friday* (directed by Howard Hawks) and in 1974 as *The Front Page* (directed by Billy Wilder) with little change in characterization of psychiatrist/alienist.

The Gay Intruders (1948) Ray McCarey. Married psychiatrists fail to cure quarreling stage couple—end up more confused than patients.

The Gingerbread Man (1998) Robert Altman. Dr. Bernice Sampson (Rosemary Newcott) is a faceless forensic psychiatrist who appears briefly to declare Robert Duvall's character mentally incompetent.

Girl at Bay (1919) Tom Mills. "Criminal psychologist" wrongly accuses heroine of murder.

Girl of the Night (1960) Joseph Cates. Psychoanalyst Lloyd Nolan saves Anne Francis from a life of prostitution and then rescues her from her pimp.

Glen or Glenda? (1953) Edward D. Wood, Jr. Psychiatrist provides jargonistic introduction in attempt to legitimize this lame exploitation of transvestitism. A cult classic.

The Gnomemobile (1967) Robert Stevenson. Rationalist foil Jerome Cowan tells Walter Brennan that real-life gnomes are actually imaginary.

Golden Eye (1995) Martin Campbell. Fergie look-alike psychologist is sent to evaluate 007 only to succumb to his irresistible charm in the front seat of his Aston Martin.

The Good Mother (1988) Leonard Nimoy. Court psychiatrist is physically unattractive but testifies that newly sexualized heroine (Diane Keaton) deserves custody of her child. Although the judge does not accept his opinion, the film clearly does.

The Good Son (1993) Joseph Ruben. Kindly elderly therapist tells her young patient (Elijah Wood) that she doesn't believe in evil. He replies, "You should." And the movie confirms his view.

Good Will Hunting (1997) Gus van Sant. Robin Williams gains the trust of young tormented genius (Matt Damon) and then cures him by repeating over and over again, "It's not your fault." In a twist that is unusual for male therapists, Damon also cures Williams, inspiring him to leave the profession and live a more satisfying life.

Grace Quigley (1985) Anthony Harvey. Chip Zien is a hip psychiatrist who tolerates—nay, rationalizes—the work of professional hit man Nick Nolte.

Grosse Pointe Blank (1997) George Armitage. Alan Arkin reveals his countertransference terror in treating a hit man (John Cusack).

Groundhog Day (1993) Harold Ramis. What can a poor shrink do for a patient who is inexplicably doomed to live the same day over repeatedly?

The Group (1966) Sidney Lumet. Shirley Knight's first lover (Hal Holbrook) is hopelessly dependent on his manipulative analyst, but she eventually finds a good husband in James Broderick, an anti-Freudian hospital psychiatrist.

The Guilt of Janet Ames (1947) Henry Levin. Melvyn Douglas is a heavy-drinking newspaperman who nevertheless understands how to cure Rosalind Russell's hysterical paralysis. In one of several dream sequences, Sid Caesar broadly burlesques psychoanalysts.

Hairspray (1988) John Waters. Director Waters, in a cameo as a parody of a repressive shrink, uses a psychedelic cattle prod on a rebellious teenage girl who insists on dating a black man.

Halloween (1978) John Carpenter. Unlike almost everyone else in this film, Donald Pleasence knows the Bogeyman when he sees him.

Hannah and Her Sisters (1986) Woody Allen. A silent therapist appears only briefly, but his patient (Michael Caine) appears to have benefited from the treatment.

Happiness (1998) Todd Solondz. We hear a voiceover when we first see Dylan Baker with a patient. This tells us that he is not concentrating and that he's probably not a very good psychiatrist. But before this pitch black comedy is over, Baker's character has turned out to be a pedophile who drugs and then rapes the friends of his eleven-year-old son.

Hard to Hold (1984) Larry Peerce. Child psychologist (Janet Eilber) is mostly competent and witty, but her relationship with rock star (Rick Springfield) is often more than she can handle.

Harold and Maude (1971) Hal Ashby. Absurd psychiatrist (G. Wood) cannot appreciate young Bud Cort's very real need to marry octogenarian Ruth Gordon.

Harvey (1950) Henry Koster. James Stewart as the lovable drunk with the giant invisible rabbit who is saved at the last minute from the psychiatric interventions of Charles Drake and Cecil Kellaway.

Harvey Middleman, Fireman (1965) Ernest Pintoff. Mrs. Koogleman (Hermione Gingold) is too involved with her own sexual escapades to help hero.

Haunted Honeymoon (1986) Gene Wilder. Paul L. Smith is a ghoulish psychiatrist from the mad scientist tradition who believes he can cure Gene Wilder's wedding night jitters by scaring the wits out of him.

Heartburn (1986) Mike Nichols. Maureen Stapleton plays no-nonsense leader of Meryl Streep's therapy group.

The Hero and the Terror (1988) William Tannen. Detective hero is living with female therapist who treated him after a traumatic experience with a maniac killer.

High Anxiety (1977) Mel Brooks. Hitchcock send-up casts Brooks as psychiatrist with vertigo.

High Wall (1947) Curtis Bernhardt. Audrey Totter functions as detective and lawyer as well as psychiatrist in order to save Robert Taylor from frame-up.

His Girl Friday (1940) Howard Hawks. See *The Front Page.*

Holiday for Lovers (1959) Henry Levin. Clifton Webb must supervise four troublesome daughters while on vacation in South America.

Hollow Triumph (1948) Steve Sekely. Paul Henreid kills a look-alike psychologist and then assumes his identity with initial success. Later released as *The Scar.*

Home Before Dark (1958) Mervyn LeRoy. Psychiatry is the solution to Jean Simmons's problems, but her unfaithful husband (Dan O'Herlihy) has other ideas.

Home Free All (1984) Stewart Bird. Daniel Benzalli is therapist who cancels treatment when antihero (Allan Nicholls) cannot pay his bills. It is just as well since Nicholls's problems are blamed on society.

Home of the Brave (1949) Mark Robson. Oracular Jeff Corey cures black serviceman (James Edwards) of hysterical paralysis.

The Hospital (1971) Arthur Hiller. David Hooks appears briefly at beginning so that George C. Scott can establish his character in a long confession.

Hot Shots (1991) Jim Abrahams. Valeria Golino stamps Charlie Sheen's file with large red letters "Paternal Anxiety Syndrome." She later becomes his lover, but her profession quickly ceases to have much resonance in this send-up of Tom Cruise movies.

House of Cards (1969) John Guillerman. Insufferably pompous psychiatrist (Keith Michell) is one of several right-wing conspirators. Heroine (Inger Stevens) refers to him as "the man who polices my psyche."

House of Games (1987) David Mamet. Writer-director Mamet probably intended to make a movie about the games of life, the various levels on which it is played, and the psychology of the players. For our purposes, he has reactivated the old myths about (1) the ease with which psychiatrists can be manipulated and (2) the compatibility of the profession with murderous impulses.

The Howling (1981) Joe Dante. Patrick Macnee seems like a good psychiatrist, but he is actually a werewolf.

The Hudsucker Proxy (1994) Joel Coen. In an over-the-top parody, a Viennese quack gleefully celebrates ECT and the permanent confinement of patients to prisonlike institutions.

Hunk (1987) Lawrence Bassoff. Another female therapist (Rebecca Bush) falls in love with her male patient (John Allen Nelson). The only twist to this recycling of the Faust story is that the doctor is in cahoots with the devil.

Husbands and Wives (1992) Woody Allen. Barnard undergraduate (Juliette Lewis) has an affair with her middle-aged psychiatrist, who pursues her to an apartment and accuses her of "leading him on."

If Lucy Fell (1996). Eric Shaeffer. When the therapist (Sarah Jessica Parker) learns that her boyfriend is enamored of Elle McPherson, she says, "I'd love to get her into therapy and fuck her up real good."

I Love My . . . Wife (1970) Mel Stuart. Elliot Gould is a wealthy surgeon who seeks help from a dour analyst for his problems with women.

I'm Dancing as Fast as I Can (1982) Jack Hofsiss. Dianne Wiest saves Jill Clayburgh after bad male psychiatrist (Joseph Maher) hooks her on Valium.

The Impossible Years (1968) Michael Gordon. University psychiatrist David Niven cannot control his teenage daughter.

Impulse (1990) Sondra Locke. Black female therapist is introduced early on to establish that sexy cop (Theresa Russell) may be a little kinky. But faceless therapist is soon forgotten, left in the dust as Russell goes off to new adventures and an upbeat Hollywood ending.

I Never Promised You a Rose Garden (1977) Anthony Page. A character based on Frieda Fromm-Reichmann (Bibi Andersson) struggles to save Kathleen Quinlan. One of the few sympathetic psychiatrists in 1970s' films.

In Person (1935) William A. Seiter. Having cured movie star (Ginger Rogers) of agoraphobia, handsome George Brent succeeds where the woman's psychiatrist had failed.

Inside Daisy Clover (1966) Robert Mulligan. Faceless psychiatrist willingly submits to studio boss (Christopher Plummer) who exploits child star (Natalie Wood).

Interiors (1978) Woody Allen. E. G. Marshall and Diane Keaton deliver monologues to unseen psychiatrists.

The Interns (1962) David Swift. J. Edward McKinley is so eminent a psychiatrist that intern Michael Callan is willing to lie and cheat in order to study with him.

Invasion of the Body Snatchers (1956) Don Siegel. One psychiatrist (Whit Bissell) saves the world from alien invaders, while another (Larry Gates) is their agent. Remade by Philip Kaufman in 1978 with Leonard Nimoy as "pod" psychiatrist but without savior psychiatrist.

I, the Jury (1953) Harry Essex. Mickey Spillane's Mike Hammer is seduced but not outwitted by murderous psychoanalyst Charlotte Manning (Peggie Castle). 1982 remake directed by Richard T. Heffron transformed Miss Manning into a sex therapist (Barbara Carrera).

It's My Turn (1980) Claudia Weill. Briefly glimpsed psychiatrist at a party is a pompous boor.

I Was a Teenage Werewolf (1957) Gene Fowler, Jr. "Consulting psychologist" (Whit Bissell) unleashes the beast in Michael Landon.

Jackknife (1989) David Jones. Group therapy session among working-class Vietnam war survivors is led by black vet in a wheelchair. You know that he can help.

Jade (1995) William Friedkin. Another sexy psychiatrist (Linda Fiorentino) who may or not be a psychotic killer.

Jagged Edge (1985) Richard Marquand. Bearded, rumpled psychiatrist appears briefly and offers a diagnosis of murder suspect that turns out to be wrong.

Kings Row (1941) Sam Wood. On the one hand, saintly Parris Mitchell (Robert Cummings) overflows with the romance of medicine, goes to turn-of-the-century Vienna for medical school, and chooses psychiatry as his specialty. Claude Rains, on the other hand, is a troubled psychiatrist who murders his schizophrenic daughter.

Klute (1971) Alan J. Pakula. Female psychiatrist Vivian Nathan gives Jane Fonda an opportunity to do some method acting, but she's not there when heroine needs her most.

Knock on Wood (1954) Norman Panama, Melvin Frank. Danny Kaye cures beautiful Mai Zetterling of her need to be a psychiatrist.

Kotch (1971) Jack Lemmon. Lovable old widower Walter Matthau submitted to absurd tests by young female psychologist.

Lady in a Jam (1942) Gregory La Cava. Heiress Irene Dunne convinces psychiatrist Patrick Knowles that he can cure her only by marrying her.

Lady in the Dark (1944) Mitchell Leisen. Barry Sullivan tells Ginger Rogers how to be a woman but mostly provides frame for production numbers.

The Last Embrace (1979) Jonathan Demme. Hitchcockian suspense/thriller includes brief scene with Jacqueline Brookes as white-coated therapist helping Roy Scheider recover from breakdown after his wife's death.

The Last Gentleman (1934) Sidney Lanfield. Greedy son calls in an alienist to declare that his rich but eccentric father (George Arliss) is incompetent, but the alienist likes the old man and announces that the son has delusions.

Leave It to Beaver (1997) Andy Cadiff. School psychologist is just as helpless as everyone else in trying to clean up the Beaver's messy life.

Leaving Las Vegas (1995) Mike Figgis. Entire narrative is the confession of a call girl (Elizabeth Shue) as she speaks from the couch of an invisible therapist.

Lethal Weapon (1987) Richard Donner. Female police psychologist says that Mel Gibson is psychotic and suicidal, but later the film implies that he is suffering a legitimate grief reaction to his wife's death.

Lethal Weapon II (1989) Richard Donner. She's back! Mel Gibson calls her "Ms. Sigmund Fraud."

Lethal Weapon III (1991) Richard Donner. This time the men hide when they see her coming.

Let's Live a Little (1948) Richard Wallace. When "neuropsychiatrist" Hedy Lamarr falls for patient Robert Cummings, she acquires the same symptoms of love madness that once belonged to Cummings.

Let There Be Light (1946) John Huston. Documentary casts psychiatry as nearly infallible panacea for troubled veterans after World War II.

The Lieutenant Wore Skirts (1956) Frank Tashlin. When his wife (Sheree North) joins the Army, Tom Ewell does everything he can to bring her home, including an elaborate scheme to get her a psychiatric discharge.

Lifeforce (1985) Tobe Hooper. Body of dour sanitarium director is temporarily invaded by naked lady vampire from outer space.

Lilith (1964) Robert Rossen. Warren Beatty plays a novice therapist who loses his heart and then his mind over a patient (Jean Seberg).

Little Man Tate (1991) Jodie Foster. Like Bibi Andersson in *I Never Promised You a Rose Garden*, Dianne Wiest is a repressed, childless spinster working with children, in this case gifted ones. And although her "patient" is only a six-year-old boy, he functions like many other male patients with female therapists by inspiring her to get in touch with her feminine side.

Little Tough Guys in Society (1938) Erle C. Kenton. When a society woman (Mary Boland) discovers that her son will not get out of bed, she hires Dr. Trenkle (Mischa Auer), who recommends bringing in the Dead End Kids to cure the son of his self-absorption.

Lizzie (1957) Hugo Haas. Richard Boone cures Eleanor Parker of multiple personality. Released a few months before *The Three Faces of Eve.*

The Locket (1946) John Brahm. Reflecting ambivalence typical of the 1940s, Laraine Day's psychiatrist husband (Brian Aherne) is first her victim, then her savior.

The Lonely Guy (1984) Arthur Hiller. Steve Martin speaks with his therapist exclusively through an intercom.

Lord Love a Duck (1966) George Axelrod. Sarah Marshall flies into hysterics because Roddy McDowall refuses to say that her Rorschach blots are dirty. She tells him he is being "hostile."

Lost Angels (1989) Hugh Hudson. Donald Sutherland has problems with his family, and his treatment of a delinquent boy is not exactly professional. But he cares.

Love at First Bite (1979) Stan Dragoti. Richard Benjamin treats girlfriend Susan St. James only to find out if she is seeing other men.

Lover Come Back (1961) Delbert Mann. Richard Deacon dominates neurotic analysand (Tony Randall).

Lovesick (1983) Marshall Brickman. Dudley Moore is cute, but numerous other members of his profession are savaged.

Lust for Life (1956) Vincente Minnelli. Vincent Van Gogh (Kirk Douglas) is committed to an institution presided over by a concerned director with an English accent. Later, he is entrusted to Dr. Gasché (of the famous $38 million portrait), who is more interested in bragging of his connections with famous painters than in actually helping Vincent.

Made for Each Other (1971) Robert B. Bean. Norman Shelly is caricatured therapist for couple who meet at an encounter group session.

Mad Love (1995) Antonia Bird. Sensible young black therapist might have been able to help manic Drew Barrymore, but her boyfriend whisks her away so that the film can become a road movie.

Magic in the Water (1995) Rick Stevenson. Mark Harmon and Harley Jane Kozak are charming and beautiful therapists, but they are as surprised as everyone by the local sea monster.

The Magus (British; 1968) Guy Green. Anthony Quinn may or may not be a psychiatrist treating Michael Caine.

The Manchurian Candidate (1962) John Frankenheimer. Good-humored black psychiatrist is part of the team trying to figure out why a group of American soldiers were elaborately "brainwashed" during the Korean War.

Manhunter (1986) Michael Mann. University of Chicago psychiatrist cautions cop (William L. Petersen) about dangers of taking his job too seriously. The cannibal psychiatrist Hannibal Lecter, played here by Brian Cox, makes his first film appearance.

Man Made Monster (1941) George Waggner. Rationalist foil thinks a man has committed murder because of traumatic incidents in his youth, when in fact a mad scientist has filled the killer full of electric rays.

The Man Who Loved Women (1983) Blake Edwards. Julie Andrews somehow falls for neurotic womanizer Burt Reynolds.

The Man Who Saw Tomorrow (1922) Alfred E. Green. Psychologist hypnotizes patient so that he can see what his life would be like with each of two women he is considering marrying.

Many Happy Returns (1934) Norman McLeod. Dr. Otto von Strudel (Egon Brecher) recommends that Gracie Allen marry George Burns (both appearing as themselves) in order to cure Gracie of her obsessive meddling.

Marat/Sade (British; 1967) Peter Brook. Although the action takes place in a primitive nineteenth-century madhouse, treatment of patients is not unlike that shown in other films from this period.

The Mark (British; 1961) Guy Green. Rod Steiger cures Stuart Whitman of child-molesting and then saves him from those who would resurrect the past.

The Marriage of a Young Stockbroker (1971) Lawrence Turman. Patricia Barry wishes to emasculate healthy, normal American males.

Martians Go Home (1990) David Odell. Martian invaders, who can read anyone's secret thoughts, reveal that voluptuous radio psychiatrist (Anita Morris) used to be a gypsy fortune-teller.

Marvin's Room (1996) Jerry Zaks. Sympathetic female psychiatrist does her best to convince Meryl Streep that she needs to change her relationship with her son (Leonardo DiCaprio).

The Mask (1994) Charles Russell. Ben Stein, typically dour and pontifical, briefly appears on a television talk show to set up the show's premise—that in one way or another we all conceal our id behind masks. Of course, he can have no idea what happens when Jim Carrey puts on his mask.

The Master Mind (1920) Kenneth Webb. Obsessed psychologist plans elaborate revenge on D.A. for role in his brother's death. He uses his psychological skills to arrange for the D.A. to fall in love with and then marry a woman fresh out of jail in hopes of exposing her criminal background when the D.A. runs for governor. But when he sees that the D.A. and the woman really love each other, he relents.

The Medusa Touch (British; 1978) Jack Gold. Lee Remick eventually commits suicide after failing to destroy demons within the mind of Richard Burton.

The Menace (1918) John Stuart Robertson. Psychologist (Herbert Prior) adopts son of imprisoned man in order to prove that criminality is an inherited trait. He seems to be succeeding until he learns that the boy is in fact his own son.

The Men's Club (1986) Peter Medak. This film is not clear about why the seven men in the club are so confused about women, but there is no question that the most confused of them all is Kramer (Richard Jordan), a psychotherapist.

Million Dollar Dollies (1918) Leonce Perret. A maharajah is bamboozled by a hypnotist, and even a psychologist cannot snap him out of it.

Ministry of Fear (1944) Fritz Lang. In wartime London, Alan Napier is author of "The Psychoanalysis of Nazism" and an advisor to the Ministry of Home Security. He turns out to be a Nazi spy as well.

Miracle on 34th Street (1947) George Seaton. In one of cinema's first attempts to distinguish psychologists from psychiatrists, Kris Kringle (Edmund Gwenn) scolds department store psychologist (Porter Hall) for practicing psychiatry.

Mirage (1965) Edward Dmytryk. Hostile psychiatrist (Robert H. Harris) is no help to amnesiac Gregory Peck.

Moment to Moment (1966) Mervyn LeRoy. Jean Seberg drifts into a disastrous affair because psychiatrist husband (Arthur Hill) neglects her.

Movie Star, American Style or LSD, I Hate You (1966) Albert Zugsmith. Renegade headshrinker Del Moore gives lysergic acid to his patients.

Mr. Deeds Goes to Town (1936) Frank Capra. Gary Cooper realizes his humanitarian goals in spite of Viennese quack (Wyrley Birch) who testifies that he is crazy.

Mr. Frost (1990) Philip Setbon. Kathy Baker, a psychiatrist in a European hospital, tries to treat Jeff Goldblum, a psychopathic killer with the power to inspire others to do his killing for him.

Mr. Jealousy (1998) Noah Baumbach. Eric Stoltz, a jealous lover, signs up for group therapy (led by Peter Bogdanovich) to find out more about his girlfriend's ex-beau, who is also a patient.

Mr. Jones (1993) Mike Figgis. Lena Olin falls for manic depressive played by Richard Gere.

Mr. Skeffington (1944) Vincent Sherman. Bette Davis is quite put out when psychoanalyst impatiently interrupts her first session monologue and tells her to go back to her husband, which, of course, she eventually does.

Mrs. Parker and the Vicious Circle (1994) Alan Rudolph. Bearded analyst who talks about Tolstoi at a party is briefly cornered by Dorothy Parker (Jennifer Jason Leigh) so that the audience can know what she's really thinking. Needless to say, he has no effect on her alcoholism, suicidal tendencies, and disastrous object relations.

Murder, My Sweet (1945) Edward Dmytryk. Hard-boiled Philip Marlowe (Dick Powell) has to cope with quack Otto Kruger.

My Blue Heaven (1990) Herbert Ross. FBI agent's wife is a sports therapist who elopes with her baseball player patient.

My Favorite Wife (1940) Garson Kanin. Pedro de Cordoba appears briefly as a meddlesome psychiatrist, complete with goatee, rimless glasses, foreign accent, and the wrong diagnosis of why Cary Grant has been avoiding Gail Patrick.

The Myth of Fingerprints (1997) Bart Freundlich. Brian Kerwin plays another incompetent and emotionally unstable psychotherapist.

The Naked Face (1984) Bryan Forbes. Roger Moore is a grieving widower, devoted to his patients, but unlike James Bond, he needs help when a Mafia don decides to silence him.

The Net (1995) Irwin Winkler. Dennis Miller is especially aggressive in violating his boundaries with Sandra Bullock.

New York Stories (1989) Woody Allen segment, "Oedipus Wrecks." After Allen's mother materializes as a gigantic specter hovering over Manhattan, even the hero's analyst suggests that he see a spiritualist.

Next Stop Wonderland (1998) Brad Anderson. Thanks to an ad in the personals, a beautiful but choosy nurse (Hope Davis) dates a stream of narcissistic talkaholics. When she finally meets a man who lets her talk, she opens up and tells him (and the audience) her life story. After she apologizes for monopolizing the conversation and asks her date to talk about himself, she's disturbed to learn that he's a therapist; he's never seen again.

Nice Girls Don't Explode (1987). Chuck Martinez. Supercilious rationalist foil (William Kuhlke) appears briefly to interpret telekinetic fire-setting as unconscious anger.

Nightmare Alley (1947) Edmund Goulding. Unscrupulous psychologist Helen Walker eventually turns "mentalist" Tyrone Power into a geek.

The Night Porter (Italian; 1974) Liliana Cavani. Psychiatrist is one of several ex-Nazis living secretly in postwar Vienna. They regularly meet for mock trials in which the defendant is "purged" of his guilt by denying accusations.

Nine Months (1995) Chris Columbus. Hugh Grant is a child psychiatrist overwhelmed with the thought of becoming a father himself.

The Ninth Configuration (1980). See *Twinkle, Twinkle, Killer Kane*.

Now, Voyager (1942) Irving Rapper. Saintly Claude Rains shows Bette Davis how to live.

Nuts (1987) Martin Ritt. Barbra Streisand chews the scenery as still another vital, nonconformist heroine victimized by her parents as well as a shrink (Eli Wallach) who cannot overcome his countertransferential resentment.

Oh, God! Book II (1980) Gilbert Cates. Anthropomorphic god (George Burns) tries to enlighten a team of grossly caricatured psychiatrists.

Oh, Men! Oh, Women! (1957) Nunnally Johnson. Psychoanalyst David Niven is a great marriage counselor, but his dizzy fiancée (Barbara Rush) thinks him out of touch with his emotions.

Old Boyfriends (1979) Joan Tewkesbury. Stern-faced psychiatrist (John Houseman) is justified when he scolds psychologist (Talia Shire) for her disastrous attempts to treat Keith Carradine.

The Omen (1976) Richard Donner. Lee Remick goes to pompous John Strike for help, and although he arrives at a perfectly plausible diagnosis of her "fantasies," the patient's real problem is her son, Satan, who eventually kills her.

On a Clear Day You Can See Forever (1970) Vincente Minnelli. Yves Montand sets up production numbers when he discovers that Barbra Streisand can recall past lives.

Once You Kiss a Stranger (1969) Roger Sparr. Ubiquitous Whit Bissell wants to commit psychopath (Carol Lynley), but she engineers to have him killed by professional golfer (Paul Burke), whose archrival she murders à la *Strangers on a Train*.

One Fine Day (1996) Michael Hoffman. Unable to find a sitter for his young daughter, George Clooney takes her with him to a session with Robert Klein. The coded language they improvise to exclude the child is just as confusing to the analyst and the patient.

One Flew Over the Cuckoo's Nest (1975) Milos Forman. Christlike sociopathic nonconformists beware! Lobotomy is the punishment for your attempts to bring salvation to emasculated males.

One Glorious Day (1922) James Cruze. Will Rogers is psychology professor who attempts to leave his body but is instead invaded by a mischievous spirit.

Ordinary People (1980) Robert Redford. Judd Hirsch hugs Timothy Hutton back to sanity.

Overboard (1988) Garry Marshall. Effete analyst would rather play cocktail piano than treat his idle rich patients.

Parenthood (1989) Ron Howard. In a world in which nothing is weird except not having children, a meddlesome school psychologist can't possibly understand Steve Martin's bizarre children as well as Dad does.

Parents (1989) Bob Balaban. School psychologist (Sandy Dennis) is ungainly, but child trusts her because "you're not a real grown-up." As in *The Stepfather*, however, when she attempts to help the child, the father intervenes murderously.

Park Avenue Logger (1936) David Howard. When a patient in a therapy session says that he is concerned about his son's lack of manliness, the psychiatrist suggests sending the boy to a logging camp.

Penelope (1966) Arthur Hiller. Dick Shawn is quack treating Natalie Wood.

The People Next Door (1970) David Greene. Nehemiah Persoff leads frustrating group therapy sessions for neurotic parents and their hippie children.

The Perfect Furlough (1958) Blake Edwards. Like most women who dare to practice psychiatry in fifties' films, Army psychologist (Janet Leigh) suffers several humiliations before Tony Curtis decides she is worthy of his affections.

Phobia (1980) John Huston. Paul Michael Glaser wants to cure his patients of their fears, but when he fails, he kills them.

Pillow Talk (1959) Michael Gordon. Tony Randall, betrayed by his best friend, says, "I should have listened to my psychiatrist. He told me never to trust anyone but him."

Pink Panther, and sequels. Blake Edwards. Inspector Clouseau (Peter Sellers) drives his boss (Herbert Lom) to therapy, and in one episode, institutionalization.

Plastered in Paris (1928) Benjamin Stoloff. "Famous specialist" fails to cure World War I veteran's kleptomania caused by war wound.

Poltergeist III (1988) Gary Sherman. The ultimate rationalist foil! Psychologist and associates witness indisputably supernatural event, then dismiss it as "mass hypnosis."

Portnoy's Complaint (1972) Ernest Lehman. Psychiatrists are an essential part of modern life even though they never speak. One is called "Harpo."

Possessed (1947) Curtis Bernhardt. Oracular Stanley Ridges restores Joan Crawford's mental health after Van Heflin drives her crazy.

The President's Analyst (1967) Theodore J. Flicker. Eponymous hero (James Coburn) is not up to the assignment.

Pressure Point (1962) Hubert Cornfield. No other actor could have completed the early sixties' trend toward idealization of the psychiatrist as well as Sidney Poitier.

Primal Fear (1996) Gregory Hoblit. Like everyone else, court-appointed psychiatrist (Frances McDormand) can't tell that Edward Norton is only pretending to be a multiple personality case.

The Prince of Tides (1991) Barbra Streisand. Most of the clichés of the genre are present here: simple derepression of one traumatic incident and a female therapist's unprofessional but unproblematic love make the hero a happy man. Although Streisand's therapist is in a miserable marriage, she is among the very few female movie psychiatrists married to someone other than a former patient.

Private Worlds (1935) Gregory La Cava. The complicated lives of an institution's staff. Claudette Colbert is one of the few female psychiatrists in the movies who is permitted to practice her trade after falling in love.

Problem Child (1990) Dennis Dugan. Child psychologist intervenes impotently in comic version of *The Bad Seed*.

The Promise (1979) Gilbert Cates. Bibi Besch is pleasant enough, but she has only a small role in restoring Kathleen Quinlan to happiness.

Promise Her Anything (1966) Arthur Hiller. Bob Cummings is a prissy child psychologist who hates children and sucks his thumb.

Psycho (1960) Alfred Hitchcock. Simon Oakland is so extraordinarily astute and self-confident in his analysis of Anthony Perkins's psychosis that some critics believe Hitchcock intended the entire scene as a joke.

Psycho (1998) Gus van Sant. In this remake of the classic, Robert Forster presents his psychodynamic formulation of Norman Bates with approximately 10% of the conviction that Simon Oakland displayed in the original.

Psycho II (1983) Richard Franklin. Robert Loggia lets Anthony Perkins out of custody a little too early and pays for the mistake with his life.

Psycho III (1986) Anthony Perkins. Priest/psychiatrist is well-meaning but almost completely inconsequential.

Raising Arizona (1987) Joel Coen. Prison psychologist supplies escaping convicts with psychobabble to explain their departure.

Raising Cain (1992) Brian De Palma. John Lithgow plays both the father who abuses his son in order to induce multiple personalities and the son who in fact has several selves, at least one of which is homicidal.

Relentless (1989) William Lustig. When detective in search of psychotic killer consults police psychiatrist, the diagnosis is "Maybe he's just crazy." When detective says, "I coulda said that," the doc laughs diabolically and says, "But I get paid for it."

Return of the Terror (1934) Howard Bretheron. Murder and intrigue at a sanitarium.

Return to Oz (1985) Walter Murch. Nicol Williamson plays villainous Nome King as well as a psychiatrist about to subject the helpless Dorothy to ECT.

Reunion in Vienna (1933) Sidney Franklin. Viennese psychiatrist (Frank Morgan) represents enlightened alternative to decadent past when charming but overbearing Habsburg nobleman (John Barrymore) returns from exile to resume a romance with Diana Wynyard, now married to Morgan.

Revolution (1968) Jack O'Connell. Documentary about hippies pokes fun at psychiatrists' pious pronouncements.

Saint, Devil and Woman (1916) Frederic Sullivan. Wayne Arey plays a daring young psychologist who saves a wealthy woman from the trances of a hypnotist and then marries her.

The Santa Clause (1994) John Pasquin. Even the highly rational Judge Reinhold eventually has to acknowledge that Tim Allen has become Santa Claus.

The Scar (1948). See *Hollow Triumph.*

Scenes from a Mall (1991) Paul Mazursky. Bette Midler is introduced as a successful psychologist and author of books on how to stay married. Then we watch her marriage fall apart.

Schizoid (1980) David Paulsen. Klaus Kinski sleeps with his patients, but, contrary to expectation, he is not the one who is murdering them.

Scissors (1991) Frank De Felitta. A *very* evil psychiatrist (Ronny Cox) kills his wife's lover and then sets up a disturbed patient (Sharon Stone) to take the blame.

The Scout (1994) Michael Ritchie. Baseball scout Albert Brooks discovers talented pitcher (Brendan Fraser) but needs the help of Dianne Wiest to cure him of the lingering trauma of an abusive father.

The Secret Diary of Sigmund Freud (1984) Danford B. Greene. Although this account of Freud's early years is played broadly as farce, the filmmakers are surprisingly savvy about the details of Freud's life.

The Secret Fury (1950) Mel Ferrer. When villains attempt to drive Claudette Colbert to insanity, a female therapist (Elisabeth Risdon) treats her in an institution not unlike the one in *The Snake Pit*.

Secrets of a Soul (German; 1926) G. W. Pabst. First serious treatment of psychoanalysis in film history, complete with German Expressionism, sophisticated dream analysis, and talking cure supervised by Freud's disciples Abraham, Kaufmann, and Sachs.

See You in the Morning (1989) Alan J. Pakula. WASPs in love: in idealized account of romance among the haute bourgeoisie, hero (Jeff Bridges) just happens to be a psychiatrist.

The Sender (1982) Roger Christian. Kathryn Harrold is concerned and competent, but she cannot solve the supernatural problems of Zeljko Ivanek.

Serial (1980) Bill Persky. Peter Bonerz is a laid-back Marin County therapist who smiles helplessly through a child's hostile attacks.

The Serpent and the Rainbow (1988) Wes Craven. Beautiful Haitian (Cathy Tyson) practices among voodoo specialists. She falls in love with hero and generally provides a rationalist foil for voodoo pyrotechnics.

The Seven-Per-Cent Solution (1976) Herbert Ross. Mildly satirized version of Sigmund Freud (Alan Arkin) helps greatly deromanticized version of Sherlock Holmes to kick the cocaine habit and then joins him in detective work.

The Seventh Veil (British; 1945) Compton Bennett. Herbert Lom speaks with unquestioned authority as he directs the life of concert pianist Ann Todd.

The Seventh Victim (1943) Mark Robson, produced by Val Lewton. As in *Cat People* (also produced by Lewton), Tom Conway plays a smooth-talking psychiatrist with evil intentions.

The Seven Year Itch (1955) Billy Wilder. Creepy Oscar Homolka arrives early for an appointment, explaining nonchalantly that a patient just cut short his analytical hour by jumping out of the window.

Sex and the Single Girl (1964) Richard Quine. In spite of a doctorate in psychology, Helen Gurley Brown (Natalie Wood) quickly succumbs to the bogus charms of Tony Curtis.

sex, lies, and videotape (1988) Steve Soderbergh. Although it was promoted as a departure from Hollywood clichés, this film brings in a faceless analyst at the beginning almost entirely for the sake of exposition.

The Shadow (1994) Russell Mulcahy. When Lamont Cranston overpowers the evil Khan, he sends the villain to a psychiatrist who performs a frontal lobotomy, thus depriving Khan of his power to cloud men's minds. (Telekinetic powers reside in the frontal lobes, we are told.)

Shadow on the Wall (1950) Patrick Jackson. Nancy Davis solves crime by helping traumatized child recall murder.

The Shaggy Dog (1959) Charles Barton. Disney farce includes another psychiatrist as rationalist foil. In this case he interprets Tommy Kirk's canine transformations as the "submerged second self" of his father (Fred MacMurray).

She's Gotta Have It (1986) Spike Lee. Black heroine, who's gotta have it (sex), goes to black female psychiatrist, who tells her that the most erogenous part of her body is between her ears.

She's Out of Control (1989) Stan Dragoti. Tony Danza, suffering from a reverse Oedipus, ends up on the couch of pipe-smoking, pompous Wallace Shawn, who has written a book about the problem entitled *Daddy's Little Girl*, which he tries to peddle to his patients.

She's So Lovely (1997) Nick Cassavetes. Neither the thoughtful young black psychologist nor the social worker played by Gena Rowlands can keep the psychotic but free-spirited lovers (Sean Penn and Robin Wright) apart.

She Wouldn't Say Yes (1946) Alexander Hall. Rosalind Russell is another inadequate female therapist until she meets Lee Bowman.

Shining Victory (1941) Irving Rapper. Beautiful assistant (Geraldine Fitzgerald) to "nerve specialist" (James Stephenson) dies saving his important data from fire.

Shock (1946) Alfred L. Werker. Vincent Price kills wife and then uses psychiatric armamentarium to destroy witness.

Shock Corridor (1963) Samuel Fuller. In search of a murderer, journalist Peter Breck enters mental institution where maltreatment eventually drives him to psychosis. He does, however, win the Pulitzer Prize.

Shockproof (1949) Douglas Sirk (script by Samuel Fuller). Good/bad heroine (Patricia Knight) thinks she has outsmarted middle-aged female psychiatrist, but lady doc can tell that the girl has a good soul.

Shock Treatment (1964) Denis Sanders. Unscrupulous Lauren Bacall runs an institution for illicit financial gain but ends up a patient.

The Shrike (1955) José Ferrer. Most psychiatrists in a big-city institution are little more than jailers, but one oracular therapist saves the day for beleaguered hero.

The Silence of the Lambs (1991) Jonathan Demme. As in *Manhunter* (see above), the diabolical Dr. Lecter (Anthony Hopkins) uses his substantial intelligence and cunning to commit mayhem. As the film ends, he sets out to eat a prison psychiatrist who had taunted him.

Silent Fall (1994) Bruce Beresford. Highly sympathetic psychiatrist (Richard Dreyfuss) is deeply dedicated to his autistic patient, fends off sexual overtures from the patient's sister (Liv Tyler), and solves a murder mystery. The treatment of his patient, though, is both unorthodox and unbelievable.

Silent Madness (1985) Simon Nuchtern. The psychiatrist as damsel in distress.

Silent Rage (1982) Michael Miller. Ron Silver plays the therapist among a team of doctors who create a genetically engineered killer. Like Donald Pleasence in the original *Halloween* (1978), Silver alone realizes the destructive potential of the monster, who is fortunately no match for Chuck Norris.

Since You Went Away (1944) John Cromwell. Supremely compassionate Viennese psychiatrist, bearing the formidable name Sigmund Gottlieb Golden, heals returning servicemen and consoles Jennifer Jones over the loss of her fiancé.

Skin Deep (1989) Blake Edwards. Michael Kidd plays yet another sour-faced analyst, except that this time he provides the advice that leads alcoholic, womanizing hero (John Ritter) to what the film suggests is a complete recovery.

The Sleeping Tiger (British; 1954) Joseph Losey. Alexander Knox reforms young criminal (Dirk Bogarde), but he fails miserably as Alexis Smith's husband.

Sleepless in Seattle (1993) Nora Ephron. Radio therapist is responsible for bringing Tom Hanks and Meg Ryan together.

Sleep, My Love (1948) Douglas Sirk. George Coulouris is malevolent photographer posing as a psychiatrist in Don Ameche's plan to drive his wife (Claudette Colbert) to insanity. Ralph Morgan appears briefly but ineffectually as real psychiatrist.

Sliver (1993) Philip Noyce. An analyst is one of several briefly glimpsed characters watched over by voyeurist William Baldwin, who owns an apartment building that is also a panopticon.

Smile (1975) Michael Ritchie. Bruce Dern needs help, but his perfectly normal son is taken to the psychiatrist.

Smorgasbord (1985) Jerry Lewis. See *Cracking Up.*

The Snake Pit (1948) Anatole Litvak. Leo Genn cures Olivia de Havilland in spite of appalling conditions in New York institution.

Some Kind of Hero (1982) Michael Pressman. Faceless psychiatrist is insensitive to mammoth problems of returning prisoner of war Richard Pryor.

Soul Man (1986) Steve Miner. At the urging of his absurd therapist (Max Wright), a father refuses to pay his son's law school tuition, thus inspiring the son (C. Thomas Howell) to masquerade as a black man in order to win a scholarship intended for minority students.

So Young, So Bad (1950) Bernard Vorhaus. Humane Paul Henreid overcomes forces of reaction at a girls' reform school.

Space Jam (1997). A succession of NBA stars are seen reclined on an analyst's couch ventilating their problems for no apparent reason other than a sight gag related to their height.

Spellbound (1945) Alfred Hitchcock. Love for Gregory Peck transforms Ingrid Bergman from a mousy therapist into intrepid sleuth of the mind. Michael Chekhov is her irascible but lovable training analyst, and Leo G. Carroll is the psychiatrist/villain.

Sphere (1998) Barry Levinson. Although Dustin Hoffman has committed a long list of ethical violations, he nevertheless solves the mystery (something about aliens causing humans to live out their unconscious fears).

Splendor in the Grass (1961) Elia Kazan. Burgeoning adolescent sexuality drives Natalie Wood crazy—only psychiatry can help her.

Stardust Memories (1980) Woody Allen. Several gags about psychiatrists, including the classic line addressed to monster by Victor Truro: "I'm a psychoanalyst. This is my pipe."

Starting Over (1979) Alan J. Pakula. Burt Reynolds's psychiatrist brother (Charles Durning) sees him through a premarital crisis in a furniture store.

The Stepfather (1987) Joseph Ruben. Extremely sympathetic therapist (Charles Lanyer) attempts to help teenage girl who thinks that her stepfather is crazy. She's right. Stepfather (Terry O'Quinn) beats the doctor to death with a two-by-four.

The Stepford Wives (1975) Bryan Forbes. Brief scene with female psychiatrist (Carol Rosson) who appears to be part of the conspiracy to replace suburban wives with automatons.

Still of the Night (1982) Robert Benton. Roy Scheider is either a typical Hitchcockian hero or a troubled psychiatrist out of control in a countertransference reaction.

St. Ives (1975) J. Lee Thompson. After an outburst that activates an analysand's worst fears, Maximilian Schell murders his only patient, a wealthy millionaire (John Houseman).

The Stone Killer (1973) Michael Winner. Officious psychiatrist lectures tough cop (Charles Bronson) on how Vietnam war teaches American boys to be "psychopaths."

Straight Talk (1992) Barnet Kellman. Dolly Parton masquerades as a radio therapist and is a smashing success, even without training or knowledge.

Strait Jacket (1964) William Castle. Joan Crawford's psychiatrist (Mitchell Cox) is victim of ax murderer.

The Subterraneans (1960) Ranald MacDougall. Nymphomaniac Leslie Caron frequents Bohemian scene in San Francisco in between visits to female therapist who is patient and doesn't say much; mostly she offers Caron a chance to overact. She does, however, pronounce Caron cured at the end in order to make way for the happy ending.

Suddenly, Last Summer (1959) Joseph L. Mankiewicz. Brain surgeon Montgomery Clift uses talking cure to save Elizabeth Taylor from villains wishing to lobotomize her.

Supernatural (1933) Victor Halperin. While quack spiritualist relies on tricks to convince Carole Lombard that her dead sister is trying to reach her, a real psychologist (H. B. Warner) actually does get in touch with the spirit world.

Surviving the Game (1994) Ernest Dickerson. Gary Busey is a lunatic psychiatrist trying to track down and kill an innocent homeless man for the sheer sport of it.

Take the Money and Run (1969) Woody Allen. In parody of analyst, Don Frazier delivers elaborate psychosexual explanation for why hero (Allen) desires to play the cello. Earlier, Allen flunks Navy admission test when a Rorschach blot reminds him of two elephants having sex with a glee club.

Taking Off (1971) Milos Forman. Two scenes with psychiatrists are designed to drive home the message that middle-class adults are much stranger than their hippie children.

Teacher's Pet (1958) George Seaton. Gig Young, a psychology professor who seems to know everything without being pompous, helps Clark Gable get together with Doris Day.

Teahouse of the August Moon (1956) Daniel Mann. Humane Army psychiatrist (Eddie Albert), more interested in horticulture than psychotherapy, goes native in postwar Japan.

10 (1980) Blake Edwards. Solemn therapist is no help to Dudley Moore in midlife crisis.

Tender Is the Night (1962) Henry King. Although Jason Robards, Jr., is a competent analyst, he never recovers from a countertransference reaction to the lovable Jennifer Jones.

The Terminal Man (1974) Mike Hodges. Team of doctors, including emotionally incompetent female psychiatrist (Joan Hackett), operates on mind of George Segal with disastrous results.

The Terminator (1984) James Cameron. Ridiculous "criminal psychologist" refuses to understand that man from the future is here to save humanity from Arnold Schwarzenegger.

Terminator II: Judgment Day (1991) James Cameron. The same psychologist from the original reappears—once again as the rationalist foil—but this time he is also the vindictive jailer of the heroine.

The Testament of Dr. Mabuse (German; 1933) Fritz Lang. Lang's last German film before the ascendancy of Hitler was about a power-mad psychiatrist.

That Old Feeling (1997) Marital therapist (David Rasche) is married to a former patient.

That Touch of Mink (1962) Delbert Mann. Alan Hewitt treats Gig Young primarily for tips on the stock market.

That Uncertain Feeling (1941) Ernst Lubitsch. Blandly incompetent Alan Mowbray encourages Merle Oberon to question her marriage with Melvyn Douglas. Husband is preoccupied with business, but he eventually succeeds in regaining the affections he never deserved to lose.

There Goes the Groom (1937) Joseph Santley. Sanitarium director (Onslow Stevens) attempts to cure Burgess Meredith's amnesia by staging a football game with a former schoolmate.

There's Something About Mary (1998) Bobby Farrelly and Peter Farrelly. Ben Stiller's analyst slips out for a bite of lunch during their session.

They Might Be Giants (1971) Anthony Harvey. Joanne Woodward is a frumpy psychiatrist named Dr. Watson who finds fulfillment as the helpmate to George C. Scott, a schizophrenic who believes that he is Sherlock Holmes.

The Thin Blue Line (1988) Errol Morris. Stylized documentary of wrong man convicted of murder was originally about the "killer shrink" who administers twenty minutes of superficial tests and then testifies that offenders should be executed.

Third of a Man (1962) Robert Lewin. Whit Bissell saves institutionalized Simon Oakland from mob violence and then helps Oakland's brother understand problems of the mentally ill.

The Three Faces of Eve (1957) Nunnally Johnson. Joanne Woodward has the part of a lifetime, but psychiatry and its domain remain mysterious. Though sympathetic, Lee J. Cobb is largely superfluous.

Three Kids and a Queen (1935) Edward Ludwig. Eccentric recluse (May Robson) is declared insane by the Lunacy Commission when she buys an entire plot of land for her dog.

Three Loves Has Nancy (1938) Richard Thorpe. Good-natured psychiatrist (Lester Matthews) tells Nancy (Janet Gaynor) and Malcolm (Robert Montgomery) what the audience has known all along—they're in love.

Three Men and a Little Lady (1990) Emile Ardolino. Black psychologist warns little lady's parents about the dangers of "unconventional" living arrangements.

Three Nuts in Search of a Bolt (1964) Tommy Noonan. Three impoverished "nuts" in need of treatment send one person reporting symptoms of all three. Psychiatrist Ziva Rodann thinks she has found rare multiple personality case.

Three on a Couch (1966) Jerry Lewis. Janet Leigh is Ph.D., M.D., but her patients only need boyfriends.

The Thrill of It All (1963) Norman Jewison. Guidance counselor psychiatrist Paul Hartman provides James Garner with strategy for regaining the attentions of his wife (Doris Day).

'Til There Was You (1997) Scott Winant. One of three thirty-something women in a powder room announces, "I won't phone a man who's not in therapy. Life's too short."

A Time to Kill (1996) Joel Schumacher. M. Emmet Walsh and Anthony Heald are dueling forensic psychiatrists. Walsh has committed statutory rape; Heald is a grandiose buffoon who has never declared anyone not guilty by reason of insanity.

Tin Cup (1996) Ron Shelton. Having fallen for therapist René Russo when he first sees her at his driving range, free-spirited golfer Kevin Costner appears at her office asking for therapy. Although she makes the usual protestations, Russo is soon completely devoted to her would-be patient.

Titicut Follies (1967) Frederick Wiseman. Grim documentary on conditions in Massachusetts mental hospital.

Tomorrow and Tomorrow (1932) Richard Wallace. Viennese psychologist (Paul Lukas) falls in love with married woman (Ruth Chatterton) and conceives a son by her. But he unselfishly leaves the woman to her husband (Robert Ames) when he realizes how much the man wants to have a son.

Trial and Error (1997) Jonathan Lynn. Pompous forensic psychiatrist disputes validity of the insanity defense in a wildly insane courtroom.

12 Monkeys (1995) Terry Gilliam. Beautiful psychiatrist (Madeleine Stowe), part rationalist foil, part unfulfilled woman, falls in love with time-traveling Bruce Willis.

Twinkle, Twinkle, Killer Kane (1980) William Peter Blatty. Stacy Keach runs weird mental hospital for shell-shocked marines. Also released as *The Ninth Configuration.*

Twister (1996) Jan de Bont. Bill Paxton's fiancée is "reproductive therapist" Jami Gertz. She wears business clothes and mouths platitudes about feelings and is thus no match for Paxton's first wife, the free-spirited, tornado-chasing Helen Hunt.

The Undead (1957) Roger Corman. Hypnotherapist (Richard Garland) enters into the past lives of his patient.

Underworld (1997) Roger Christian. In this gangster film self-consciously imbued with oedipal themes, Annabella Sciorra actually delivers a summary of Freud's argument in *Totem and Taboo.* Earlier, Denis Leary says that he took a degree in psychotherapy while he was in prison: "Given my own nature, I consider myself the only working psychopathic psychotherapist in all of psychopathology."

An Unmarried Woman (1978) Paul Mazursky. Real-life psychologist Penelope Russianoff helps Jill Clayburgh face the troubling realities of modern relationships.

Used People (1992). Beeban Kidron. Marcia Gay Hardin drips hot, molten wax on child therapist Joe Pantoliano to make him reveal what her kid told him in therapy.

Vampire's Kiss (1989) Robert Bierman. Elizabeth Ashley can't stop the decompensation of Nicolas Cage, who is convinced that he's a vampire. Nevertheless, the lady may be the only female therapist in the movies to be shown with a male lover who's not a patient. In fact, he's a young stud half her age.

Vertigo (1958) Alfred Hitchcock. Psychiatrists patch up James Stewart after his breakdown, but his obsessions are beyond therapy.

A Very Special Favor (1965) Michael Gordon. Leslie Caron is a successful but unfulfilled therapist until she falls for Rock Hudson and motherhood.

Voyage to the Bottom of the Sea (1961) Irwin Allen. Joan Fontaine misinterprets scientific genius Walter Pidgeon and then attempts to sabotage submarine on its mission to save the world.

Walking and Talking (1996) Nicole Holofcener. Ann Heche is a trainee therapist who struggles with erotic countertransference but—amazingly—does not act on her feelings.

What About Bob? (1991) Frank Oz. Bill Murray is a wildly borderline patient who drives his therapist (Richard Dreyfuss) into a homicidal psychotic rage.

What a Way to Go! (1964) J. Lee Thompson. Bob Cummings, whose office includes a hydraulic couch, faints when he learns that Shirley MacLaine's wild stories are true.

What's New, Pussycat? (1965) Clive Donner. Peter Sellers with Viennese accent and Prince Valiant haircut is only interested in chasing women and running from his Wagnerian wife.

When the Clouds Roll By (1919) Victor Fleming. "Doctor of the mind" (Herbert Grimwood) turns out to be an escaped lunatic.

Where Were You When the Lights Went Out? (1968) Hy Averback. Terry-Thomas's analyst (Parley Baer) blandly responds "What do you think?" to his patient's questions but also manages to suggest that he is homosexual.

Whirlpool (1950) Otto Preminger. Neurotic wife (Gene Tierney) of renowned psychoanalyst (Richard Conte) is prey to evil hypnotist (José Ferrer) until Conte uses his scientific skills to save her.

Whispers in the Dark (1992) Christopher Crowe. Annabelle Sciorra falls in love with her patient's boyfriend in a preposterous thriller.

Who Is Harry Kellerman and Why Is He Saying Those Terrible Things About Me? (1971) Ulu Grosbard. Psychiatrist Jack Warden is just another of rock singer Dustin Hoffman's delusions.

Who's Been Sleeping in My Bed? (1963) Daniel Mann. Martin Balsam cures Dean Martin of women problems.

Whose Life Is It, Anyway? (1981) John Badham. The doctors, nurses, physical therapists, and orderlies in this hospital are all dedicated, personable, and/or highly professional. Only the psychiatrists are caricatures.

Wild in the Country (1961) Philip Dunne. If you can accept Elvis Presley as a young Faulkner, you can accept Hope Lange as a successful therapist who saves her patient with a suicide attempt.

Willie and Phil (1980) Paul Mazursky. This homage to Jules and Jim includes scene with oddball army psychiatrist at induction center.

Willy Wonka and the Chocolate Factory (1971) Mel Stuart. Brief scene with psychiatrist who is so anxious to find prize in chocolate bar that he interrogates a patient who dreams that he found it.

Woman Times Seven (1967) Vittorio De Sica. Shirley MacLaine's strange behavior leads psychiatrist Robert Morley to recommend long-term institutionalization, but Shirley is just trying to win her husband's attentions.

A Woman Under the Influence (1974) John Cassavetes. Eccentric housewife (Gena Rowlands) is institutionalized and given ECT, but her supposedly normal husband (Peter Falk) exhibits a more destructive kind of craziness.

Worth Winning (1989) Will Mackenzie. Because of envy (?), the friend/therapist of Mark Harmon bets that Harmon cannot charm three women into consenting to marry him during a three-month period.

The Wrong Man (1956) Alfred Hitchcock. Werner Klemperer is competent and self-assured in brief scene with Henry Fonda.

Young Man with a Horn (1950) Michael Curtiz. Lauren Bacall plays a society vamp studying psychoanalysis who almost ruins the life of trumpet-playing genius (Kirk Douglas).

Zelig (1983) Woody Allen. Mia Farrow parodies female psychiatrist in love. Newspaper headline reads: "Chameleon cured by woman doctor. She's pretty, too!"

Zotz! (1962) William Castle. Tom Poston has magic powers that his therapist (James Millholin) is unable to appreciate.

Chronology

1906
Dr. Dippy's Sanitarium

1909
The Criminal Hypnotist

1916
Saint, Devil and Woman

1918
The Menace
Million Dollar Dollies

1919
The Cabinet of Dr. Caligari
Girl at Bay
When the Clouds Roll By

1920
Fixed By George
The Master Mind

1921
The Case of Becky

1922
The Man Who Saw Tomorrow
One Glorious Day

1925
The Boomerang

1926
Secrets of a Soul

1928
Plastered in Paris

1930
Free Love

1931
Dracula
The Front Page

1932
Tomorrow and Tomorrow

1933
Reunion in Vienna
Supernatural
The Testament of Dr. Mabuse

1934
The Black Cat
The Last Gentleman
Many Happy Returns
The Return of the Terror

1935
The Flame Within
In Person
Private Worlds
Three Kids and a Queen

1936

After the Thin Man
Desire
Dracula's Daughter
Mr. Deeds Goes to Town
Park Avenue Logger

1937

Death in the Air
There Goes the Groom

1938

The Amazing Dr. Clitterhouse
Bluebeard's Eighth Wife
Bringing Up Baby
Carefree
Charlie Chan in Honolulu
Condemned Women
Little Tough Guys in Society
Three Loves Has Nancy

1939

Blind Alley
Bridal Suite
Children of Loneliness
Everybody's Baby

1940

His Girl Friday
My Favorite Wife

1941

Kings Row
Man Made Monster
Shining Victory
That Uncertain Feeling

1942

Cat People
Lady in a Jam
Now, Voyager

1943

Calling Dr. Death
Captive Wild Woman
Crime Doctor
The Seventh Victim

1944

Arsenic and Old Lace
Dark Waters
Lady in the Dark
Ministry of Fear
Mr. Skeffington
Since You Went Away

1945

Bewitched
Conflict
Murder, My Sweet
The Seventh Veil
Spellbound

1946

Angel on My Shoulder
Bedlam
The Dark Mirror
Dead of Night
Let There Be Light
The Locket
She Wouldn't Say Yes
Shock

1947

The Bachelor and the Bobby Soxer
Dark Delusion

Dishonored Lady
The Guilt of Janet Ames
High Wall
Miracle on 34th Street
Nightmare Alley
Possessed

1948

The Dark Past
The Gay Intruders
Hollow Triumph (The Scar)
Let's Live a Little
Sleep, My Love
The Snake Pit

1949

The Accused
Caught
Home of the Brave
Shockproof

1950

Dial 1119
Harvey
The Secret Fury
Shadow on the Wall
So Young, So Bad
Whirlpool
Young Man with a Horn

1951

Bedtime for Bonzo
Fourteen Hours

1953

The Beast from 20,000 Fathoms
Glen or Glenda?
I, the Jury

1954

The Caine Mutiny
Knock on Wood
The Sleeping Tiger

1955

The Cobweb
The Seven Year Itch
The Shrike

1956

Invasion of the Body Snatchers
The Lieutenant Wore Skirts
Lust for Life
Teahouse of the August Moon
The Wrong Man

1957

Fear Strikes Out
I Was a Teenage Werewolf
Lizzie
Oh, Men! Oh, Women!
The Three Faces of Eve
The Undead

1958

Home Before Dark
The Perfect Furlough
Teacher's Pet
Vertigo

1959

Anatomy of a Murder
Compulsion
Holiday for Lovers
Pillow Talk
The Shaggy Dog
Suddenly, Last Summer

1960

Butterfield 8
From the Terrace
Girl of the Night
Psycho
The Subterraneans

1961

Lover Come Back
The Mark
Splendor in the Grass
Voyage to the Bottom of the Sea
Wild in the Country

1962

The Cabinet of Caligari
The Chapman Report
The Couch
David and Lisa
Freud
The Interns
The Manchurian Candidate
Pressure Point
Tender Is the Night
That Touch of Mink
Third of a Man
Zotz!

1963

Call Me Bwana
Captain Newman, M.D.
The Caretakers
A Child Is Waiting
Shock Corridor
The Thrill of It All
Who's Been Sleeping in My Bed?

1964

Bedtime Story
Lilith
Sex and the Single Girl
Shock Treatment
Strait Jacket
Three Nuts in Search of a Bolt
What a Way to Go!

1965

Brainstorm
Day of the Nightmare
Harvey Middleman, Fireman
Mirage
A Very Special Favor
What's New, Pussycat?

1966

Blindfold
Dead Heat on a Merry-Go-Round
A Fine Madness
The Group
Inside Daisy Clover
Lord Love a Duck
Moment to Moment
Movie Star, American Style or LSD,
  I Hate You
Penelope
Promise Her Anything
Three on a Couch

1967

Chafed Elbows
The Gnomemobile
Marat/Sade
The President's Analyst
Titicut Follies
Woman Times Seven

1968

The Bliss of Mrs. Blossom
The Boston Strangler
Coogan's Bluff
The Detective
The Impossible Years
The Magus
Revolution
Where Were You When the Lights
  Went Out?

1969

Alice's Restaurant
The Arrangement
Bob and Carol and Ted and Alice
Coming Apart
House of Cards
Once You Kiss a Stranger
Take the Money and Run

1970

Diary of a Mad Housewife
End of the Road
I Love My . . . Wife
On a Clear Day You Can See Forever
The People Next Door

1971

A Clockwork Orange
Doctors' Wives
Harold and Maude
The Hospital
Klute
Kotch
Made for Each Other
The Marriage of a Young Stockbroker
Taking Off
They Might Be Giants

Who Is Harry Kellerman and Why Is
  He Saying Those Terrible Things
  About Me?
Willy Wonka and the Chocolate
  Factory

1972

Daughters of Satan
Deep Throat
Portnoy's Complaint

1973

Blume in Love
The Exorcist
The Stone Killer

1974

The Front Page
The Night Porter
The Terminal Man
A Woman under the Influence

1975

One Flew Over the Cuckoo's Nest
St. Ives
Smile
The Stepford Wives

1976

Face to Face
The Omen
The Seven-Per-Cent Solution

1977

Annie Hall
The Demon Seed
Equus
Exorcist II: The Heretic

High Anxiety
I Never Promised You a Rose Garden

1978

Big Wednesday
The Deer Hunter
The End
The Evil
Halloween
Interiors
Invasion of the Body Snatchers
The Medusa Touch
An Unmarried Woman

1979

The Bell Jar
The Last Embrace
Love at First Bite
Old Boyfriends
The Promise
Starting Over

1980

Bad Timing: A Sensual Obsession
Bronco Billy
Coast to Coast
Dressed to Kill
The Fifth Floor
It's My Turn
Oh, God! Book II
Ordinary People
Phobia
Schizoid
Serial
Stardust Memories
10
Twinkle, Twinkle, Killer Kane
  (*The Ninth Configuration*)
Willie and Phil

1981

The Howling
Whose Life Is It, Anyway?

1982

Airplane II: The Sequel
Death Wish II
Frances
I'm Dancing as Fast as I Can
I, the Jury
The Sender
Silent Rage
Some Kind of Hero
Still of the Night

1983

Cracking Up
The Entity
Lovesick
The Man Who Loved Women
Psycho II
Zelig

1984

Cold Feet
Crimes of Passion
Hard to Hold
Home Free All
The Lonely Guy
The Naked Face
The Secret Diary of Sigmund Freud
The Terminator

1985

Agnes of God
Birdy
Grace Quigley
Jagged Edge

Lifeforce
Return to Oz
Silent Madness
Smorgasbord

1986

Bedroom Eyes
The Boy Who Could Fly
Down and Out in Beverly Hills
Duet for One
From Beyond
Hannah and Her Sisters
Haunted Honeymoon
Heartburn
Manhunter
The Men's Club
Psycho III
She's Gotta Have It
Soul Man

1987

Angel Heart
The Believers
Beyond Therapy
The Couch Trip
Critical Condition
Dead of Winter
House of Games
Hunk
Lethal Weapon
Nice Girls Don't Explode
Nuts
Raising Arizona
The Stepfather

1988

Another Woman
Bad Dreams
Bird

Casual Sex?
Child's Play
The Dead Pool
The Good Mother
Hairspray
The Hero and the Terror
Overboard
Poltergeist III
The Serpent and the Rainbow
sex, lies, and videotape
The Thin Blue Line

1989

Bill and Ted's Excellent Adventure
Chances Are
Communion
Dead Bang
Dead Man Out
The Dream Team
Jacknife
Lethal Weapon II
Lost Angels
New York Stories
Parenthood
Parents
Relentless
See You in the Morning
She's Out of Control
Skin Deep
Vampire's Kiss
Worth Winning

1990

Chattahoochee
Crazy People
Edward Scissorhands
Exorcist III
Impulse
Martians Go Home

Mr. Frost
My Blue Heaven
Problem Child
Three Men and a Little Lady

1991
The Butcher's Wife
Dead Again
Drop Dead Fred
Hot Shots
Lethal Weapon III
Little Man Tate
The Prince of Tides
Scenes from a Mall
Scissors
The Silence of the Lambs
Terminator II: Judgment Day
What About Bob?

1992
Article 99
Basic Instinct
Death Becomes Her
Final Analysis
Husbands and Wives
Raising Cain
Straight Talk
Used People
Whispers in the Dark

1993
Amos and Andrew
Attack of the 50 Ft. Woman
Benny and Joon
The Crush
Fearless
The Good Son
Groundhog Day
Mr. Jones

Sleepless in Seattle
Sliver

1994
Ace Ventura, Pet Detective
Blue Sky
Bulletproof Heart
Color of Night
The Hudsucker Proxy
The Mask
Mrs. Parker and the Vicious Circle
The Santa Clause
The Scout
The Shadow
Silent Fall
Surviving the Game

1995
Batman Forever
Don Juan DeMarco
Dracula: Dead and Loving It
Dr. Jekyll and Ms. Hyde
Golden Eye
Jade
Leaving Las Vegas
Mad Love
Magic in the Water
The Net
Nine Months
12 Monkeys

1996
The Chamber
The Evening Star
Faithful
The First Wives' Club
If Lucy Fell
Marvin's Room
One Fine Day

Primal Fear
A Time to Kill
Tin Cup
Twister
Walking and Talking

1997

As Good As It Gets
*Austin Powers: International Man of
  Mystery*
Bliss
Conspiracy Theory
Deconstructing Harry
Donnie Brasco
Everyone Says I Love You
Female Perversions
Good Will Hunting
Grosse Pointe Blank
Leave It to Beaver
The Myth of Fingerprints

She's So Lovely
Space Jam
That Old Feeling
'Til There Was You
Trial and Error
Underworld

1998

Antz
Armageddon
Celebrity
Disturbing Behavior
Doctor Doolittle
Happiness
Mr. Jealousy
Next Stop Wonderland
Psycho
Sphere
There's Something About Mary

References

Agee, J. (1958). *Agee on film*. New York: McDowell Obolensky.

Alloway, L. (1971). *Violent America: The movies, 1946–64*. New York: Museum of Modern Art.

Althusser, L. (1971). Ideology and ideological state apparatuses (notes towards an investigation). In *Lenin and philosophy and other essays*. Translated by Ben Brewster. London: New Left Books.

———. (1976). Marxism and humanism. In *For Marx*. Translated by Ben Brewster. London: New Left Books.

Altman, C. (1976). Psychoanalysis and the cinema: The imaginary discourse. *Quarterly Review of Film Studies* 2:257–72.

Ansen, D. (1983). Manhattan transfer. *Newsweek*, 21 February, 61.

———. (1986). Manhattan serenade. *Newsweek*, 3 February, 67–68.

Anzieu, D. (1976). "L'enveloppe sonore du soi." *Nouvelle revue de psychanalyse* 13:161–79.

Appelo, T. (1996). He's good for what ails flicks. *Entertainment Weekly* 63.

Bak, R. (1968). The phallic woman: The ubiquitous fantasy in perversions. *Psychoanalytic Study of the Child* 23:15–36.

Barthes, R. (1972). *Mythologies*. Translated by Annette Lavers. New York: Hill and Wang.

Basinger, J. (1993). *A woman's view: How Hollywood spoke to women, 1930–1960*. New York: Alfred A. Knopf.

Becker, E. (1973). *The denial of death*. New York: Free Press.

Behlmer, R. (1982). *America's favorite movies*. New York: Ungar.

Benjamin, J. (1988). *The bonds of love: Psychoanalysis, feminism, and the problem of domination*. New York: Pantheon.

———. (1998). *The shadow of the other*. New York: Routledge.

Bergstrom, J. (1979). Alternation, segmentation, hypnosis: Interview with Raymond Bellour. *Camera Obscura* 3–4:71–103.

Berman, J. (1985). *The talking cure: Literary representations of psychoanalysis*. New York: New York University Press.

Bingham, D. (1994). *Acting male: Masculinities in the films of James Stewart, Jack Nicholson, and Clint Eastwood*. New Brunswick, N.J.: Rutgers University Press.

Blum, H. (1969). A psychoanalytic view of *Who's afraid of Virginia Woolf? Journal of the American Psychoanalytic Association* 17:888–903.

Bordwell, D. (1985). *Narration in the fiction film*. Madison: University of Wisconsin Press.

———. (1989). *Making meaning: Inference and rhetoric in the interpretation of cinema.* Cambridge, Mass.: Harvard University Press.

Bordwell, D., J. Staiger, and K. Thompson. (1985). *The classical Hollywood cinema: Film style and mode of production to 1960.* New York: Columbia University Press.

Bram, A. (1997). Perceptions of psychotherapy and psychotherapists: Implications from a study of undergraduates. *Professional Psychology: Research and Practice* 28:170–78.

Braudy, L. (1968). Hitchcock, Truffaut, and the irresponsible audience. *Film Quarterly* 21:21–27.

———. (1977). *The world in a frame.* New York: Doubleday.

Brenner, C. (1982). *The mind in conflict.* New York: International Universities Press.

Brewster, B. (1998). *Theatre to cinema: Stage pictorialism and the early feature film.* New York: Oxford University Press.

Brown, G. (1990). With fans like this . . . . *Village Voice Film Supplement,* December, 21.

Bruccoli, M. (1963). *The composition of "Tender is the night."* Pittsburgh: University of Pittsburgh Press.

Brunswick, R. (1940). The preoedipal phase of the libido development. *Psychoanalytical Quarterly* 9:239–319.

Buhle, M. (1998). *Feminism and its discontents.* Cambridge, Mass.: Harvard University Press.

Burnham, J. (1978). The influence of psychoanalysis upon American culture. In *American psychoanalysis: Origins and development.* Edited by J. Quen and E. Carlson, 52–72. New York: Brunner/Mazel.

———. (1979). From avant-garde to specialism: Psychoanalysis in America. *Journal of the History of the Behavioral Sciences* 15:128–34.

———. (1982). American medicine's golden age: What happened to it? *Science* 215:1474–79.

Butler, J. (1990). *Gender trouble.* New York: Routledge.

Cagin, S., and P. Dray. (1984). *Hollywood films of the seventies: Sex, drugs, violence, rock 'n' roll and politics.* New York: Harper and Row.

Canham, K. (1973). *Hollywood professionals.* New York: A. S. Barnes.

Carroll, N. (1981). Nightmare and the horror film: The symbolic biology of fantastic beings. *Film Quarterly* 34:16–25.

———. (1988). *Mystifying movies: Fads and fallacies in contemporary film theory.* New York: Columbia University Press.

Cavell, S. (1981a). *North by northwest. Critical Inquiry* 7:761–76.

———. (1981b). *Pursuits of happiness: The Hollywood comedy of remarriage.* Cambridge, Mass.: Harvard University Press.

Chasseguet-Smirgel, J. (1970). Feminine guilt and the Oedipus complex (1964). In *Female sexuality.* Edited by J. Chasseguet-Smirgel, 94–134. Ann Arbor: University of Michigan Press.

Ciment, M. (1977). Entretien avec Robert Altman. *Positif* 197 (September):13–20.

Clover, C. (1992). *Men, women and chainsaws*. Princeton, N.J.: Princeton University Press.

Cohan, S. (1993). "Feminizing" the song-and-dance man: Fred Astaire and the spectacle of masculinity in the Hollywood musical. In *Screening the male: Exploring masculinities in Hollywood cinema*. Edited by S. Cohan and I. Hark, 46–69. New York: Routledge.

Coltrera, J. (1981). Lives, events, and other players: Directions in psychobiography. In *Lives, events, and other players: Directions in psychobiography*. Edited by J. Coltrera, 3–73. New York: Jason Aronson.

Corliss, R. (1974). *Talking pictures*. Woodstock: Overlook Press.

Crowther, B. (1946). Review of *Shock*. *New York Times*, 9 March, 10.

Davidson, V. (1976). Psychiatry's problem with no name: Therapist-patient sex. *American Journal of Psycho-analysis* 37:43–50.

Dayan, D. (1976). The Tutor code of classical cinema. In *Movies and methods: An anthology*, edited by Nichols B., 438–51, Berkeley: University of California Press.

de Lauretis, T. (1984). *Alice doesn't: Feminism, semiotics, cinema*. Bloomington: Indiana University Press.

Demby, B. (1976). Robert Altman talks about his life and his art. *New York Times*, 19 June, sec. 2.

Dervin, D. (1985). *Through a Freudian lens deeply*. Hillsdale, N.J.: Analytic Press.

DiPiero, T. (1991). "The patriarch is not (just) a man." *Camera Obscura* 25–26: 101–24.

Doane, M. (1982). Film and the masquerade: Theorizing the female spectator. *Screen* 23(3–4):74–87.

———. (1986). *The desire to desire: The woman's film of the 1940s*. Bloomington: Indiana University Press.

Doherty, T. (1996). Genre, gender and the *Aliens* trilogy. In *The dread of difference: Gender and the horror film*. Edited by B. K. Grant, 181–99. Austin: University of Texas Press.

DuPont, J. (1988). *The clinical diary of Sàndor Ferenczi*. Translated by M. Balint and N. Jackson. Cambridge, Mass.: Harvard University Press.

Durgnat, R. (1982). Review of *The imaginary signifier: Psychoanalysis and cinema*, by Christian Metz. *Film Quarterly* 36(2):58–64.

Eber, M., and J. O'Brien. (1982). Psychotherapy in the movies. *Psychotherapy: Theory, Research and Practice* 19:116–20.

Ebert, R. (1978). Beyond narrative: The future of the feature film. In *The great ideas today*. Edited by M Adler, 176–215. Chicago: Encyclopaedia Britannica.

Eberwein, R. (1984). *Film and the dream screen*. Princeton, N.J.: Princeton University Press.

Eckert, C. (1974a). The anatomy of a proletarian film: Warner's *Marked woman*. *Film Quarterly* 27:10–24.

———. (1974b). Shall we deport Lévi-Strauss? *Film Quarterly* 27:63–65. Reprinted in Nichols (1985), 426–29.

Eco, U. (1985). *Casablanca:* Cult movies and intertextual collage. *Sub-Stance* 47:3–12.

Editors of *Cahiers du cinéma*. (1985). John Ford's *Young Mr. Lincoln*. In *Film theory and criticism*. 3rd ed. Edited by G. Mast and M. Cohen, 695–740. New York: Oxford University Press.

Ehrenburg, I. (1931). *Die Traumfabrik: Chronik des Films*. Berlin: Malik.

Eigen, M. (1974). On pre-oedipal castration anxiety. *International Review of Psychoanalysis* 1:489–98.

Ellenberger, H. (1955). A comparison of European and American psychiatry. *Bulletin of the Menninger Clinic* 19:43–51.

Faludi, S. (1991). *Backlash: The undeclared war against American women*. New York: Crown.

Feldstein, R. (1985). The dissolution of the self in *Zelig*. *Literature/Film Quarterly* 13:155–60.

Felman, S. (1982). *Literature and psychoanalysis: The question of reading: Otherwise*. Baltimore: Johns Hopkins University Press.

Feuer, J. (1982). *The Hollywood musical*. Bloomington: Indiana University Press.

Fink, P. (1983). The enigma of stigma and its relation to psychiatric education. *Psychiatric Annals* 13:669–90.

Fish, S. (1976). Interpreting the variorum. *Critical Inquiry* 2:465–85.

Fitzgerald, F. (1934). *Tender is the night*. New York: Charles Scribner's Sons.

Forrester, J. (1997). *Dispatches from the Freud wars*. Cambridge, Mass.: Harvard University Press.

Frank, B., and B. Krohn. (1983). Entretien avec Martin Scorsese. *Cahiers du cinéma* 347:10–17.

Freedman, O., and R. Gordon. (1973). Psychiatry under siege: Attacks from without. *Psychiatric Annals* 3:10–34.

Freud, S. (1900). The interpretation of dreams. *S.E.* 4 and 5, 1953.

———. (1910). Leonardo da Vinci and a memory of his childhood. *S.E.* 11:57–137, 1957.

———. (1914). On narcissism: An introduction. *S.E.* 14:67–102, 1963.

———. (1914). On the history of the psycho-analytic movement. *S.E.* 14:1–66, 1963.

———. (1915). Observations on transference-love. *S.E.* 12:157–73, 1958.

———. (1916). Some character-types met with in psycho-analytic work. *S.E.* 14:309–33, 1963 (specifically, "Those wrecked by success," 316–31).

———. (1920). Beyond the pleasure principle. *S.E.* 18:1–64, 1955.

———. (1923). The ego and the id. *S.E.* 19:1–66, 1961.

———. (1925a). Some additional notes on dream interpretation as a whole. *S.E.* 19:123–38, 1961.

———. (1925b). Some psychical consequences of the anatomical distinction between the sexes. *S.E.* 19:241–58, 1961.

———. (1927). Fetishism. *S.E.* 21:147–57, 1961.

———. (1939). Moses and monotheism: Three essays. *S.E.* 23:1–137, 1964.

———. (1940). Splitting of the ego in the process of defence. *S.E.* 23:271–78, 1964.

Frye, N. (1957). *The anatomy of criticism.* Princeton, N.J.: Princeton University Press.

Fussell, P. (1983). *Class: A guide through the American status system.* New York: Summit Press.

Gabbard, G. (1979). Stage fright. *International Journal of Psychoanalysis* 60:383–92.

———. (1983). Further contributions to the understanding of stage fright: Narcissistic issues. *Journal of the American Psychoanalytic Association* 31:423–41.

———. (1989). *Sexual exploitation in professional relationships.* Washington, D.C.: American Psychiatric Press.

Gabbard, G., and E. Lester. (1995). *Boundaries and boundary violations in psychoanalysis.* New York: Basic Books.

Gabbard, G., S. Twemlow, and F. Jones. (1981). Do "near-death experiences" occur only near death? *Journal of Nervous and Mental Disease* 169:374–77.

Gabbard, K. (1988). *Aliens* and the new family romance. *Post Script* 8(1):29–42.

Gach, J. (1980). Culture and complex: On the early history of psychoanalysis in America. In *Essays in the history of psychiatry.* Edited by E. Wallace and L. Pressley, 142–57. Columbia, S.C.: William S. Hall Psychiatric Institute of the South Carolina Department of Mental Health.

Gibson, W. (1954). *The cobweb.* New York: Alfred A. Knopf.

Goldberger, M., and D. Evans. (1985). On transference manifestations in male patients with female analysts. *International Journal of Psycho-Analysis* 66:295–309.

Gorbman, C. (1987). *Unheard melodies: Narrative film music.* Bloomington: Indiana University Press.

Greenberg, H. (1975). *The movies on your mind.* New York: Dutton.

———. (1983). The fractures of desire: Psychoanalytic notes on *Alien* and the contemporary "cruel" horror film. *Psychoanalytic Review* 70:241–67.

———. (1989). *Working girl:* Leveraged sell-out. *Journal of Popular Film and Television* 17(1):20–23.

———. (1993). *Screen memories: Hollywood cinema on the psychoanalytic couch.* New York: Columbia University Press.

———. (1998). "8½" baked. *Projections.* 12:15–19.

Greenson, R. (1966). That "impossible" profession. *Journal of the American Psychoanalytic Association* 14:9–27.

Grinfeld, M. (1998). Psychiatry and mental illness: Are they mass media targets? *Psychiatric Times,* 15 March (3):1.

Grob, G. (1985). *The inner world of American psychiatry, 1890–1940.* New Brunswick, N.J.: Rutgers University Press.

Guthmann, H. (1969). The characterization of the psychiatrist in American fiction, 1859–1965. Ph.D. diss., University of Southern California.

Halliwell, L. (1983). *Halliwell's film guide.* New York: HarperCollins.

Hansen, M. (1991). *Babel and Babylon : Spectatorship in American silent film.* Cambridge, Mass.: Harvard University Press.

Haskell, M. (1974). *From reverence to rape: The treatment of women in the movies.* New York: Holt, Rinehart and Winston.

———. (1987). *From reverence to rape: The treatment of women in the movies.* 2nd ed. Chicago: University of Chicago Press.

Heath, S. (1981). *Questions of cinema.* Bloomington: Indiana University Press.

Heller, S. (1990). Once-theoretical scholarship on film is broadened to include history of movie-industry practices. *Chronicle of Higher Education,* 21 March, A6.

Henderson, B. (1980–81). *The Searchers:* An American dilemma. *Film Quarterly* 34(2):12–27.

Henry, M. (1983). Entretien avec Martin Scorsese. *Positif* 267 (May):14–19.

Hillier, J., ed. (1985). *Cahiers du cinéma: The 1950s: Neo-realism, Hollywood, new wave.* Cambridge, Mass.: Harvard University Press.

Hirschberg, L. (1997). Woody Allen and Martin Scorsese. *New York Times Magazine,* 16 November, 91–96.

Hoberman, J: Kiss-kiss of death. *The Village Voice,* 24 November, 1998.

Hoberman, J., and J. Rosenbaum. (1983). *Midnight movies.* New York: Harper and Row.

Holden, S. (1998). In a rush of new films, some unsung virtues (and cautions). *New York Times,* 9 January, B1, B12.

Holland, N. (1959). Psychiatry in pselluloid. *Atlantic Monthly,* February, 105–7.

Huss, R. (1986). *The mindscapes of art: Dimensions of the psyche in fiction, drama, and film.* Rutherford, N.J.: Fairleigh Dickinson University Press.

Huston, J. (1980). *An open book.* New York: Alfred A. Knopf.

Jacobs, D. (1982). . . . *But we need the eggs: The magic of Woody Allen.* New York: St. Martin's Press.

James, H. (1934). *The art of the novel.* New York: Charles Scribner's Sons.

James, W. (1958). *Varieties of religious experience: A study in human nature* (1902). New York: New American Library (Mentor ed.).

Jameson, R., and K. Murphy. (1976). They take on their own life. *Movietone News,* 16 September, 2–12.

Jaques, E. (1965). Death and the mid-life crisis. *International Journal of Psycho-Analysis* 46:502–14.

Jones, A. (1991). "She was bad news": Male paranoia and the contemporary new woman. *Camera Obscura* 25/26:297–320.

Jones, E. (1964). *Hamlet and Oedipus.* New York: Anchor.

Kael, P. (1973). Movieland—the bum's paradise. *New Yorker,* 22 October, 133–39.

———. (1980). The frog who turned into a prince, the prince who turned into a frog. *New Yorker,* 27 October, 183–90.

Kaminsky, S. (1978). *John Huston: Maker of magic.* Boston: Houghton-Mifflin.

Kaplan, D. (1988). The psychoanalysis of art: Some ends, some means. *Journal of the American Psychoanalytic Association* 36:280–91.

Kaplan, E. A., ed. (1989). *Women in film noir*. Rev. ed. London: British Film Institute.

Kaplan, E. A. (1994). Film and history: Spectatorship, transference, and race. In *History and . . . : Histories within the human sciences*. Edited by R. Cohen and M. Roth, 179–208. Charlottesville: University of Virginia Press.

Karme, L. (1979). The analysis of the male patient by a female analyst: The problem of the negative oedipal transference. *International Journal of Psycho-Analysis* 60:253–261.

Kawin, B. (1978). *Mindscreen: Bergman, Godard, and first-person film*. Princeton, N.J.: Princeton University Press.

Kernberg, O. (1965). Notes on countertransference. *Journal of the American Psychoanalytic Association* 13:38–56.

———. (1974). Further contributions to the treatment of narcissistic personalities. *International Journal of Psycho-Analysis* 55:215–40.

———. (1975). *Borderline conditions and pathological narcissism*. New York: Jason Aronson.

———. (1980). *Internal world and external reality*. New York: Jason Aronson.

Kinder, M. (1980). The adaptation of cinematic dreams. *Dreamworks* 1:54–68.

Kirk, G. (1970). *Myth: Its meaning and functions in ancient and other cultures*. Cambridge, U.K.: Cambridge University Press.

Knee, A. (1996). The American science fiction film and fifties culture. Ph.D. diss., New York University.

Knight, A. (1963). Who's morbid? *Saturday Review*, 10 August, 34.

Kohut, H. (1971). *The analysis of the self*. New York: International Universities Press.

———. (1977). *The restoration of the self*. New York: International Universities Press.

———. (1984). *How does analysis cure?* Chicago: University of Chicago Press.

Kramm, J. (1952). *The shrike*. New York: Random House.

Krutnik, F. (1991). *In a lonely street: Film noir, genre, masculinity*. New York: Routledge.

Kuhn, A. (1982). *Women's pictures: Feminism and the cinema*. London: Routledge and Kegan Paul.

Kulish, N. (1986). Gender and transference: The screen of the phallic mother. *International Review of Psycho-Analysis*. 13:393–404.

Lacan, J. (1976). *Ecrits: A selection*. Translated by Alan Sheridan. New York: Norton.

Lahr, J. (1996). The imperfectionist: Why is Woody Allen singing in his new movie, and how did he survive the scandal? *New Yorker*, 9 December, 68–83.

Laplanche, J., and J. Pontalis. (1973). *The language of psychoanalysis*. Translated by Donald Nicholson-Smith. New York: Norton.

Lasch, C. (1979). *The culture of narcissism*. New York: Norton.

Leamer, L. (1986). *As time goes by: The life of Ingrid Bergman*. New York: Harper and Row.

Leaming, B. (1986). *Orson Welles: A life.* New York: Viking.

Lear, J. (1998). *Open minded: Working out the logic of the soul.* Cambridge, Mass.: Harvard University Press.

Lehman, P. (1992). "Don't blame this on a girl": Female rape-revenge films. In *Screening the male: Exploring masculinities in the Hollywood cinema.* Edited by S. Cohan and I. Hark. New York: Routledge.

———. (1993). *Running scared: Masculinity and the representation of the male body.* Philadelphia: Temple University Press.

Lehmann, H. (1980). Unusual psychiatric disorders, atypical psychoses, and brief reactive psychoses. In *Comprehensive textbook of psychiatry.* 3rd ed. Edited by H. Kaplan, A. Freedman, and B. Sadock, 1986–2002. Baltimore: Williams and Wilkins.

Lerner, H. (1974). Early origins of envy and devaluation of women: Implications for sex role stereotypes. *Bulletin of the Menninger Clinic* 38:538–53.

Lester, E. (1985). The female analyst and the erotized transference. *International Journal of Psycho-Analysis* 66:283–93.

Lévi-Strauss, C. (1975). *The raw and the cooked: Introduction to a science of mythology: I.* Translated by J. Weightman and D. Weightman. New York: Harper and Row.

Linter, J. (1979). Reflections on the media and the mental patient. *Hospital and Community Psychiatry* 30:415–16.

Lundberg, F., and M. Farnham. (1946). *Modern woman: The lost sex.* New York: Harper.

Lurie, L. (1981–82). The construction of the castrated woman in psychoanalysis and cinema. *Discourse* 4:52–74.

MacCabe, C. (1976). Theory and film: Principles of realism and pleasure. *Screen* 17.3:7–9. Reprinted in C. MacCabe. (1985). *Tracking the signifier.* Minneapolis: University of Minnesota Press.

Mast, G., and B. Kawin. (1996). *A short history of the movies.* 4th ed. New York: Bobbs-Merrill.

Mast, G., M. Cohen, and L. Braudy. (1992). *Film theory and criticism: Introductory readings.* 4th ed. New York: Oxford University Press.

Mayer, E., and D. De Marneffe. (1992). When theory and practice diverge: Gender-related patterns of referral to psychoanalysts. *Journal of the American Psychoanalytic Association* 40:551–86.

McNeil, A. (1980). *Total television.* New York: Penguin.

Melosh, B. (1983). Doctors, patients, and "big nurse": Work and gender in the postwar hospital. In *Nursing history: New perspectives, new possibilities.* Edited by E. Lagemann, 157–79. New York: Teachers College Press.

Menaker, D. (1998). *The treatment.* New York: Alfred A. Knopf.

Metz, C. (1982). *The imaginary signifier: Psychoanalysis and the cinema.* Translated by Celia Britton et al. Bloomington: Indiana University Press.

Michaels, L., ed. (1993). "Interpretations, Inc." Special issue of *Film Criticism* 17 (Winter/Spring):2–3.

Miller, M., and R. Sprich. (1981). The appeal of *Star Wars:* An archetypal-psychoanalytic view. *American Imago* 38:203–19.

Modleski, T. (1988). *The women who knew too much: Hitchcock and feminist theory.* New York: Methuen.

Monaco, J. (1979). *American film now.* New York: Oxford University Press.

———. (1998). *How to read a film: The world of movies, media, and multimedia art: Technology, language, history, theory.* 3rd ed. New York: Oxford University Press.

Moss, R. (1980). Woody Allen. *Saturday Review*, November, 40–44.

Mulvey, L. (1975). Visual pleasure and narrative cinema. *Screen* 16(3):6–18.

———. (1989). *Visual and other pleasures.* Bloomington: Indiana University Press.

Münsterberg, H. (1970). *The film: A psychological study* (1916). New York: Dover.

Myers, H. (1986). How do women treat men? In *The psychology of men.* Edited by G. Fogel, 262–75, New York: Basic Books.

Nichols, B., ed. (1976). *Movies and methods: An anthology.* Berkeley: University of California Press.

———. (1985). *Movies and methods*, Vol. II. Berkeley: University of California Press.

Nielsen, A. (1980). Choosing psychiatry: The importance of psychiatric education in medical school. *American Journal of Psychiatry* 137:428–31.

Niver, K. (1971). *Biograph Bulletins, 1896–1908.* Los Angeles: Artisan Press.

Oudart, J. (1978). Cinema and suture. *Screen* 18(4):35–47.

Pardes, H., and H. Pincus. (1983). Challenges to academic psychiatry. *American Journal of Psychiatry* 140:1117–26.

Penley, C. (1995). *NASA/Trek: Popular science and sex in America.* New York: Verso.

Petro, P. (1989). *Joyless streets: Women and melodramatic representation in Weimar Germany.* Princeton, N. J.: Princeton University Press.

Piersall, J., and A. Hirshberg. (1955). *Fear strikes out.* Boston: Little, Brown.

Plank, R. (1956). Portraits of fictitious psychiatrists. *American Imago* 13:259–67.

Polan, D. (1986). *Power and paranoia: History, narrative, and the American cinema, 1940–1950.* New York: Columbia University Press.

Pope, K., and J. Bouhoutsos. (1986). *Sexual intimacy between therapists and patients.* New York: Praeger.

Rand, N., and M. Torok. (1997). *Questions for Freud: The secret history of psychoanalysis.* Cambridge, Mass.: Harvard University Press.

Ray, R. (1985). *A certain tendency of the Hollywood cinema, 1930–1980.* Princeton, N. J.: Princeton University Press.

Rickey, C. (1982). Frances Farmer's dark victory. *Village Voice*, 30 November, 73ff.

Rieff, P. (1966). *The triumph of the therapeutic.* New York: Harper and Row.

Riviere, J. (1966). Womanliness as masquerade (1929). In *Psychoanalysis and female sexuality.* Edited by H. M. Ruitenbeek. New Haven, Conn.: College and University Press.

Rodowick, D. N. (1991). *The difficulty of difference: Psychoanalysis, sexual difference, and film theory.* New York: Routledge.

Roheim, G. (1945). Aphrodite or the woman with a penis. *Psychoanalytic Quarterly* 25:515–29.

Rosen, P., ed. (1986). *Narrative, apparatus, ideology: A film theory reader.* New York: Columbia University Press.

Rosolato, G. (1974). La Voix: Entre corps et langage. *Revue française de psychanalyse* 38(1):75–94.

Russ, H. (1993). Erotic transference through countertransference: The female therapist and the male patient. *Psychoanalytic Psychology* 10:393–406.

Russo, V. (1981). *The celluloid closet: Homosexuality in the movies.* New York: Harper and Row.

Samuels, L. (1985). Female psychotherapists as portrayed in film, fiction, and nonfiction. *Journal of the American Academy of Psychoanalysis* 13:367–78.

Sarris, A. (1968). *The American cinema: Directors and directions, 1929–1968.* New York: Dutton.

———. (1980). Woody doesn't rhyme with Federico. *Village Voice,* 1–7 October, 49.

———. (1988). Auteurism turns silver. *Village Voice,* 7 June, 66.

Sartre, J. (1986). *The Freud scenario.* Edited by J. Pontalis; translated by Quintin Hoare. Chicago: University of Chicago Press.

Sayre, N. (1982). *Running time: Films of the cold war.* New York: Dial Press.

Schatz, T. (1982). "Annie Hall" and the issue of modernism. *Literature/Film Quarterly* 10:180–88.

Schickel, R. (1973). "Some nights in Casablanca." In *Favorite movies: Critics' choice.* Edited by P. Nobile, 114–25. New York: Macmillan.

Schneider, I. (1977). Images of the mind: Psychiatry in the commercial film. *American Journal of Psychiatry* 134:613–20.

———. (1985). The psychiatrist in the movies: The first fifty years. In *The Psychoanalytic study of literature.* Edited by J. Reppen and M. Charney, 53–67. Hillsdale, N.J.: Analytic Press.

Segal, H. (1964). *Introduction to the work of Melanie Klein.* New York: Basic Books.

Self, R. (1984). Review of *American skeptic: Robert Altman's genre-commentary films,* by Norman Kagan. *Wide Angle* 6(1):66–68.

———. (1985). Robert Altman and the theory of authorship. *Cinema Journal* 25(1):3–11.

Sharpe, E. (1937). *Dream analysis.* New York: Brunner/Mazel.

Silverman, K. (1983). *The subject of semiotics.* New York: Oxford University Press.

———. (1988). *The acoustic mirror: The female voice in psychoanalysis and cinema.* Bloomington: Indiana University Press.

———. (1992). *Male subjectivity at the margins.* New York: Routledge.

Sizemore, C. (1977). *I'm Eve.* Garden City, N.Y.: Doubleday.

Sklar, R. (1975). *Movie-made America.* New York: Random House.

Spoto, D. (1983). *The dark side of genius: The life of Alfred Hitchcock.* Boston: Little, Brown.

Steinberg, C. (1980). *Film facts.* New York: Facts on File, Inc.

Stine, W. (1974). *Mother Goddam.* New York: Hawthorn Books.

Stoller, R. (1975). *Perversion: The erotic form of hatred.* New York: Pantheon.

Straayer, C. (1992). Redressing the "natural": The temporary transvestite film. *Wide Angle* 14(1):36–55.

Studlar, G. (1988). *In the realm of pleasure: von Sternberg, Dietrich, and the masochistic aesthetic.* Urbana: University of Illinois Press.

———. (1989). Midnight s/excess: Cult configurations of "femininity" and the perverse. *Journal of Popular Film and Television* 17(1):2–14.

Taubin, A. (1998). Star glazing. *Village Voice,* 12 April, 67.

Thomas, A., and S. Chess. (1984). Genesis and evolution of behavioral disorders from infancy to early adult life. *American Journal of Psychiatry* 141:1–9.

Thomson, D. (1998). Shoot the actor. *Film Comment* 34(2):12–19.

Truffaut, F. (1984). *Hitchcock.* Rev ed. New York: Simon and Schuster.

Turim, M. (1989). *Flashbacks in film: Memory and history.* New York: Routledge.

Tyson, P. (1986). "The female analyst and the male analysand." Presentation to the San Francisco Psychoanalytic Institute, February.

Vernet, M. (1975). Freud: Effects spéciaux/mise en scène: U.S.A. *Communications* 23:223–34.

Walsh, A. (1984). *Women's film and female experience, 1940–1950.* New York: Praeger.

Ward, M. (1946). *The snake pit.* New York: Random House.

Weissman, S. (1987). Chaplin's "The kid." In *Images in our souls: Cavell, psychoanalysis, and cinema.* Edited by J. Smith and W. Kerrigan, 183–186. Baltimore: Johns Hopkins University Press.

Whitemore, D., and P. Cecchettini. (1976). *Passport to Hollywood: Film immigrants.* New York: McGraw-Hill.

Williams, L. (1981). *Figures of desire: A theory and analysis of surrealist film.* Urbana: University of Illinois Press.

———. (1989). *Hard core: Power, pleasure, and the "frenzy of the visible."* Berkeley: University of California Press.

Winick, C. (1963). The psychiatrist in fiction. *Journal of Nervous and Mental Disease* 136:43–57.

Wolfenstein, M., and N. Leites. (1970). *The movies: A psychological study.* New York: Atheneum.

Wood, M. (1975). *America at the movies.* New York, Basic Books.

Wood, R. (1977). *Hitchcock's films.* Cranbury, N.J.: A. S. Barnes.

———. (1986). *Hollywood from Vietnam to Reagan.* New York: Columbia University Press.

Wouk, H. (1951). *The Caine mutiny: A novel of World War II.* Garden City, N.Y.: Doubleday.

Wrye, H. (1993). Erotic terror: Male patients' horror of the early maternal erotic transference. *Psychoanalytic Inquiry* 13:240–57.

Yager, J., K. Lamotte, A. Nielsen, and J. Eaton. (1982). Medical students' evaluation of psychiatry: A cross-country comparison. *American Journal of Psychiatry* 139:1003–9.

Yager, J., and S. Scheiber. (1981). Why psychiatry is recruiting fewer residents: The opinions of medical school deans and psychiatric department chairmen. *Journal of Psychiatric Education* 5:258–68.

Zizek, S., ed. (1992). *Everything you always wanted to know about Lacan (but were afraid to ask Hitchcock)*. New York: Verso.

Zizek, S. (1993). "The thing that thinks": The Kantian background of the noir subject. In *Shades of noir*. Edited by J. Copjec, 211–31. New York: Verso.

Zizek, S. (1994). *The metastases of enjoyment: Six essays on woman and causality*. New York: Verso.

Subject Index

Page numbers printed in **boldface** *type refer to tables or plates.*

Abbott, Diahnne, 255
Accuracy of film portrayals of
    psychiatry, 173–176
Adams, Joe, 88
Adam's Rib (1949), 13
Adler, Alfred, 43
Adult films, 24–25
Adventures of Robin Hood (1938), 214
After the Thin Man (1936), 49
Agee, James, 65
Agnes of God (1985), 18, 138–139,
    164–165
Aiello, Danny, 267, **269**
Albert, Eddie, 102
Alcoholism, 25, 56, 95, 104–105
Alda, Alan, 105, 249, 290
Alex in Wonderland (1971), 234
Alien (1979), 277, 280–291, **285, 286,**
    295–296, 301
Alien: Resurrection (1997), 290, 302
Aliens (1986), 289–290, 295, 302
All That Jazz (1979), 233–238, **237,**
    238, 241, 242, 244–247
Allen, Irwin, 91
Allen, Nancy, 109, 110
Allen, Woody, 16, 124–127, 131–133,
    140, 157, 159, 218, 234, 238–244,
    240, 246–250, **247,** 253, 262–265,
    263, 267–275, 282, 310
Alley, Kirstie, 127, 159
Alloway, Lawrence, 79
Allyson, June, 68
Alternative therapies, 128
Althusser, Louis, 5, 190, 196–198,
    201

Altman, Robert, 22, 129, 140, 221–223,
    230, 232, 311
Amadeus (1984), 135
The Amazing Dr. Clitterhouse (1938),
    49
American Graffiti (1973), 210
American Psychoanalytic Association,
    184
Anatomy of a Murder (1959), 78–79
Andersson, Bibi, **138,** 164
Andrews, Dana, 5
Andrews, Julie, 157
Angel Heart (1987), 140
Angels with Dirty Faces (1938), 214,
    215
Annie Hall (1977), 124, 125, 244, 246,
    273
Another Woman (1988), 126
Ansen, David, 140
Anspach, Susan, 129
Anti-Semitism, 60–61
Ants in Your Pants of 1939, 239
Antz (1998), 133
Anzieu, Didier, 212
Arbus, Alan, 105
Archer, Anne, 297
Arkin, Alan, 137, 143
Armitage, George, 143
Armstrong, Curtis, 218
Arthur (1981), 105
Arthur, Robert Alan, 234
As Good as It Gets (1997), 143,
    180–181
Ashby, Hal, 135
Ashley, Elizabeth, 113, 164

"Assertions of the self," 4
Astaire, Fred, 14, 47–49, **48,** 200, 272
Auteur theory of cinema, 190, 213–214
Autobiographical films, 233–250
　　All That Jazz, 233–238, **237, 238,**
　　　　244–246
　　death and, 245–250
　　8½, 234–235
　　midlife crisis and, 242–245
　　narcissistic object relations in,
　　　　235–242
　　Stardust Memories, 124, 234–235,
　　　　238–244, **240,** 246–247, **247**
Avakian, Aram, 17, 136
Averback, Hy, 313
The Awful Truth (1937), 47
Ayres, Lew, 59, **60,** 66, 79

Babel and Babylon (Hansen), 198
Bacall, Lauren, 70, 71, 116
The Bachelor and the Bobby Soxer
　　(1947), **163**
Back Street (1941), 13
The Bad and the Beautiful (1952), 69
Bad Dreams (1988), **162**
Bak, R., 294–295
Baker, Elliot, 119
Baldwin, Alec, 301
Balsam, Martin, 102
Bananas (1971), 244
Bancroft, Anne, 104
The Band Wagon (1953), 69
Barkin, Ellen, 297–299, 301, 302, 306
Barrault, Marie-Christine, 241
The Barretts of Wimpole Street (1934),
　　43
Barry, Patricia, 112–113, 137
Barrymore, John, 41
Barth, John, 120
Barthes, Roland, 5–6, 13, 190
Bartlett, Hall, 103
Basic Instinct (1992), 159, **162,**
　　305–306

Basinger, J., 148, 151
Bates, Kathy, 293, 296, 306
Batman Returns (1992), 296
Baxter, Warner, 8
Bean, Orson, 78–79
Beatrice: Life of the Party, 105
Beatty, Warren, 76, 116, 262
"Beauty and the Beast," 221, 231
Becker, Ernest, 251–252, 261
Bedelia, Bonnie, 304
Bedlam (1946), 63
Bedroom Eyes (1986), 157, **162**
Bedtime for Bonzo (1951), 66
Bell, Alexander Graham, 6
The Bell Jar (1979), 120
Bellamy, Ralph, 17, 31, 44–45, **46,** 47,
　　51, 77, 122
Bellour, Raymond, 209
Bellow, Saul, 120, 262, 265, 266
Ben Casey, 313
Benjamin, Jessica, 167
Benjamin, Richard, 20, 111, 112,
　　137
Bennett, Joan, 43
Benny and Joon (1993), 143
Benton, Robert, 139
Bergen, Polly, 103
Bergman, Ingrid, 4, 19, 21, 53–54, 59,
　　117, 139, 147, 149, **150,** 156, 206,
　　207, 209, 211, 213, 219, 228
Bergmann, Martin, 126
Berkeley, Busby, 195
Berman, Jeffrey, 120
Bernhard, Sandra, 256, 260
Bernhardt, Curtis, 6, 59
The Best Years of Our Lives (1946), 5
Bettelheim, Bruno, 262, 264–265
Beverly Hills Cop (1984), 219
Beverly Hills Cop II (1987), 219
Bewitched (1945), **163**
Beyond Therapy (1987), 140, **162**
Biehn, Michael, 290
The Big Fix (1978), 128

A Bill of Divorcement (1932 and 1940), 40–41
Bingham, Dennis, 200
Birch, Wyrley, 50
Bisexuality, 132, 159, 165, 200
Bissell, Whit, 66, 72, 73, 75, 78–79, 85
"Black film" (film noir), 56–59, 75, 296
Black psychiatrists in films, 88, 136–137, 143
Blade Runner (1982), 201, 282–284, 296, 300
Blair, Linda, 279
Blind Alley (1939), 17, 23, 30–31, 44–46, **46,** 51, 52, 55, 59, 71, 99, 105, 122, 125
Blindfold (1966), 21, 23, 117
Bliss (1997), **162**
Bloom, Claire, 25
Blow Out (1981), 110
Blue Sky (1994), 17
Bluebeard's Eighth Wife (1938), 49
Blum, John Morton, 262, 265
Blume in Love (1973), 127, 129–131, 313, 314
Bob and Carol and Ted and Alice (1969), 127–130, 313, 314
Body Double (1984), 110
Bogart, Humphrey, 4, 72, 118, 200, 206, 209, 215, 216, 219
Bonnie and Clyde (1967), 119
Boomerang (1925), 37–38
Boorman, John, 24, 137
Borderline personality disorder, 178
Bordwell, David, 197–198, 201
Bosco, Philip, 301
The Boston Strangler (1968), 23, 122–123
Bottome, Phyllis, 43
Boyer, Charles, 43, 70, 71, 152
Branagh, Kenneth, 273, 274
Brando, Marlon, 141
Braudy, Leo, 22
Breathless (1961), 119

Breen Office, 41, 42
Brenner, Charles, 174
Brewster, Ben, 198
Brickman, Marshall, 19, 92, 107, 139
Bridges, Jeff, 79
Bridges, Lloyd, 30
Brigadoon (1954), 69
Brill, A. A., 76
Bringing Up Baby (1938), 18, **20,** 49, 122
Broderick, James, 118
Bronson, Charles, 114, 119
Brooks, Dean, 133, 312–313
Brooks, James, 143
The Brother from Another Planet (1984), 268
Brothers, Joyce, 169
Brown, Georgia, 293
Browning, Tod, 23
"Buddy films," 211, 299
Buffalo Bill and the Indians, or Sitting Bull's History Lesson (1976), 223
Bunston, Herbert, 23
Burnham, John, 44, 76–77, 106, 115, 130
Burrow, Trigant, 76
Burton, Richard, 24, 136
Butch Cassidy and the Sundance Kid (1969), 119, 299
Butler, Judith, 200
Buttafuoco, Mary Jo, 274
Butterfield 8 (1960), **163**

Caan, James, 293, 296
The Cabinet of Dr. Caligari (1919 and 1962), 37, 55, 73, 90, **163**
Cahiers du cinéma, 190–191, 194, 197
Caine, Michael, 19, 108, 110, 126, 179
The Caine Mutiny (1954), 72–73, 75–76, 79, 89, 118
Call Me Bwana (1963), 92
Callan, Michael, 85
Callenbach, Ernest, 101

Cambridge, Godfrey, 121
Camera Obscura, 191, 198
Cameron, James, 289, 295
Canham, Kingsley, 214
Cannon, Dyan, 128, 314
Capgras's syndrome, 280, 287
Capra, Frank, 6, 49–50, 56, 67
Captain Blood (1935), 214
Captain Newman, M.D. (1963), 18, 102–103, 105
Carefree (1938), 22, 47–49, **48, 162, 163**
The Caretakers (1963), 103
Caron, Leslie, 117, 152, 156
Carpenter, John, 24, 268, 277, 279, 280, 287
Carrera, Barbara, 66
Carrie (1976), 111
Carroll, Leo G., 54
Carroll, Noël, 197–198, 277
Carson, Johnny, 254, 255, 313
Casablanca (1942), 4–5, 73, 205–219
   "centering" techniques in, 215–216
   cult status of, 218–219
   director of, 213–215
   as expression of American ideology, 215–218
   Lacanian reading of, 209–210
   music in, 212–213
   oedipal conflict in, 207–209
   reasons for enduring appeal of, 205–206
The Case of Becky (1921), 37
Cassavetes, John, 86
Castle, Peggie, 19, 66
Castle, William, 92, 116
Castration anxiety, 168, 195, 210, 294–295
Cat People (1942), 21, 23
Catch-22 (1970), 300
Categories of films, 21–27
Cates, Gilbert, 18
Cates, Joseph, 85

Cathartic cure
   claimed by actual patients from watching films, 181–182
   in films, 27–34, 52, 71, 95, 141, 178
Cavell, Stanley, 197
Cavett, Dick, 254, 255
Cecchettini, Philip Alan, 205
Celebrity, 241–242, 251–275, 312–314
   films providing insight into, 253
      Allen's "celebrity tetralogy," 267
      Celebrity, 273–274
      The King of Comedy, 254–262, **257**
      The Purple Rose of Cairo, 267–275, **269, 271**
      Zelig, 262–267, **263, 264**
   grief reactions to death of, 261
   heroism and, 251–252
   political, 252–253
   relationship between fan and, 241–242
   substance behind image of, 252–253
Celebrity (1998), 127, 267, 273–274
Chabrol, Claude, 190
Chafed Elbows (1967), 121
Chaplin, Charlie, 214, 242
The Chapman Report (1962), 25, 86
Chekhov, Michael, 53–54, 94, 147, 149, **150**
Cher, 133
A Child Is Waiting (1963), 72
Child sexual abuse, 85
Children of Loneliness (1939), 50–51
Christ figures, 269
Christie, Julie, 161
Chrobak, Rudolf, 166
Chronicle of Higher Education, 198
Ciment, Michel, 222
Cimino, Michael, 11, 137
Citizen Kane (1941), 218
Clark, Kendall, 68
Classic film period, 4
Clayburgh, Jill, 131–132, 138, 165

Clifford, Graeme, 17, 171
Clift, Montgomery, 95, **98,** 99, 118, 194–195
Clinical implications, 171–185
 accuracy of film portrayals, 173–176
 countertransference issues, 19, 22, 88, 93, 94, 137, 139, 140, 143, 148–164, **162,** 171–172
 reactions of patients to film portrayals, 172–173, 176–182
 transference reactions, 28, 57, 108, 138, 150, 153, 154, 157, 171, 174–180, 260, 271–272
Close, Glenn, 297, 304, 306
Close-up shots, 283–284
Clover, Carol, 200
Cobb, Lee J., 28, 31, 81–82, **82**
Coburn, James, 121, 122, 137
The Cobweb (1955), 68–71, 78, 79, 83–84, 92, 104
The Cocktail Party (Eliot), 120
Cohan, Steven, 200
Colbert, Claudette, 14, 43–44, **45,** 90
Coltrera, Joseph, 202–203
Comedy, 21–22, 92
 psychoanalytic, 124–126
 romantic, 21, 22
 slapstick, 36–37
Coming Apart (1969), 19
Communications, 191
Condemned Women (1938), **162, 163**
Connery, Sean, 119, 155, 283
Conrad, Joseph, 284
Conspiracy Theory (1997), 141
Conte, Richard, 21
Conti, Tom, 140
Conversion symptoms, 28
Conway, Tom, 21, 23
Cooke, Alistair, 81
Cool Hand Luke (1967), 118, 119
Cooper, Gary, 6, 49
Coppola, Francis, 129
Corbman, Claudia, 212

Corey, Jeff, 30
Corliss, Richard, 207, 209
Cornfield, Hubert, 88
Cort, Bud, 135
Corti, Axel, 98
Costner, Kevin, 159
The Couch Trip (1987), 140
Countertransference issues, 19, 22, 88, 93, 94, 137, 139, 140, 143, 171–172
 female psychiatrists and countertransference love, 148–164, **162,** 171
Cracking Up (1983), 32
Crampton, Barbara, 157
Crawford, Joan, 6–7, 14, 103, 116
Crews, Frederick, 199
Crichton, Michael, 146
Cries and Whispers (1972), 228
Crime-and-detective films, 22–23
Crimes and Misdemeanors (1989), 126, 249
Crimes of Passion (1984), 17
Crocodile Dundee (1986), 302, 303
Cromwell, John, 17
Cross-dressing, 302
Crossfire (1947), 60
Crouse, Lindsay, 140
Crowther, Bosley, 63
Cruise, Tom, 177
Cukor, George, 25, 86
Culp, Robert, 128
Cult films, 218–219, 303
Cultural studies, 201
Cummings, Robert, 116
Curtis, Tony, 102, 122, 153, **153,** 156
Curtiz, Michael, 205, 207, 213–215
Cusack, John, 143

da Silva, Howard, 86, **87,** 88, 111, 138
da Vinci, Leonardo, 294–296
Dailey, Dan, 83, **84**
Damita, Lily, 215

Damon, Matt, 144, **145,** 179
Dane, Clarence, 40
Daniels, Jeff, 268, **269,** 270, **271**
Darin, Bobby, 88–90, **89,** 102
Dark Delusion (1947), **163**
The Dark Mirror (1946), 23, 59–60, **60,** 66, 74, 79, 105, **162**
The Dark Past (1948), 31, 59
Dark Waters (1944), **163**
David and Lisa (1962), 17, 26, 70, 86, **87,** 88, 92, 94, 101, 102, 104, 111, 112, 138, **163**
Davis, Bette, 33, 51, **52,** 86–87
Davis, Geena, 166
Davis, Judy, 127, 273, 274
Day, Doris, 92, 102
Dayan, Daniel, 194, 196
The Days of Wine and Roses (1958 and 1962), 104, 105
de Broca, Philippe, 86
de Cordova, Frederick, 66
de Havilland, Olivia, 18, 27, 59–61, **60,** **62,** 63, **64,** 92
DeMille, Cecil B., 39, 65
De Niro, Robert, 48, 254, 257, **257,** 259
De Palma, Brian, 59, 108–111, 141, 288, 302
de Salvo, Anne, **247**
de Saussure, Ferdinand, 190
Deacon, Richard, 73, 92
Dead Bang (1989), 23, 140
Dead Heat on a Merry-Go-Round (1966), 117, 122, **162**
Dead Ringer (1964), 59
Death
 grief reactions to death of celebrity, 261
 narcissism and, 245–250
Death instinct, 285
Death Wish (1974), 118, 259
Death Wish II (1982), 114, 119

Deconstructing Harry (1997), 126–127, 159, **162,** 248, 250
The Deer Hunter (1978), 11, 137
Dekker, Albert, 95, 195
Demedicalization of psychiatry in films, 20, 27, 37, 44, 76, 152
Demme, Jonathan, 141
The Demon Seed (1977), 161
Denial, 245
Derrida, Jacques, 190
Desperate Hours (1990), 296
The Detective (1968), 23
Dewhurst, Colleen, 119, 155
Diary of a Mad Housewife (1970), 14, 16, 111–112, 120
DiCaprio, Leonardo, 273
Dickinson, Angie, 18, 102, 108
The Difficulty of Difference, 200
DiPiero, Thomas, 200
Dirty Harry (1971), 118
Dishonored Lady (1947), **163**
Displacement, 5, 31, 189, 217–218, 306
Disputed Passage (1939), 44
Dissociative identity disorder. *See* Multiple personality disorder
Dive Bomber (1941), 215
Dmytryk, Edward, 72
Doane, Mary Ann, 156, 195
Doctor-patient relationship, 177–180. *See also* Countertransference issues; Transference reactions
Doherty, Tom, 290
Don Juan DeMarco (1995), 141
Donner, Clive, 20
Donner, Richard, 137
Doppelgänger effect, 245–246, 280
Douglas, Gordon, 66
Douglas, Kirk, 200
Douglas, Michael, 159, 305, 306, 312
Dourif, Brad, 135
Dow, Peggy, 22
Down and Out in Beverly Hills (1986), 127–128, 132, 313

Downey, Robert, 121
Dr. Dippy's Sanitarium (1906), 35–37
*Dr. Strangelove, or How I Learned to
    Stop Worrying and Love the Bomb*
    (1964), 115
Dracula (1931), 23
Dragoti, Stan, 20, 137
Drake, Charles, 22
Dream analysis, 197, 221–222
The Dream of a Rarebit Fiend (1906),
    37
The Dream Team (1989), 140
Dreams, 8–9, 31, 55, 83, 90, 99, 165,
    179
Dressed to Kill (1980), 19, 107–111,
    141, 179, 288, 302
Dreyfuss, Richard, 83, 141
Drury, James, 85
Duck Soup (1933), 126
"The Duellists" (Conrad), 284
Duet for One (1986), **162**
Duggan, Andrew, 25, 86
Duke, Patty, 104
Dullea, Keir, 70, 86
Dunne, Philip, 21, 90, 153
Durning, Charles, 18
Duvall, Robert, 102
Duvall, Shelley, 223, **224,** 225
Dzundza, George, 305

Eastwood, Clint, 253
Easy Rider (1969), 118, 119
Ebert, Roger, 222
Eberwein, Robert, 197
Eckert, Charles, 5, 191, 217
Eco, Umberto, 206
ECT (electroconvulsive therapy), 26,
    27, 32–33, 62, 79–81, 103,
    113–114, 134, 177
Edelman, Herb, 32
Edwards, Blake, 91, 104, 137, 140, 157,
    298
Edwards, James, 30

Edwards, Vince, 313
Ego splitting, 285
8½ (1963), 234–235, 238, 239, 241,
    248
Electroconvulsive therapy (ECT), 26,
    27, 32–33, 62, 79–81, 103,
    113–114, 134, 177
Eliot, T. S., 120
Ellenberger, Henri, 114
Elvira Madigan (1967), 32
Emasculation, 168
End of the Road (1970), 17, 136–137
The Entity (1983), 23
Equus (1977), 136, 141
Eraserhead (1978), 206
Erikson, Erik, 115
Erotic thriller films, 159
The Escaped Lunatic (1904), 35, 36
E.T. (1982), 268
Ethical issues, 19, 127, 140, 159,
    168–169, 177
European "art films," 77
European film theorists, 190–191
The Evening Star (1996), **162**
Everybody's Welcome, 213
Evil psychotherapists, 54–56, 91–92,
    116, 140, 141
"Evil twins," 59–60
The Exorcist (1973), 278, 279, 287
Exorcist II: The Heretic (1977), 24,
    137
Expert psychiatric witnesses, 173

Fail-Safe (1964), 115
Fairbanks, Douglas, 37, **38**
Faithful (1996), 133
Falk, Peter, 88–90
Fantasy films, 23
Farrow, John, 40
Farrow, Mia, 126, 249, 262, **264,** 267,
    271
Fassbinder, Rainer Werner, 200
Fatal Attraction (1987), 297, 304, 306

Fear Strikes Out (1957), 16, 26, 27, 33,
    79–81, **80,** 83, 84, 113
Fearless (1993), 141
Fears, universal, 281
Federal funding for mental health, 103,
    183
Feld, Fritz, 18, **20,** 49, 122
Fellini, Federico, 228, 234, 248
Felman, Shoshana, 209
Female psychotherapists in films, 21,
    43, 53–54, 57, 71, 90–91,
        112–113, 116–117, 119, 137, 138,
        141, 143, 147–169
    audience discomfort with, 152
    being "cured" by patient, 147, 151,
        156
    countertransference love and,
        148–164, **162**
    female patients and, 164–165
    murderous, 159
    as rationalist foil, 147
    as sex object, 148
    understanding stereotype of,
        165–169
"Feminine mystique," 13
Feminine passivity, 168
Feminist film criticism, 195, 210,
    213–214
La Femme Nikita (1990), 296
Ferenczi, Sàndor, 144
Ferrer, José, 21, 26, 67, 68, 72
Ferrer, Mel, 116
Fetishism, 294–295, 300
Feuer, Jane, 197
Ficelle role of film psychiatrist, 7, 11,
    14, 15
Field, Sally, 104
The Fifth Floor (1980), 26
Figgis, Mike, 17, 20
Film Criticism, 198
Film genres, 21–27
Film noir, 56–59, 75, 296
Film theorists, 190–191

A Fine Madness (1966), 118–120, 155,
    162
Fiorentino, Linda, 159
The First Wives' Club (1996), 159, **162**
Firth, Peter, 136
Fish, Stanley, 14
Fitzgerald, F. Scott, 92, 94
Five Easy Pieces (1970), 118
The Flame Within (1935), **162**
*Flashbacks in Film: Memory and
    History* (Turim), 192
Fleischer, Richard, 122
Fleming, Rhonda, 53, 85, 149
Fleming, Victor, 19, 37
Fletcher, Louise, 24, 134, **134**
Flicker, Theodore J., 121
Flynn, Errol, 214–215
Fonda, Henry, 48, 96, 123
Fonda, Jane, 7, 18, 25, 138, 164
Fontaine, Joan, 14, 91–93
For Whom the Bell Tolls (1943), 213
Forbes, Bryan, 137, 138
Forbidden Planet (1956), 279
Ford, Harrison, 301, 304
Ford, John, 86, 217
Foreman, Carl, 30
Forman, Milos, 18, 114, 133, 135
Forster, Robert, 97
Fortier, Robert, 223, **229**
Fosse, Bob, 233, 234, 236, 237,
    239–241, 244, 246, 247, 259
Foster, Jodie, **142,** 146
Fourteen Hours (1951), 66
Frances (1982), 26, 27, 171, 173, 177
Francis, Anne, 85
Francis, Robert, 72
Frank, Melvin, 150
Frankenstein (1931), 95
Franklin, Sidney, 41
Franz, Dennis, 108, 110
Free Love (1930), 46–47, 77
Freeman, Howard, **64**
French film theorists, 190–191

Freud (1962), 25, 64, 83, 97–101, **98, 100,** 104, 107, **163**
Freud, Anna, 99
Freud, Sigmund, 5, 9, 13, 21, 28, 38, 61, 76, 83, 126, 136, 137, 139, 151, 166, 168, 189, 191, 202–203, 222, 232, 281, 294–295
Friedkin, William, 159
From Beyond (1986), 157, **162**
The Front Page (1931, 1940, and 1974), 11, 22, 36, 39–40, 44, 46, 175
Fuller, Samuel, 113
Funding for mental health, 103, 183
Furie, Sidney J., 23
Fussell, Paul, 300
Futuristic films, 282. *See also* Science fiction films

Gach, John, 38
Gangster films, 217
Garland, Judy, 113
Garner, James, 102
Gates, Larry, 73, 78
Gavin, John, 109
The Gay Intruders (1948), 22, 63
Gazzara, Ben, 78–79
Geer, Will, 121
Geffner, Deborah, 233
Gender confusion, 302–303
Gender differences
    in sexual involvement between therapist and patient, 161, **162**
    in successful treatment of patient by opposite-sex therapist, 161, **163**
Gender prejudices, 167
Gender studies, 200
Gender Trouble, 200
Genn, Leo, 26, 61, **62,** 69, 79, 82
Gentlemen's Agreement (1947), 60
Gere, Richard, 159–160, 200
Ghost (1990), 306
Ghostbusters (1984), 301

Ghostbusters II (1989), 301
G.I. Jane, 296, 305
Gibson, Margaret Brenman, 69
Gibson, Mel, 141
Gibson, William, 69, 104
Gigi (1958), 69
Gilman, Charlotte Perkins, 120
Gingold, Hermione, 116
Girl of the Night (1960), 25, 85, **163**
Gish, Lillian, 70
Givens, Robin, 304
The Glass Menagerie, 6
Glen or Glenda? (1953), 51, 65–66
Godard, Jean-Luc, 119, 190
Gold, Jack, 137
Golden age of American cinema, 41
Golden Age of psychiatry in films (1957–1963), 3, 12, 16, 27, 34, 63, 75–106
    canonization, 84–101
    first transitional period, 78–84
    migration of a genre, 103–106
    second transitional period, 101–103
Golden Boy (1939), 119
Goldsmith, Jerry, 283
Golino, Valeria, 158–159
Gone With the Wind (1939), 37
Good Will Hunting (1997), 141, 144, **145,** 161, 179–182
Goodman, John, 297, 306
"Goodness of fit" concept, 33
Gordon, Keith, 109
Gordon, Michael, 152
Gordon, Ruth, 135
Gordon, Steve, 105
Gorman, Cliff, 244
The Graduate (1967), 115, 122
Grahame, Gloria, 69–70
Grant, Lawrence, 49
Greek mythology, 15, 240
Green, Guy, 85
Greenberg, Harvey, 12, 97, 205, 207, 210, 248, 283

Greenstreet, Sidney, 217
Griffith, D. W., 190
Griffith, Melanie, 300–301
Grimwood, Herbert, 19, 37, **38**
Grosse Pointe Blank (1997), 143
Groundhog Day (1993), 23, 141
The Group (1966), 118
Guillerman, John, 115
Guinness, Alec, 139

Hack, Shelley, 255
Haddon, Dayle, 157
Hairspray (1988), 140
Hall, Jon, 8
Halloween (1978), 24, 277
Halloween IV (1988), 200
Hamilton, Linda, 299, 304
Hands Across the Table (1935), 47
Hannah, Daryl, 296
Hannah and Her Sisters (1986),
    125–126, 249
Hansen, Miriam, 198
Hard Core: Power, Pleasure, and the
    "Frenzy of the Visible" (Williams),
    200
Harold and Maude (1971), 135
Harris, Robert H., 117
Harrold, Kathryn, 138
Hart, Moss, 8, 11
Harvey (1950), 22, 67
Harvey, Anthony, 137, 155
Harvey Middleman, Fireman (1965),
    116–117
Haskell, Molly, 12–14
Hassett, Marilyn, 120
Hawks, Howard, 18, 39, 47, 49, 118
Hays Office. *See* Breen Office
Heald, Anthony, 141
Heart of Darkness, 284
Heath, Stephen, 196, 216
Heche, Anne, 163–164
Hecht, Ben, 39
Heflin, Van, 5

Heller, Joseph, 120
Henderson, Brian, 217
Henley, Hobart, 46
Henn, Carrie, 289, 290
Henreid, Paul, 44, 51, 59, 87, 118, 208
Hepburn, Katharine, 14, **20,** 49, 95,
    122, 156
The Hero and the Terror (1988), **162**
Heroes, 251–252
    celebrity and, 251–253
    changing criteria for, 252–253
    Christ figures, 269
    in left- and right-cycle films,
        118–119
    narcissism and, 252
    outlaw vs. official, 4, 118, 219
    societal creation of, 252
Hershey, Barbara, 23, 126
Hey Hey in the Hay Loft, 238
Hi, Mom! (1970), 110
Higgins, Michael, 140
High Anxiety (1977), 22
High Noon (1952), 283
High Wall (1947), 23, 59, **162**
Hill, Arthur, 117
Hill, Lister, 103
Hill, Walter, 298
Hiller, Arthur, 7, 17
Hirsch, Judd, 18, **19,** 31–32, 145, 178,
    182
His Girl Friday (1940), 13, 39, 40, 47
Hitchcock, Alfred, 17, 19, 39, 53, 54,
    85, 90, 95–97, 107–111, 141, 148,
    195, 199, 211, 214, 288, 302
Hoberman, J., 274
Hoffman, Dustin, 48, 146, 303
Hofsiss, Jack, 138
Holbrook, Hal, 118
Holden, Stephen, 127
Holden, William, 31, 200
Hollow Triumph (1948), 59
Holm, Ian, 287
Holmes, Oliver Wendell, Sr., 36

Holmes, Taylor, 56
Holofcener, Nicole, 163
Home Before Dark (1958), 84–85, 105, **163**
Home of the Brave (1949), 26, 30, 61, 65, 72, 77, 88, 89, 201
Homoeroticism in buddy films, 299, 305
Homosexuality, 26, 51, 95, 132, 152, 200
Hooks, David, 7
Hooper, Tobe, 278
Hope, Bob, 92
Hopkins, Anthony, 141, **142**
Horror films, 23–24, 147, 200, 277–291, 310–311
Horton, Edward Everett, 39
The Hospital (1971), 7, 26
Hot Shots (1991), 158, **162**
House of Cards (1969), 115
House of Games (1987), 140, 163
Houseman, John, 68, 172
Howard, Ron, 268
Howard, Sidney, 46
Howe, Irving, 262, 272
The Howling (1981), 23
Hudson, Rock, 21, 92, 117, 152
Humanization of psychiatrists in films, 71, 82, 93
Humoresque (1946), 119
Hunk (1987), 157, **162**
Hunt, Helen, 143–144
Hupfeld, Herman, 213
Hurd, Gale Ann, 289, 295
Hurt, John, 284, **286**
Husbands and Wives (1992), 126, **162,** 249
Huss, Roy, 112
Huston, John, 25, 64–65, 97–101, 105, 107, 139
Hutton, Timothy, **19,** 31, 145, 178
Hypnosis, 6, 28, 29, 37, 99, 150

I, the Jury (1953 and 1982), 19, 23, 66–67, 92, 147
I Love You, Alice B. Toklas (1968), 313
I Never Promised You a Rose Garden (1977), 17, 103, 137, **138,** 164
I Was a Teenage Werewolf (1957), 66, 72
Ibsen, Henrik, 6, 9
Idealization of psychiatrists in films, 76, 178, 310
Idealizing transference, 260, 272
"Ideology and Ideological State Apparatuses (Notes Towards an Investigation)" (Althusser), 197
Ideology of films, 5–7
"If It's So Schmaltzy, Why Am I Weeping?" (Greenberg), 205
I'm Dancing as Fast as I Can (1982), 138, 165
Image of psychiatry, 114–115
    accuracy of film portrayals, 173–176
    funding for psychiatric research and education, 103, 183
    influence of film portrayals on, 172–173, 182–185
    patterns of referral to female analysts, 184
    prejudicial attitudes about psychotherapists, 183–184
    split view of public at large, 184–185
    trends in recruitment of medical students into specialty, 182–183
The Imaginary Signifier (Metz), 193
Imitation of Life (1959), 201
Impotence, 129
Impulse control problems, 144
In Person (1935), 47
In the Realm of Pleasure: von Sternberg, Dietrich, and the Masochistic Aesthetic (Studlar), 199
Ineffectual psychiatrists in films, 11–12, 16, 66, 116, 141

Infantile development, 284–287
Infantile fantasies, 288, 291, 294
Infantile sexuality, 100
"Inflated genre" films, 77
Inside Daisy Clover (1966), 113, 118
Insulin injection, 26, 171
Interiors (1978), 16, 244
Intermezzo (1939), 13
The Interns (1962), 26
Introjective-projective mechanisms,
    277–278, 285–287
Invaders from Mars (1953 and 1986),
    278–279
Invasion of the Body Snatchers (1956
    and 1978), 23, 72–74, 78,
    278–279, 287
Ireland, John, 154
It's My Turn (1980), 131, 175–176

Jackson, Anne, 120
Jackson, Glenda, 140
Jackson, Samuel L., 146
Jacobs, Diane, 238, 243
Jade (1995), 159
Jagged Edge (1985), 79
James, Henry, 7
James, William, 251
Jaques, Elliot, 243, 244
Jargon, 175
Jewison, Norman, 16, 102, 138
Jillian, Ann, 59
Johnny Belinda (1948), 28, 157, 211
Johnny Guitar (1954), 296
Johnny Handsome (1990), 298
Johns, Glynis, 25, 90
Johnson, Don, 140, 159, 218
Johnson, Nunnally, 28, 81, 82
Johnson, Van, 72
Jones, Amelia, 304, 305
Jones, Ernest, 208
Jones, James Earl, 17, 136
Jones, Jennifer, 17, 92
Juliet of the Spirits (1965), 228

Kael, Pauline, 222, 234
Kaplan, Donald, 206
Kaplan, E. Ann, 201
Karloff, Boris, 63
Kasdan, Lawrence, 143
Kaufman, Charles, 98
Kaufman, Philip, 23, 278
Kaufman, Sue, 111
Kawin, Bruce, 197
Kay, Roger, 90
Kaye, Danny, 150, 151, 155, 313
Kazan, Elia, 16, 76, 85
Keaton, Diane, 125, 126, 159
Keener, Catherine, 164
Keith, Ian, 56
Kelland, Clarence Budington, 49
Kellaway, Cecil, 67
The Kennel Murder Case (1933), 214
Kernberg, Otto, 235–237, 242–243,
    255, 259
Kerr, John, 69–70
Kershner, Irvin, 118, 155
Kesey, Ken, 119, 313
Khouri, Callie, 166
Kidd, Micheal, 140
Kinder, Marsha, 197
King, Henry, 19, 92
The King of Comedy (1983), 253–262,
    257, 266, 267, 272, 274
King of Hearts (1966), 86
King of New York (1990), 296
Kinsey, Alfred, 25
Kirk, G. S., 15
Kismet (1955), 69
Kitty Foyle (1940), 13, 14
Klang, 224
Klein, Melanie, 277–281, 284–285,
    287–291, 295
Klemperer, Werner, 96
Klugman, Jack, 104
Klute (1971), 7
Knee, Adam, 199
Knight, Shirley, 118

Knock on Wood (1954), 21, 66, 150–153, 155, 156, **162**
Kohut, Heinz, 235, 240, 254, 260, 272
Kopple, Barbara, 248
Koster, Henry, 22, 67
Kotch (1971), 137
Kotto, Yaphet, 283
Kramer, Stanley, 26, 30, 72, 73, 77
Kramm, Joseph, 67
Kristeva, Julia, 190
Kristofferson, Kris, 129
Krutnik, Frank, 200
Kübler-Ross, Elisabeth, 245
Kubrick, Stanley, 115, 281
Kulish, Nancy, 295
Kuriansky, Judith, 169

La Cava, Gregory, 42
"La politique d'auteur," 213
Lacan, Jacques, 190–197, 201
    concept of oedipal conflict, 193–194
    feminist/Lacanian film criticism, 195, 210
    Lacanian reading of *Casablanca*, 209–210
    revision of Freud's theories by, 192–194
Ladd, Alan, 4
Lady in a Jam (1942), **163**
Lady in the Dark (1944), 7–15, **10**, 17, 21, 33, 34, 47, 53, 55, 63, 77, 112
Lahr, John, 247, 274–275
Lake, Veronica, 239
Landau, Martin, 249
Landon, Michael, 66
Lang, Fritz, 57
Lange, Hope, 90, 153–154, **155**
Lange, Jessica, 171, 236
Langella, Frank, 111
Lasch, Christopher, 233, 253, 259, 266
The Last Embrace (1979), 161
Last Rites (1988), 296
Laugh-In, 122

Leather, Derrick, 283
Leaving Las Vegas (1995), 17
LeBeau, Madeleine, 212
Left- and right-cycle films, 118–119
Lehman, Ernest, 137
Lehman, Peter, 200
Leigh, Janet, 91, 108, 110, 117, 156, 161, 196
Leisen, Mitchell, 7, 47
Lemmon, Jack, 104–105, 137
Lennon, John, 261
Lenny (1974), 234, 244
Leno, Jay, 258
LeRoy, Mervyn, 84
Les Miserables (1935), 43
Lesbianism, 132, 200, 312
Leslie, Bethel, 102
Let There Be Light (1946), 61, 63–65, 97, 99
Lethal Weapon (1987), 219
Lethal Weapon III (1991), 296
Let's Live a Little (1948), 55, **162**
Letterman, David, 258
Levant, Oscar, 70
Lévi-Strauss, Claude, 15, 165, 190, 197, 217
Levinson, Barry, 146
Lewin, Robert, 85
Lewis, Jerry, 32, 254, 258, 261
Lewis, Juliette, 126
L'Homme Qui Aimait les Femmes (1977), 157
License to Kill (1989), 296
Lilith (1964), 116, **162**
Lincoln, Abraham, 4
Lithgow, John, 141
Little Big Man (1970), 118
Litvak, Anatole, 18, 49
Lobotomy, 26, 27, 95, 119, 134, 135, 155
The Locket (1946), **163**
Logan's Run (1976), 282
The Lonely Guy (1984), 17

The Long Kiss Goodnight (1996), 296
Lord Love a Duck (1966), 117
Lorre, Peter, 91
The Lost Weekend (1945), 104, 105
Love at First Bite (1979), 20, 137, **162**
Lover Come Back (1961), 22, 92
Loves of a Psychiatrist, 25
Lovesick (1983), 19, 22, 92–94, 107,
    139, 139–140, **162,** 173, 177
Lubitsch, Ernst, 49
Lugosi, Bela, 40, 65
Lukas, Paul, 92
Lumet, Sidney, 115, 118, 136
Lust for Life (1956), 69

MacArthur, Charles, 39
MacCabe, Colin, 196, 210, 216
MacLaine, Shirley, 116
MacMurray, Fred, 72
Macnee, Patrick, 23
Madame X (1966), 12
Magical powers attributed to
    psychiatrists, 174–175
Magnificent Obsession (1935), 44
Maher, Joseph, 138
Making Love (1982), 51
*Making Meaning: Inference and
    Rhetoric in the Interpretation of
    Cinema* (Bordwell), 197, 198
Malden, Karl, 33
Male Subjectivity at the Margins
    (Silverman), 200
Mamet, David, 140
The Man Who Loved Women (1983),
    157, **162**
The Man Who Saw Tomorrow (1922), 6,
    37
The Manchurian Candidate (1962), 88,
    141
Manhattan (1979), 244
Manhattan Murder Mystery (1993),
    126
Manic relation to objects, 245

Mankiewicz, Joseph L., 95
Mann, Daniel, 102
Mann, Delbert, 92
Manoff, Dinah, 31
Mantegna, Joe, 273
Marat/Sade (1967), 27, 121
Margolin, Janet, 70, 92
Margulies, David, 110
The Mark (1961), 26, 85
Marked Woman (1937), 217
The Marriage of a Young Stockbroker
    (1971), 112–113, 120, 137, 167
Marshall, Sarah, 117
Martin, Dean, 102
Martin, Steve, 17
Masculinity in popular media, 200
Masculinized women, 289. *See also*
    Phallic women
M*A*S*H, 105, 152
Masochism, 157, 303
Mason, Marsha, 129
Masterson, Mary Stuart, 143
Mastroianni, Marcello, 235
Maté, Rudolph, 31, 59
Matt Lincoln, 105, 313
Matthau, Walter, 137
Mazursky, Paul, 127–133, 234, 268,
    310, 312–314
McCallum, David, 99
McCarey, Leo, 47
McCarthyist politics, 278–279
McCrea, Joel, 43–44, 238
McDowall, Roddy, 117
McGovern, Elizabeth, 22, 31, 32, 139,
    139, 177
McGuire, Dorothy, 28
McKinley, J. Edward, 85
The Medusa Touch (1978), 23, 137, 147
Melodramas, 4–5, 21, 22
Melosh, Barbara, 152
Memories, repressed traumatic, 29–31
The Men (1950), 72
Men in White (1934), 26

Menaker, Daniel, 199
Men's studies, 200
Mental Health and Mental Retardation
 Act, 103
Mental illness in films, 26
Mental institution films, 26–27, 35–37,
 61–63, 68, 95, 113–114, 133–135
Metz, Christian, 190, 191, 193, 197,
 198, 212, 311–312
Miami Vice, 218
Michaels, Lloyd, 198
Midler, Bette, 132
Midlife crisis, 242–245
Midnight Cowboy (1969), 299
Mildred Pierce (1945), 214
Miles, Vera, 96, 109
Milestone, Lewis, 39, 175
Milland, Ray, 8, 9
Miller, David, 102
Miller, J. P., 104
Minnelli, Liza, 254
Minnelli, Vincente, 10, 68–69
Miracle on 34th Street (1947), 23, 63
The Miracle Worker (1962 and 1979),
 104
Mirage (1965), 23, 117
Mirror-stage concept, 193
Mirror transference, 260
Misery (1990), 293, 296, 306
Mitchum, Robert
Modleski, Tania, 198–200
Moment to Moment (1966), 118
Monaco, James, 131
Monroe, Marilyn, 99, 101, 182
Montand, Yves, 10
Moonlighting, 218
Moore, Demi, 305, 306
Moore, Dudley, 19, 22, 105, 107, 137,
 139, **139**, 177
Moore, Mary Tyler, 18, 31, 32
Moore, Norma, **80**
Moore, Roger, 138
Moranis, Rick, 157

Morgan, Dennis, 213
Morgan, Frank, 41
Morning Glory (1933), 13
Morris, Chester, 31, 45, **46**
Mortensen, Viggo, 305
Moscow on the Hudson (1984), 268
Moses, Marian, 122
Moses and Monotheism (Freud), 202
Mother, phallic, 167–168, 288,
 294–296
Mother-child relationship, 166, 167
"Mother films," 22
*Movie Star, American Style or LSD,
 I Hate You* (1966), 118
Movie stars. *See* Celebrity
Mr. Deeds Goes to Town (1936), 6,
 49–50, 61, 67
Mr. Jones (1993), 20, 141, 159–161,
 162
Mrs. Dalloway, 120
Ms. 45 (1981), 296
Muhich, Donald F., 127–130, 132,
 313–314
Mulholland Falls (1996), 168
Mulligan, Robert, 16, 79, 113
Multiple personality disorder, 28–30,
 81–82, 104, 110, 143
Mulvey, Laura, 14, 148, 195, 199–200,
 211, 294, 299
Murder, My Sweet (1945), 63, 77
Murdoch, Iris, 120
Murphy, Michael, 131
Music in films
 Alien, 280–281
 Casablanca, 212–213
 Sea of Love, 297, 298
 2001: A Space Odyssey, 281
Musicals, 8, 14, 22, 47
Mutual analysis, 144
My Blue Heaven (1990), 157–158,
 162
My Favorite Wife (1940), 63
My Six Convicts (1952), 72

Mystery of the Wax Museum (1933), 214

Mystifying Movies: Fads and Fallacies in Contemporary Film Theory (Carroll), 197

Mythology
classical Greek, 15, 240
in films, 3–6, 15, 33–34, 114, 118, 122, 165–166
functions of, 15
of phallic mother, 294–295

Nabokov, Vladimir, 120
Nagel, Conrad, 46
The Naked Face (1984), 138
Napier, Alan, 154
Narcissism, 33, 233–275, 310
as arrest of normal development of self, 260
in autobiographical films, 233–250 (*See also* Autobiographical films)
celebrity and, 241, 251–275 (*See also* Celebrity)
death and, 245–250
midlife crisis and, 242–245
object relations and, 235–242
symptomatology of patients with, 235
transferences formed by patients with, 260
Narcosynthesis, 7, 8, 61, 64
Nathan, Vivian, 7
National Institute of Mental Health, 103, 183
Nazism, 88, 89
"Near-death experience," 246
The Net (1995), **162**
Neuwirth, Bebe, 127
New York, New York (1977), 257
New York Review of Books, 199
Nichols, Mike, 300

Nicholson, Jack, 18, 118, 133–135, **134,** 143, 146, 180
Night of the Living Dead (1968), 277, 279–280
Nightmare Alley (1947), 17, 56–58, **58,** 63, 66, 91–92, 147, 167
9½ Weeks (1986), 159
Niven, David, 83, **84**
Nolan, Lloyd, 85
Nolte, Nick, **158,** 159, 168
North by Northwest (1959), 97
Novak, Kim, 96
Now, Voyager (1942), 12, 17, 32, 51–53, **52,** 61, 71, 74, 77, 82, 86–88, 157, **163,** 182
Nyby, Christian, 279

Oakland, Simon, 17, 78, 85, 96–97, 109, 111, 122
Object relations, narcissistic, 235–242
Obsession (1976), 110
Obsessive-compulsive disorder, 143
O'Connell, Arthur, 78
O'Connell, Jack, 115
Odds Against Tomorrow (1959), 86
Odets, Clifford, 154
Oedipal conflict, 99–100, 167, 168
in *Casablanca*, 207–209
Lacan's concept of, 193–194
in *3 Women*, 226–227
Oh, God! Book II (1980), 18, 23
Oh, Men! Oh, Women! (1957), 47, 82–84, **84,** 92, **163**
O'Herlihy, Dan, 84–85, 90
The Old Maid (1939), 13
Olin, Lena, 19, 141, 159–161
The Omen (1976), 137
On a Clear Day You Can See Forever (1970), 10, **163**
One Flew Over the Cuckoo's Nest (1975), 18, 26, 27, 114, 119–120, 133–135, **134,** 152, 177, 309, 312–313

One Glorious Day (1922), 37
O'Neal, Patrick, 119
O'Neal, Ryan, 133
Oracular psychiatrists in films, 17, 31, 68, 109–111, 122
Ordinary People (1980), 17, 18, **19,** 31–32, 103, 105, 107, 132, 137, 140, 144–146, 173, 178, 179, 309, 312
O'Toole, Peter, **117**
Oudart, Jean-Pierre, 194
Outland (1981), 282, 283

Pacino, Al, 297, 301, 305
Pakula, Alan J., 7, 113, 282, 304
Palminteri, Chazz, 133, 168
Panama, Norman, 150
The Parallax View (1974), 282
Parenting deficiencies, 33
Parker, Alan, 140
Patients' reactions to film portrayals of psychiatry, 172–173, 176–182
Peck, Gregory, 18, 53–55, 102, 117, 149, **150,** 156
Peerce, Larry, 120
Penelope (1966), 117
Penley, Constance, 198
Penn, Arthur, 104
The Perfect Furlough (1958), 25, 66, 91, 156, **162**
Perkins, Anthony, 33, 78–81, **80,** 108
Perkins, Millie, 154
Perry, Eleanor, 111, 112
Perry, Frank, 86, 111, 112
Persecutory anxiety, 287–289
"Personal films," 86
Peters, Werner, 119
Petro, Patrice, 197
Phallic symbols, 230–232
Phallic women, 290, 293–307, 311
　　male anxiety related to, 306–307
　　new directions in portrayals of, 303–307

phallic mother, 167–168, 288, 294–296
psychoanalysis and gender confusion, 302–303
　in *Sea of Love,* 296–299
　without maternal qualities, 296
　in *Working Girl,* 299–302
Phantom of the Paradise (1974), 111
Pharmacotherapy, 27
Pickles, Vivian, 135
Pidgeon, Walter, 91, 279
Pillow Talk (1959), 92, 102, 115
Pink Flamingos (1972), 206, 303
Pinky (1947), 60
Pitt, Brad, 166
Plan 9 from Outer Space (1959), 65
Plastered in Paris (1928), 38
Plath, Sylvia, 120
Play It Again, Sam (1972), 218
Playhouse 90, 104
Pleasence, Donald, 24
Plimpton, George, 141
Plummer, Christopher, 113
Pnin (Nabokov), 120
Poitier, Sidney, 88–90, **89**
Polan, Dana, 197
Politics and politicians, 4, 252–253
Pollack, Sydney, 282
Porter, Edwin S., 37
Portnoy's Complaint (1972), 137
Possessed (1947), 6, 8, 53, 61, **163**
Poston, Tom, 92
Powell, William, 49
Power, Tyrone, 56, 57, **58**
Preminger, Otto, 21, 71, 78
The President's Analyst (1967), 121–122, 137
Presley, Elvis, 91, 153–154, **155,** 261
Pressman, Michael, 11
Pressure Point (1962), 26, 72, 88–90, **89,** 94, 101, 102, 104, 136
Presumed Innocent (1990), 304–305
Pretty Woman (1990), 306

Price, Vincent, 63
Primal Fear (1996), 141
The Prince of Tides (1991), 141, 158,
    158, 159, 161, **162**
Private Worlds (1935), 41–43, **45,**
    45–46, 54, 69, 81, 90, 161
Problem Child (1990), 141
Problems in films, 4, 12
Production Code, 24, 41, 43, 81, 154
Prostitution, 85, 127, 159, 268, 303
Pryor, Richard, 11
The Psychiatrist, 105
Psychiatrists in films, 3, 6, 15–21,
    309–310
    after the Golden Age, 107–146
    as alienists, 39–40
    attribution of magical powers to,
        174–175
    black, 88, 136–137, 143
    crime-and-detective films, 22–23
    devaluation of, 116–118, 121, 310
    eccentric, 18
    emotional, 18–19
    faceless, 11, 12, 16, 26, 122, 138
    female, 21, 43, 53–54, 57, 71,
        90–91, 112–113, 116–117,
        119, 137, 138, 141, 143,
        147–169
    ficelle role of, 7, 11, 14, 15
    films of Allen and Mazursky,
        123–133
    functions of, 309
    in the Golden Age (1957–1963),
        75–106
    humanization of, 71, 82, 93
    idealized, 76, 178, 310
    ideological function of, 6
    importance of being familiar with
        images of, 178–179
    ineffectual, 11–12, 16, 66, 116, 141
    as lone antihero, 121–122
    mental institution films, 26–27
    musicals and romantic comedies, 22

neutral attitude affected by, 10
oracular, 17, 31, 68, 109–111, 122
paired stereotypes of "good" versus
    "bad," 15–17, **16**
played by real analysts, 127–132,
    312–314
as plot expediter, 6–7, 116
as rationalist foil, 147
in the 1920s, 37–39
in the 1930s, 39–51, 77
in the 1940s, 51–65, 77
in the 1950s, 65–74, 77
in the 1960s, 114–123
in the 1970s, 133–137
in the 1980s, 137–141
in the 1990s, 141–146
science fiction, horror, and fantasy
    movies, 23–24
self-disclosure by, 144, 180–181
sexual, 19–21
sexual films, 24–25
as social agents, 17–18, 135–136
social problem films, 25–26
stereotypes of, 11, 18, 36, 310
on television, 104, 105
victimizing role of, 111–113, 120
viewed as archetypes, 174
as villains, 54–56, 91–92, 116, 140,
    141
Psychiatry in films, 27–34
    accuracy of portrayals of, 173–176
    ambivalence toward, 5, 36, 62,
        131–132, 146
    cathartic cure, 27–34, 52, 71, 95,
        141, 178
    continuity in images of, 3
    demedicalization of, 20, 27, 37, 44,
        76, 152
    film genres and, 21–27
    reactions of patients to, 172–173,
        176–182
    related to historical periods, 34
    trivialization of, 100–101

Psychiatry in literature, 119–120
Psycho (1960 and 1998), 17, 78, 85, 90,
    96–97, 107–111, 122–123,
    194–196, 201, 288, 302
Psychoanalysis, 5, 28–31, 38–39, 55, 58,
    62, 75, 76, 86, 115, 118, 120, 128,
    129, 191
Psychoanalytic film criticism, 189–203
    of *Alien* and horror/science fiction
        films, 277–291
    applied to issues of race and class,
        201
    boundaries of current trends in, 192
    Carroll's and Bordwell's attacks on
        "SLAB theory," 197–198
    of *Casablanca*, 205–219
    controversy about, 191
    current status in university studies,
        199
    defections from in early 1990s,
        198–199
    feminist/Lacanian theory, 195
    gender confusion and,
        302–303
    gender studies, 200
    influence of Lacan's theories on,
        192–194
    methodological problems in,
        202–203
    of narcissism, 233–275
        autobiographical films, 233–250
        celebrity, 251–275
    operation of suture within film,
        194–196
    of phallic women, 290, 293–307
    potential for pluralism in, 201–202
    semiotics, 194
    of *3 Women*, 221–232
Psychoanalytic humor, 124–126
Psychological thrillers, 21
Psychopharmacology, 143–144
The Purple Rose of Cairo (1985), 253,
    267–275, **269, 271**

Quine, Richard, 153
Quinlan, Kathleen, **138,** 164

Racial issues, 25–26, 30, 85, 88–89, 201
A Rage in Harlem (1991), 296, 304
Ragina's Secrets, 25
Raging Bull (1980), 257
Rains, Claude, 32, 51, **52,** 61, 82, 182
Raising Cain (1992), 110, 141
Rambo III (1988), 219
Rampling, Charlotte, 241
Randall, Tony, 83, 92
Rape, 130, 177
Ratings system for films, 24–25
Ray, Robert, 4, 15, 26, 73, 77, 83, 97,
    118, 189, 197, 215–217, 259
Reagan, Ronald, 66, 213, 253, 255
Rebecca (1940), 211
Recruitment of medical students into
    psychiatry, 182–183
Red River (1948), 118
Redford, Robert, 178
Reds (1981), 262
Reefer Madness (1936), 51
Reinhardt, Max, 98
Reinhardt, Wolfgang, 98
Reinking, Ann, 236
Reiser, Paul, 290
Remick, Lee, 137
Repressed traumatic memories, 29–31
Reunion in Vienna (1933), 41–42, 45,
    47, **163**
Revill, Clive, 119
Revolution (1968), 115
Reynolds, Burt, 18, 157
Richardson, Tony, 17
Rifkin, Ron, 126
Right- and left-cycle films, 118–119
Riskin, Robert, 49
Ritchie, Michael, 140
Ritter, John, 140
Rivette, Jacques, 190
Riviere, Joan, 200

Robards, Jason, Jr., 19, 92, 94
Roberts, Eric, 259
Robson, Mark, 30, 65
The Rocky Horror Picture Show (1975), 206, 303
Rodowick, D. N., 200
Rogers, Ginger, 8, **10,** 14, 22, 47–49, **48,** 83, **84,** 272
Rogers, Will, 37
Roheim, Geza, 295
Rohmer, Eric, 190
Role reversal, 147, 151, 156
Romantic comedies, 21, 22
Romero, George, 279
Rosmersholm, 9
Rosolato, Guy, 212
Ross, Herbert, 137
Rossellini, Roberto, 207
Roth, Philip, 137
Rowe, Bill, 283
Rowlands, Gena, 126
The Royal Family of Broadway (1930), 13
Rule, Janice, 222, 223
Rush, Barbara, 83
Russell, Ken, 16
Russell, Kurt, 280
Russell, Rosalind, 40, 156
Russianoff, Penelope, 131–132, 165, 312, 313
Russo, René, 141, 159
Russo, Vito, 95
Ryan, Robert, 61

Sadomasochism, 157
Safra, Jaqui, **247**
Sanders, Denis, 113
Sandrick, Mark, 22
The Santa Clause (1994), 22
Sarafian, Richard, 104
Sarah T.—Portrait of a Teenage Alcoholic, 105
Sarandon, Susan, 166

Sarris, Andrew, 205, 234
Sartre, Jean-Paul, 97–99
Sayles, John, 268
Scacchi, Greta, 304
The Scar (1948), 59
Scenes from a Mall (1991), 132
Scheider, Roy, 139, 233, 234, **238**
Schell, Maximilian, 19, 172
Schenck, Aubrey, 63
Schickel, Richard, 205
Schizoid (1980), **163**
Schizophrenia, 143
Schlesinger, John, 140
Schneider, Irving, 35
Science fiction films, 23–24, 147, 199, 277–291, 310–311
Scorsese, Martin, 129, 248, 253–259
Scott, George C., 7, 155–156
Scott, Ridley, 166, 277, 281–284, 287, 289, 305, 310
Screen, 191, 196–198, 216
The Sea Hawk (1940), 214
Sea of Love (1990), 294, 296–299, 305–307
The Searchers (1956), 217
Sears, Heather, 28
Seberg, Jean, 116, 118, 119, 155
Segal, George, 129
Segal, Hanna, 284–286, 288, 295
Seize the Day, 120
Sekely, Steve, 59
Self, Robert, 222–223
Self-absorption, 233
Self-censorship of films, 41. *See also* Production Code
Self-consciousness, 233–234
Self-disclosure by therapist, 144, 180–181
Sellers, Peter, 20, 71, 116, **117**
Selznick, David O., 54
Semiotics, 190–191, 194
Semi-Tough (1977), 128
The Sender (1982), 23, 138, 147

A Sensitive, Passionate Man, 105
The Serpent and the Rainbow (1988), 147
The Seven-Per-Cent Solution (1976), 137, **163**
The Seven Year Itch (1955), 66
The Seventh Veil (1945), 53
A Severed Head (Murdoch), 120
Sex and the Single Girl (1964), 21, 25, 116, 153, **153,** 155, 156, **162**
Sexual involvement between therapist and patient, 161, **162.** *See also* Countertransference issues
Sexuality, 24–25, 41
infantile, 100
Seymour, Jane, 59
Shadow on the Wall (1950), **162**
Shadows (1960), 86
Shaffer, Peter, 136
Shaid, Nick, **45**
Shane (1953), 215
Shaw, Anabel, 63
Shaw, George Bernard, 269
Shawn, Dick, 117, 152
She Wouldn't Say Yes (1946), **162**
Sheen, Charlie, 159
Sheridan, Ann, 213
Sherwood, Robert E., 41
Shields, Jim, 283
Shimkus, Joanna, 113
Shock (1946), 63, 65
Shock Corridor (1963), 26, 113
Shock Treatment (1964), 26, 92, 113–114, 116
Short Cuts (1993), 201
The Shrike (1955), 26–27, 67–68, 73, 78, **163**
Siegel, Don, 23, 73
The Silence of the Lambs (1991), 141, **142,** 146, 296, 303–304
Silent Night, Deadly Night (1984), 280
Silkwood (1983), 300
Silver, Ron, 23

Silverman, Kaja, 192, 200–201, 211
Simmons, Jean, 84–85
Simon, Simone, 21, 23
The Sin of Madelon Claudet (1931), 12
Sinatra, Frank, 88
Since You Went Away (1944), 12, 17, 53, 74, 75, **163**
Siodmak, Robert, 59
Sisters (1973), 59, 110
60 Minutes, 247
Skerritt, Tom, 280
Skin Deep (1989), 140–141
Sklar, Robert, 5–6, 41, 42, 49, 50
"SLAB theory," 198
Slapstick comedy, 36–37
Sleeper (1973), 282
The Sleeping Tiger (1954), 71
Sleeping with the Enemy (1991), 296, 304
Smith, Kent, 21
Smith, Lane, 17, 171
The Snake Pit, 18, 26, 27, 60–63, **62, 64,** 67, 71, 79, 82, 92, 95, 102, 157, **163**
Snodgrass, Carrie, 14, 111, 112
So Young, So Bad (1950), **163**
Social criticism, 130
Social problem films, 25–26, 39, 60, 75, 104–105, 115
Some Kind of Hero (1982), 11
Some Like It Hot (1959), 302
Something Wild (1987), 300
Sontag, Susan, 262, 265
Sound in films, 281, 283
Spacek, Sissy, 223, **224,** 225, **229**
Spellbound (1945), 12, 19, 21, 39, 53–55, 57, 59, 61, 63, 74, 81, 94, 96, 139, 147–149, **150,** 156, 157, **162,** 309
Sphere (1998), 146, **162**
Spielberg, Steven, 268
Spillane, Micky, 147
The Spiral Staircase (1946), 28, 211

Splash (1984), 268
Splendor in the Grass (1961 and 1981), 16, 25, 76, 85, 104, 105, **163**
Spock, Benjamin, 75
St. Ives (1975), 19, 171–172
Stack, Robert, 103
Stanton, Harry Dean, 283
Star 80 (1983), 259–260
Star Trek, 198
Star Wars (1977), 215, 219, 282
Stardust Memories (1980), 124, 234–235, 238–244, **240,** 246–247, **247,** 267, 270, 273
Starman (1984), 268
Starting Over (1979), 18, 137
Steiger, Rod, 85, 138
Steiner, Max, 212, 213
Stella Dallas (1937), 13, 22, 32
The Stepfather (1987), **163**
The Stepford Wives (1975), 137
Stevens, George, 4
Stevens, Inger, 115
Stevens, Mark, 62
Stewart, James, 49, 67, 78–79, 96, 199, 200
Stewart, Patrick, 141
Still of the Night (1982), 23, 139
Stoller, R., 295
Stone, George E., 39
Stone, Sharon, 146, 296, 305–306
The Story of Esther Costello (1957), 28
The Story of Louis Pasteur (1936), 44
Stowe, Madeleine, 21, 141, 159, **160**
Stradner, Rose, **46**
Strait Jacket (1964), 116
Stranger-in-a-strange-land theme, 268
Strasberg, Susan, 70, 92
Streisand, Barbra, 10, 141, 158, **158,** 159
Stromboli (1950), 207
Studies of Hysteria (Freud), 28
Studlar, Gaylyn, 199
Sturges, Preston, 238

Suburbia Confidential, 25
Sudden Impact (1983), 296
Suddenly, Last Summer (1959), 95, 96, **163,** 194–195
Suicide, 7, 31, 135
Sullivan, Barry, 8, 10, **10, 11**
Sullivan's Travels (1941), 238–239
Survivor guilt, 31, 151
Suture within film, 194–196
Swift, David, 85
Switch (1991), 298
Sybil, 104

Take the Money and Run (1969), 244, 262
A Tale of Two Cities (1935), 43
Talking cure, 27–28, 55–56
Taubin, Amy, 249
Taxi Driver (1976), 255, 258–259
Taylor, Elizabeth, 95, 194–195
Taylor, Robert, 59
Tea and Sympathy (1956), 69
Telephone conversations in films, 6
Television programs, 22, 59, 104, 105, 169, 313
10 (1980), 137
Tender Is the Night (1962), 19, 92, 94–95, 101, **162, 163**
The Terminator (1984), 23, 289
Terminator II (1991), 296, 299, 304
Testimony by expert psychiatric witnesses, 173
The Texas Chainsaw Massacre (1974), 200, 277
That Old Feeling (1997), **162**
That Touch of Mink (1962), 92, 102
That Uncertain Feeling (1941), 63
Thelma and Louise (1991), 166, 296, 304, 305
Them! (1954), 66
"Thematic paradigm," 5
They Might Be Giants (1971), 137, 155–157, **162**

The Thing (1951 and 1982), 279, 280, 287
Third of a Man (1962), 72, 85
Thompson, J. Lee, 116, 171
Thomson, David, 249
Three Days of the Condor (1975), 282
The Three Faces of Eve (1957), 17, 26, 28–30, 33, 81–83, **82,** 104, **163,** 182
Three Nuts in Search of a Bolt (1964), 25
Three on a Couch (1966), 117, 161
Three Warriors, 313
3 Women (1977), 221–232, **224, 229,** 311
The Thrill of It All (1963), 16, 102
Thunderbolt and Lightfoot (1974), 299
Tierney, Gene, 21
Tilly, Meg, 18, 138, 164–165
Tin Cup (1996), 141, 159, **162**
Titanic (1997), 289
Titicut Follies (1967), 27, 121
To Each His Own (1946), 13
Tobin, Genevieve, 46
Together Again (1944), 13
Tootsie (1982), 302, 303
Top Gun (1986), 177, 219
Torn, Rip, 19
Total Recall (1990), 296, 300
Totter, Audrey, 59
Tourneur, Jacques, 21, 23
Transference reactions, 28, 57, 108, 138, 150, 153, 154, 157, 171, 174–180
    as fascination with fatality of human condition, 261
    formed by narcissistic patients, 260
    idealizing transference, 260, 272
    mirror transference, 260
    reality vs., 271–272
Transvestism, 65, 295
Traumatic memories, repressed, 29–31
Travers, Henry, 42

The Treatment (Menaker), 199
Trippelhorn, Jeanne, 159
Trivialization of psychiatry in films, 100–101
Truffaut, François, 157, 190
Trump, Donald, 274
Truro, Victor, 124
Turim, Maureen, 192
Turman, Lawrence, 112, 137
Turner, Kathleen, 304
Turow, Scott, 305
12 Monkeys (1995), 21, 141, 159, **160, 162**
The Twisted Sex, 25
2001: A Space Odyssey (1968), 281, 282

Un Chien andalou (1928), 55
Under the Volcano (1984), 105
An Unmarried Woman (1978), 103, 131–132, 137, 165, 312

V. I. Warshawski (1991), 304
Vampire's Kiss (1989), 164
Van Dyke, W. S., 49
van Sant, Gus, 97
Van Sloan, Edward, 23
Vanlint, Derek, 284
Veidt, Conrad, 4, 208
Verdon, Gwen, 234
Vereen, Ben, 246
Vertigo (1958), 96, 199–200
A Very Special Favor (1965), 21, 25, 117, 152, 156, **162**
Victor/Victoria (1982), 302
Vidor, Charles, 17, 30
Vinson, Helen, 43
"Visual Pleasure and Narrative Cinema" (Mulvey), 195, 199, 294
Voice-overs, 211
von Eltz, Theodore, **45**
von Sternberg, Josef, 195, 199
von Sydow, Max, 249

Voyage to the Bottom of the Sea (1961), 91

Voyeurism in cinematic experience, 311–312

Walken, Christopher, 11, 137
Walker, Helen, 56, **58**
Walking and Talking (1996), 163–164
Walking Tall (1973), 118
Wallace, Irving, 25
Wallis, Hal, 213
Walsh, Andrea, 13, 14
Wanger, Walter, 42
War films, 4, 30
Washington, George, 4
Waters, John, 140
Wayne, David, 81
Wayne, John, 48, 118, 182
Weaver, Sigourney, 281, 289, 290, 300–302
Weill, Claudia, 131, 175
Weld, Tuesday, 154
Wengraf, John, 83
West, Adam, 113
Westerns, 21
What a Way to Go! (1964), 116
What About Bob? (1991), 141
What's New, Pussycat? (1965), 20, 71, 116, **117, 162**
When the Clouds Roll By (1919), 19, 36–38, **38**
Whirlpool (1950), 21, 71
Whispers in the Dark (1992), 163
Whitaker, Forest, 304
Whitemore, Don, 205
Whitman, Stuart, 85
Who's Been Sleeping in My Bed? (1963), 25, 102
Whose Life Is It, Anyway? (1981), 83
Widmark, Richard, 69–70, 79, 83
Wiest, Dianne, 138, 165
The Wild Duck (Ibsen), 6

Wild in the Country (1961), 90–91, 153–155, **155, 162**
Wild Man Blues (1998), 248–249
Wilder, Billy, 36, 104
Williams, Adam, 16, 79, **80**
Williams, Linda, 200
Williams, Robin, 144, 146, 179–181
Williams, Tennessee, 6, 95
Williamson, Nicol, 138
Willie and Phil (1980), 127, 313
Willis, Austin, 122, 123
Willis, Bruce, 159, **160**
Wilson, Dooley, 210
Winner, Michael, 114, 258
Winters, Shelley, 25
Wise, Robert, 86
The Wizard of Oz (1939), 12, 37, 90
"Womanliness as Masquerade" (Riviere), 200
Women, masculinized, 289. *See also* Phallic women
Women's films, 12, 53, 85, 156–157
  "sacrifice" category of, 12–13, 22
  television melodramas, 22
  in which achievement and femininity are compatible, 13
Women's movement, 157
Women's roles, 12–14, 135, 147–148
Women's studies, 200
Wood, Edward D., Jr., 65
Wood, G., 136
Wood, Michael, 3–5, 12, 15, 48, 215
Wood, Natalie, 25, 76, 85, 113, 116, 117, 128, 153, **153,** 155, 156
Wood, Robin, 24, 32, 41, 96, 197, 299
Woodward, Joanne, 28–29, 81, **82,** 104, 137, 155–156
Woolf, Virginia, 120
Working Girl (1988), 294, 299–302, 307
Wouk, Herman, 72
The Wrong Man (1956), 96
Wyman, Jane, 28

Wynyard, Diana, 41

Yankee Doodle Dandy (1942),
    214
"The Yellow Wallpaper" (Gilman),
    120
York, Susannah, 25, **98,** 99
Young Dr. Freud (1977), 98
Young Mr. Lincoln (1939),
    86

Zaentz, Saul, 312
Zelig (1983), 157, **162, 163,** 253,
    262–267, **263, 264,** 270, 272, 274
Zetterling, Mai, 150, 151, 155, 156
Zieff, Howard, 140
Zimbalist, Efrem, Jr., 85
Zimmerman, Paul D., 254, 258, 259
Zizek, Slavoj, 201
Zotz! (1962), 23, 92
Zucco, George, 49

Film Index

*Page numbers printed in **boldface** type refer to tables or plates.*

Adam's Rib (1949), 13

Adventures of Robin Hood (1938), 214

After the Thin Man (1936), 49

Agnes of God (1985), 18, 138–139,
    164–165

Alex in Wonderland (1971), 234

Alien (1979), 277, 280–291, **285, 286,**
    295–296, 301

Alien: Resurrection (1997), 290, 302

Aliens (1986), 289–290, 295, 302

All That Jazz (1979), 233–238, **237,**
    238, 241, 242, 244–247

Amadeus (1984), 135

The Amazing Dr. Clitterhouse (1938),
    49

American Graffiti (1973), 210

Anatomy of a Murder (1959), 78–79

Angel Heart (1987), 140

Angels with Dirty Faces (1938), 214,
    215

Annie Hall (1977), 124, 125, 244, 246,
    273

Another Woman (1988), 126

Ants in Your Pants of 1939, 239

Antz (1998), 133

Arthur (1981), 105

As Good as It Gets (1997), 143,
    180–181

The Awful Truth (1937), 47

The Bachelor and the Bobby Soxer
    (1947), **163**

Back Street (1941), 13

The Bad and the Beautiful (1952), 69

Bad Dreams (1988), **162**

Bananas (1971), 244

The Band Wagon (1953), 69

The Barretts of Wimpole Street (1934),
    43

Basic Instinct (1992), 159, **162,**
    305–306

Batman Returns (1992), 296

Bedlam (1946), 63

Bedroom Eyes (1986), 157, **162**

Bedtime for Bonzo (1951), 66

The Bell Jar (1979), 120

Benny and Joon (1993), 143

The Best Years of Our Lives (1946), 5

Beverly Hills Cop (1984), 219

Beverly Hills Cop II (1987), 219

Bewitched (1945), **163**

Beyond Therapy (1987), 140, **162**

The Big Fix (1978), 128

A Bill of Divorcement (1932 and 1940),
    40–41

Blade Runner (1982), 201, 282–284,
    296, 300

Blind Alley (1939), 17, 23, 30–31,
    44–46, **46,** 51, 52, 55, 59, 71, 99,
    105, 122, 125

Blindfold (1966), 21, 23, 117

Bliss (1997), **162**

Blow Out (1981), 110

Blue Sky (1994), 17

Bluebeard's Eighth Wife (1938), 49

Blume in Love (1973), 127, 129–131,
    313, 314

Bob and Carol and Ted and Alice
    (1969), 127–130, 313, 314

Body Double (1984), 110

Bonnie and Clyde (1967), 119
Boomerang (1925), 37–38
The Boston Strangler (1968), 23,
    122–123
Breathless (1961), 119
Brigadoon (1954), 69
Bringing Up Baby (1938), 18, **20,** 49,
    122
The Brother from Another Planet (1984),
    268
*Buffalo Bill and the Indians, or Sitting
    Bull's History Lesson* (1976), 223
Butch Cassidy and the Sundance Kid
    (1969), 119, 299
Butterfield 8 (1960), **163**

The Cabinet of Dr. Caligari (1919 and
    1962), 37, 55, 73, 90, **163**
The Caine Mutiny (1954), 72–73,
    75–76, 79, 89, 118
Call Me Bwana (1963), 92
Captain Blood (1935), 214
Captain Newman, M.D. (1963), 18,
    102–103, 105
Carefree (1938), 22, 47–49, **48, 162,
    163**
The Caretakers (1963), 103
Carrie (1976), 111
Casablanca (1942), 4–5, 73, 205–219
The Case of Becky (1921), 37
Cat People (1942), 21, 23
Catch-22 (1970), 300
Celebrity (1998), 127, 267, 273–274
Chafed Elbows (1967), 121
The Chapman Report (1962), 25, 86
A Child Is Waiting (1963), 72
Children of Loneliness (1939), 50–51
Citizen Kane (1941), 218
The Cobweb (1955), 68–71, 78, 79,
    83–84, 92, 104
Condemned Women (1938), **162,
    163**
Conspiracy Theory (1997), 141

Cool Hand Luke (1967), 118, 119
The Couch Trip (1987), 140
Cracking Up (1983), 32
Cries and Whispers (1972), 228
Crimes and Misdemeanors (1989), 126,
    249
Crimes of Passion (1984), 17
Crocodile Dundee (1986), 302, 303
Crossfire (1947), 60

Dark Delusion (1947), **163**
The Dark Mirror (1946), 23, 59–60, **60,**
    66, 74, 79, 105, **162**
The Dark Past (1948), 31, 59
Dark Waters (1944), **163**
David and Lisa (1962), 17, 26, 70, 86,
    87, 88, 92, 94, 101, 102, 104, 111,
    112, 138, **163**
The Days of Wine and Roses (1958 and
    1962), 104, 105
Dead Bang (1989), 23, 140
Dead Heat on a Merry-Go-Round
    (1966), 117, 122, **162**
Dead Ringer (1964), 59
Death Wish (1974), 118, 259
Death Wish II (1982), 114, 119
Deconstructing Harry (1997), 126–127,
    159, **162,** 248, 250
The Deer Hunter (1978), 11, 137
The Demon Seed (1977), 161
Desperate Hours (1990), 296
The Detective (1968), 23
Diary of a Mad Housewife (1970), 14,
    16, 111–112, 120
Dirty Harry (1971), 118
Dishonored Lady (1947), **163**
Disputed Passage (1939), 44
Dive Bomber (1941), 215
Don Juan DeMarco (1995), 141
Down and Out in Beverly Hills (1986),
    127–128, 132, 313
Dr. Dippy's Sanitarium (1906),
    35–37

Dr. Strangelove, or How I Learned to Stop Worrying and Love the Bomb (1964), 115
Dracula (1931), 23
The Dream of a Rarebit Fiend (1906), 37
The Dream Team (1989), 140
Dressed to Kill (1980), 19, 107–111, 141, 179, 288, 302
Duck Soup (1933), 126
Duet for One (1986), **162**

Easy Rider (1969), 118, 119
8½ (1963), 234–235, 238, 239, 241, 248
Elvira Madigan (1967), 32
End of the Road (1970), 17, 136–137
The Entity (1983), 23
Equus (1977), 136, 141
Eraserhead (1978), 206
The Escaped Lunatic (1904), 35, 36
E.T. (1982), 268
The Evening Star (1996), **162**
The Exorcist (1973), 278, 279, 287
Exorcist II: The Heretic (1977), 24, 137

Fail-Safe (1964), 115
Faithful (1996), 133
Fatal Attraction (1987), 297, 304, 306
Fear Strikes Out (1957), 16, 26, 27, 33, 79–81, **80,** 83, 84, 113
Fearless (1993), 141
La Femme Nikita (1990), 296
The Fifth Floor (1980), 26
A Fine Madness (1966), 118–120, 155, **162**
The First Wives' Club (1996), 159, **162**
Five Easy Pieces (1970), 118
The Flame Within (1935), **162**
For Whom the Bell Tolls (1943), 213
Forbidden Planet (1956), 279
Fourteen Hours (1951), 66
Frances (1982), 26, 27, 171, 173, 177

Frankenstein (1931), 95
Free Love (1930), 46–47, 77
Freud (1962), 25, 64, 83, 97–101, **98, 100,** 104, 107, **163**
From Beyond (1986), 157, **162**
The Front Page (1931, 1940, and 1974), 11, 22, 36, 39–40, 44, 46, 175

The Gay Intruders (1948), 22, 63
Gentlemen's Agreement (1947), 60
Ghost (1990), 306
Ghostbusters (1984), 301
Ghostbusters II (1989), 301
G.I. Jane, 296, 305
Gigi (1958), 69
Girl of the Night (1960), 25, 85, **163**
Glen or Glenda? (1953), 51, 65–66
Golden Boy (1939), 119
Gone With the Wind (1939), 37
Good Will Hunting (1997), 141, 144, **145,** 161, 179–182
The Graduate (1967), 115, 122
Grosse Pointe Blank (1997), 143
Groundhog Day (1993), 23, 141
The Group (1966), 118

Hairspray (1988), 140
Halloween (1978), 24, 277
Halloween IV (1988), 200
Hands Across the Table (1935), 47
Hannah and Her Sisters (1986), 125–126, 249
Harold and Maude (1971), 135
Harvey (1950), 22, 67
Harvey Middleman, Fireman (1965), 116–117
Heart of Darkness, 284
The Hero and the Terror (1988), **162**
Hey Hey in the Hay Loft, 238
Hi, Mom! (1970), 110
High Anxiety (1977), 22
High Noon (1952), 283
High Wall (1947), 23, 59, **162**

His Girl Friday (1940), 13, 39, 40, 47
Hollow Triumph (1948), 59
Home Before Dark (1958), 84–85, 105,
    163
Home of the Brave (1949), 26, 30, 61,
    65, 72, 77, 88, 89, 201
The Hospital (1971), 7, 26
Hot Shots (1991), 158, **162**
House of Cards (1969), 115
House of Games (1987), 140, 163
The Howling (1981), 23
Humoresque (1946), 119
Hunk (1987), 157, **162**
Husbands and Wives (1992), 126, **162,**
    249

I, the Jury (1953 and 1982), 19, 23,
    66–67, 92, 147
I Love You, Alice B. Toklas (1968), 314
I Never Promised You a Rose Garden
    (1977), 17, 103, 137, **138**, 164
I Was a Teenage Werewolf (1957), 66,
    72
I'm Dancing as Fast as I Can (1982),
    138, 165
Imitation of Life (1959), 201
In Person (1935), 47
Inside Daisy Clover (1966), 113, 118
Interiors (1978), 16, 244
Intermezzo (1939), 13
The Interns (1962), 26
Invaders from Mars (1953 and 1986),
    278–279
Invasion of the Body Snatchers (1956
    and 1978), 23, 72–74, 78,
    278–279, 287
It's My Turn (1980), 131, 175–176

Jade (1995), 159
Jagged Edge (1985), 79
Johnny Belinda (1948), 28, 157, 211
Johnny Guitar (1954), 296
Johnny Handsome (1990), 298

Juliet of the Spirits (1965), 228

The Kennel Murder Case (1933), 214
The King of Comedy (1983), 253–262,
    257, 266, 267, 272, 274
King of Hearts (1966), 86
King of New York (1990), 296
Kismet (1955), 69
Kitty Foyle (1940), 13, 14
Klang, 224
Klute (1971), 7
Knock on Wood (1954), 21, 66,
    150–153, 155, 156, **162**
Kotch (1971), 137

Lady in a Jam (1942), **163**
Lady in the Dark (1944), 7–15, **10,** 17,
    21, 33, 34, 47, 53, 55, 63, 77, 112
The Last Embrace (1979), 161
Last Rites (1988), 296
Leaving Las Vegas (1995), 17
Lenny (1974), 234, 244
Les Miserables (1935), 43
Let There Be Light (1946), 61, 63–65,
    97, 99
Lethal Weapon (1987), 219
Lethal Weapon III (1991), 296
Let's Live a Little (1948), 55, **162**
L'Homme Qui Aimait les Femmes
    (1977), 157
License to Kill (1989), 296
Lilith (1964), 116, **162**
Little Big Man (1970), 118
The Locket (1946), **163**
Logan's Run (1976), 282
The Lonely Guy (1984), 17
The Long Kiss Goodnight (1996),
    296
Lord Love a Duck (1966), 117
The Lost Weekend (1945), 104, 105
Love at First Bite (1979), 20, 137, **162**
Lover Come Back (1961), 22, 92
Loves of a Psychiatrist, 25

Lovesick (1983), 19, 22, 92–94, 107, **139,** 139–140, **162,** 173, 177
Lust for Life (1956), 69

Madame X (1966), 12
Magnificent Obsession (1935), 44
Making Love (1982), 51
The Man Who Loved Women (1983), 157, **162**
The Man Who Saw Tomorrow (1922), 6, 37
The Manchurian Candidate (1962), 88, 141
Manhattan (1979), 244
Manhattan Murder Mystery (1993), 126
Marat/Sade (1967), 27, 121
The Mark (1961), 26, 85
Marked Woman (1937), 217
The Marriage of a Young Stockbroker (1971), 112–113, 120, 137, 167
The Medusa Touch (1978), 23, 137, 147
The Men (1950), 72
Men in White (1934), 26
Midnight Cowboy (1969), 299
Mildred Pierce (1945), 214
Miracle on 34th Street (1947), 23, 63
The Miracle Worker (1962 and 1979), 104
Mirage (1965), 23, 117
Misery (1990), 293, 296, 306
Moment to Moment (1966), 118
Morning Glory (1933), 13
Moscow on the Hudson (1984), 268
Movie Star, American Style or LSD, I Hate You (1966), 118
Mr. Deeds Goes to Town (1936), 6, 49–50, 61, 67
Mr. Jones (1993), 20, 141, 159–161, **162**
Ms. 45 (1981), 296
Mulholland Falls (1996), 168
Murder, My Sweet (1945), 63, 77

My Blue Heaven (1990), 157–158, **162**
My Favorite Wife (1940), 63
My Six Convicts (1952), 72
Mystery of the Wax Museum (1933), 214

The Naked Face (1984), 138
The Net (1995), **162**
New York, New York (1977), 257
Night of the Living Dead (1968), 277, 279–280
Nightmare Alley (1947), 17, 56–58, **58,** 63, 66, 91–92, 147, 167
9½ Weeks (1986), 159
North by Northwest (1959), 97
Now, Voyager (1942), 12, 17, 32, 51–53, **52,** 61, 71, 74, 77, 82, 86–88, 157, **163,** 182

Obsession (1976), 110
Odds Against Tomorrow (1959), 86
Oh, God! Book II (1980), 18, 23
Oh, Men! Oh, Women! (1957), 47, 82–84, **84,** 92, **163**
The Old Maid (1939), 13
The Omen (1976), 137
On a Clear Day You Can See Forever (1970), 10, **163**
One Flew Over the Cuckoo's Nest (1975), 18, 26, 27, 114, 119–120, 133–135, **134,** 152, 177, 309, 312–313
One Glorious Day (1922), 37
Ordinary People (1980), 17, 18, **19,** 31–32, 103, 105, 107, 132, 137, 140, 144–146, 173, 178, 179, 309, 312
Outland (1981), 282, 283

The Parallax View (1974), 282
Penelope (1966), 117
The Perfect Furlough (1958), 25, 66, 91, 156, **162**

Phantom of the Paradise (1974), 111
Pillow Talk (1959), 92, 102, 115
Pink Flamingos (1972), 206, 303
Pinky (1947), 60
Plan 9 from Outer Space (1959), 65
Plastered in Paris (1928), 38
Play It Again, Sam (1972), 218
Portnoy's Complaint (1972), 137
Possessed (1947), 6, 8, 53, 61, **163**
The President's Analyst (1967),
    121–122, 137
Pressure Point (1962), 26, 72, 88–90,
    89, 94, 101, 102, 104, 136
Presumed Innocent (1990), 304–305
Pretty Woman (1990), 306
Primal Fear (1996), 141
The Prince of Tides (1991), 141, 158,
    158, 159, 161, **162**
Private Worlds (1935), 41–43, **45**,
    45–46, 54, 69, 81, 90, 161
Problem Child (1990), 141
Psycho (1960 and 1998), 17, 78, 85, 90,
    96–97, 107–111, 122–123,
    194–196, 201, 288, 302
The Purple Rose of Cairo (1985), 253,
    267–275, **269, 271**

A Rage in Harlem (1991), 296, 304
Ragina's Secrets, 25
Raging Bull (1980), 257
Raising Cain (1992), 110, 141
Rambo III (1988), 219
Rebecca (1940), 211
Red River (1948), 118
Reds (1981), 262
Reefer Madness (1936), 51
Reunion in Vienna (1933), 41–42, 45,
    47, **163**
Revolution (1968), 115
The Rocky Horror Picture Show (1975),
    206, 303
The Royal Family of Broadway (1930),
    13

The Santa Clause (1994), 22
The Scar (1948), 59
Scenes from a Mall (1991), 132
Schizoid (1980), **163**
The Sea Hawk (1940), 214
Sea of Love (1990), 294, 296–299,
    305–307
The Searchers (1956), 217
Semi-Tough (1977), 128
The Sender (1982), 23, 138, 147
The Serpent and the Rainbow (1988),
    147
The Seven-Per-Cent Solution (1976),
    137, **163**
The Seven Year Itch (1955), 66
The Seventh Veil (1945), 53
Sex and the Single Girl (1964), 21, 25,
    116, 153, **153**, 155, 156, **162**
Shadow on the Wall (1950), **162**
Shadows (1960), 86
Shane (1953), 215
She Wouldn't Say Yes (1946), **162**
Shock (1946), 63, 65
Shock Corridor (1963), 26, 113
Shock Treatment (1964), 26, 92,
    113–114, 116
Short Cuts (1993), 201
The Shrike (1955), 26–27, 67–68, 73,
    78, **163**
The Silence of the Lambs (1991), 141,
    142, 146, 296, 303–304
Silent Night, Deadly Night (1984), 280
Silkwood (1983), 300
The Sin of Madelon Claudet (1931),
    12
Since You Went Away (1944), 12, 17,
    53, 74, 75, **163**
Sisters (1973), 59, 110
Skin Deep (1989), 140–141
Sleeper (1973), 282
The Sleeping Tiger (1954), 71
Sleeping with the Enemy (1991), 296,
    304

The Snake Pit, 18, 26, 27, 60–63, **62, 64,** 67, 71, 79, 82, 92, 95, 102, 157, **163**

So Young, So Bad (1950), **163**

Some Kind of Hero (1982), 11

Some Like It Hot (1959), 302

Something Wild (1987), 300

Spellbound (1945), 12, 19, 21, 39, 53–55, 57, 59, 61, 63, 74, 81, 94, 96, 139, 147–149, **150,** 156, 157, **162,** 309

Sphere (1998), 146, **162**

The Spiral Staircase (1946), 28, 211

Splash (1984), 268

Splendor in the Grass (1961 and 1981), 16, 25, 76, 85, 104, 105, **163**

St. Ives (1975), 19, 171–172

Star 80 (1983), 259–260

Star Wars (1977), 215, 219, 282

Stardust Memories (1980), 124, 234–235, 238–244, **240,** 246–247, **247,** 267, 270, 273

Starman (1984), 268

Starting Over (1979), 18, 137

Stella Dallas (1937), 13, 22, 32

The Stepfather (1987), **163**

The Stepford Wives (1975), 137

Still of the Night (1982), 23, 139

The Story of Esther Costello (1957), 28

The Story of Louis Pasteur (1936), 44

Strait Jacket (1964), 116

Stromboli (1950), 207

Suburbia Confidential, 25

Sudden Impact (1983), 296

Suddenly, Last Summer (1959), 95, 96, **163,** 194–195

Sullivan's Travels (1941), 238–239

Switch (1991), 298

Take the Money and Run (1969), 244, 262

A Tale of Two Cities (1935), 43

Taxi Driver (1976), 255, 258–259

Tea and Sympathy (1956), 69

10 (1980), 137

Tender Is the Night (1962), 19, 92, 94–95, 101, **162, 163**

The Terminator (1984), 23, 289

Terminator II (1991), 296, 299, 304

The Texas Chainsaw Massacre (1974), 200, 277

That Old Feeling (1997), **162**

That Touch of Mink (1962), 92, 102

That Uncertain Feeling (1941), 63

Thelma and Louise (1991), 166, 296, 304, 305

Them! (1954), 66

They Might Be Giants (1971), 137, 155–157, **162**

The Thing (1951 and 1982), 279, 280, 287

Third of a Man (1962), 72, 85

Three Days of the Condor (1975), 282

The Three Faces of Eve (1957), 17, 26, 28–30, 33, 81–83, **82,** 104, **163,** 182

Three Nuts in Search of a Bolt (1964), 25

Three on a Couch (1966), 117, 161

Three Warriors, 313

3 Women (1977), 221–232, **224, 229,** 311

The Thrill of It All (1963), 16, 102

Thunderbolt and Lightfoot (1974), 299

Tin Cup (1996), 141, 159, **162**

Titanic (1997), 289

Titicut Follies (1967), 27, 121

To Each His Own (1946), 13

Together Again (1944), 13

Tootsie (1982), 302, 303

Top Gun (1986), 177, 219

Total Recall (1990), 296, 300

12 Monkeys (1995), 21, 141, 159, **160, 162**

The Twisted Sex, 25

2001: A Space Odyssey (1968), 281, 282

Un Chien andalou (1928), 55
Under the Volcano (1984), 105
An Unmarried Woman (1978), 103, 131–132, 137, 165, 312

V. I. Warshawski (1991), 304
Vampire's Kiss (1989), 164
Vertigo (1958), 96, 199–200
A Very Special Favor (1965), 21, 25, 117, 152, 156, **162**
Victor/Victoria (1982), 302
Voyage to the Bottom of the Sea (1961), 91

Walking and Talking (1996), 163–164
Walking Tall (1973), 118
What a Way to Go! (1964), 116
What About Bob? (1991), 141
What's New, Pussycat? (1965), 20, 71, 116, **117, 162**

When the Clouds Roll By (1919), 19, 36–38, **38**
Whirlpool (1950), 21, 71
Whispers in the Dark (1992), 163
Who's Been Sleeping in My Bed? (1963), 25, 102
Whose Life Is It, Anyway? (1981), 83
Wild in the Country (1961), 90–91, 153–155, **155, 162**
Wild Man Blues (1998), 248–249
Willie and Phil (1980), 127, 313
The Wizard of Oz (1939), 12, 37, 90
Working Girl (1988), 294, 299–302, 307
The Wrong Man (1956), 96

Yankee Doodle Dandy (1942), 214
Young Dr. Freud (1977), 98
Young Mr. Lincoln (1939), 86

Zelig (1983), 157, **162, 163**, 253, 262–267, **263, 264**, 270, 272, 274
Zotz! (1962), 23, 92